***Bartonella* and *Afipia* Species Emphasizing *Bartonella henselae***

# Contributions to Microbiology

## Vol. 1

Series Editor *Axel Schmidt*, Wuppertal

KARGER

Basel · Freiburg · Paris · London · New York ·
New Delhi · Bangkok · Singapore · Tokyo · Sydney

# *Bartonella* and *Afipia* Species Emphasizing *Bartonella henselae*

Volume Editor *Axel Schmidt*, Wuppertal

30 figures and 18 tables, 1998

KARGER

Basel · Freiburg · Paris · London · New York ·
New Delhi · Bangkok · Singapore · Tokyo · Sydney

**Contributions to Microbiology**

formerly 'Concepts in Immunopathology' and
'Contributions to Microbiology and Immunology'

**Axel Schmidt**

PD Dr. med., FIBA
Bayer AG
Pharma Research Antiinfectives
Wuppertal;
Institute for Microbiology and Virology
University Witten-Herdecke, Germany

Library of Congress Cataloging-in-Publication Data
*Bartonella* and *Afipia* species emphasizing *Bartonella henselae* / volume editor, Axel Schmidt.
(Contributions to microbiology; vol. 1)
Includes bibliographical references and indexes. (hardcover: alk. paper)
1. *Bartonella* infections. 2. *Afipia* infections. 3. Cat-scratch disease. I. Schmidt, Axel, 1962– . II. Series.
[DNLM: 1. *Bartonella* Infections – microbiology. 2. *Bartonella* Infections – diagnosis.
3. *Bartonella henselae* – isolation & purification. 4. *Bartonella henselae* – pathogenicity.
5. Gram-Negative Bacteria – isolation & purification. WC 640 B293 1998]
QR201.B (*Bartonella* infections) IN PROCESS
616′.01427–dc21
ISBN 3–8055–6649–2

Bibliographic Indices. This publication is listed in bibliographic services, including Current Contents® and Index Medicus.

Drug Dosage. The authors and the publisher have exerted every effort to ensure that drug selection and dosage set forth in this text are in accord with current recommendations and practice at the time of publication. However, in view of ongoing research, changes in government regulations, and the constant flow of information relating to drug therapy and drug reactions, the reader is urged to check the package insert for each drug for any change in indications and dosage and for added warnings and precautions. This is particularly important when the recommended agent is a new and/or infrequently employed drug.


Printed in Switzerland on acid-free paper.
ISBN 3–8055–6649–8

In Remembrance of
Hans P.R. Seeliger (1920–1997)
Clinical Bacteriologist and Mycologist

# Contents

# Preface

It is with great pleasure that I have prepared this preface to the first volume of the Karger book series *Contributions to Microbiology.* It was immensely gratifying when H. Schoenfeld (series editor, Karger book series *Antibiotics and Chemotherapy* as well as editor Karger journal *Chemotherapy*, where I have the chance to assist him on the Editorial Board) nominated me as series editor for *Contributions to Microbiology. Contributions to Microbiology* has developed from a fusion of the two Karger book series *Contributions to Microbiology and Immunology* and *Concepts in Immunopathology*, both edited by J.M. Cruse and R.E. Lewis, Jr.

In general, the series *Contributions to Microbiology* will focus on relevant topics of microbiology including aspects of bacteriology, virology, parasitology, and mycology. Special emphasis – as far as possible – will be placed on updates of emerging pathogens, and the series will try to stress the interdisciplinarity of the field including 'modern' aspects such as progress and approaches in molecular biology, clinical aspects relevant to human and veterinary medicine, and crop and plant infections and protection, as well as questions of epidemiology and prevention of infectious diseases. I shall also try and include an adequate amount of contributions to molecular targets suitable for the finding and development of new anti-infective principles and/or substances which may help fill the gap to the series *Antibiotics and Chemotherapy.* Presentations from scientific congresses, conferences and workshops on circumscribed topics are also welcome to this book series as separate volumes.

Emerging or recently classified pathogens are a great challenge in medicine. I therefore took a chance and focused the first volume on clinically relevant aspects of infections caused by the still not very well known bacterial genera *Afipia* and *Bartonella* with a special focus on *B. henselae. B. henselae* is a bacterial pathogen that has already been observed in sections of clinical specimens from patients with cat-scratch disease using special staining methods.

The first successful cultivation of the organism was in the early 1990s, and thus this organism and its medical implications are still under extensive research. Human diseases caused by *Bartonella* species and in particular by *B. henselae* are discussed, covering aspects ranging from clinics in human and veterinary medicine, and diagnostics, pathology and therapy, to new progress in research including modern molecular biological techniques. The epidemiological aspects of human and animal infections are also taken into consideration, especially the application of innovative molecular methods for the characterization of isolates for epidemiological purposes. Overall, this book especially offers a comprehensive description regarding the still relatively unknown pathogenic bacterial species *B. henselae* and will hopefully lead to a higher awareness in cases of infection with this organism.

All chapters are written by outstanding international experts in the field and I thank them all for their excellent and efficient collaboration despite their other duties and responsibilities. Further, I want to thank both R. Steinebrunner who took care of this book series in the early phase and T. Nold (both Karger) who took over his position later for their excellent collaboration and exchange of information. Also, many thanks go to Mrs. R. Gisin and Mrs. S. Willi from Karger who kindly assisted me with the preparation of the book wherever they could. Finally, I want to emphasize that in my function as series editor, I look forward to suggestions, criticism and remarks from the reader, with the hope that this 'young' book series will have a chance to be of relevance and a benefit to its readership.

Wuppertal, Germany, April 1998 *Axel Schmidt*

Schmidt A (ed): *Bartonella* and *Afipia* Species Emphasizing *Bartonella henselae*.
Contrib Microbiol. Basel, Karger, 1998, vol 1, pp 1–31

# The Genera *Afipia* and *Bartonella*

*Richard J. Birtles, Didier Raoult*

Unité des Rickettsies, CNRS UPRESA 6020, Faculté de Médecine,
Marseille, France

This chapter will review medical, veterinary, microbiological and epidemiological aspects of all but one of the species which make up the genera *Bartonella* and *Afipia*. The species missing is *Bartonella henselae*, which has been allocated a chapter of its own in this volume.

The genera *Bartonella* and *Afipia* continue to be associated solely because of the proported role of *Bartonella henselae* and *Afipia felis* in cat scratch disease (CSD). In taxonomic terms the two genera are quite distinct, and their evolutionary divergence is reflected in marked differences in the morphologies and physiologies of the organisms and in their natural cycles. If both species do indeed cause CSD it is likely that the symptoms have been induced by different pathogenic processes, thus the disease may be better considered as two quite distinct syndromes which present in an indistinguishable manner.

## General Characteristics of the Two Genera

Although *Bartonella* and *Afipia* species share some common evolutionary descent, as demonstrated by their membership of the α subdivision of the *Proteobacteria*, beyond this the two genera are not specifically related. Phylogenetic analysis of the two taxa has shown that whereas *Afipia* species share a close evolutionary relationship with the root-nodulating species *Bradyrhizobium japonicum* and the budding bacterium *Blastobacter denitrificans* [Willems and Collins, 1992], *Bartonella* species are most akin to members of the *Brucella* [Birtles et al., 1995].

*The Genus* Afipia

The genus *Afipia* was proposed by Brenner et al. [1991a] with six members, all of which are Gram-negative, oxidase-positive, nonfermentative rods and which have been shown to be motile by means of a single flagellum. All species can be grown on buffered charcoal yeast extract agar and nutrient broth, but growth is inhibited if this broth contains 6% sodium chloride. Colonies of *Afipia* species typically appear grey-white, glistening, convex, and opaque after 72 h incubation at 32 °C, are urease-positive, and turn litmus milk alkaline. Two of the six species were proposed for previously recognized but uncharacterized organisms, with *Afipia felis* representing the 'cat scratch disease bacillus' first isolated by English et al. in 1988 and *Afipia clevelandensis* representing the former 'Cleveland Clinic Foundation Strain' as described by Hall et al. [1991]. The additional four species included *Afipia bromeae*, and three unnamed genospecies. Today, 6 years after these first proposals, no additional species have been described.

Cellular fatty acid analysis has revealed that the *Afipia* species contain 11-methyl-octadec-12-enoic (Cbr19:1), cis-octadec-11-enoic (C18:1 ω7c), and generally 17- and 19-carbon acids with a cyclopropane ring as major acids. Their G + C content has been estimated as being between 61.5 and 69%. DNA: DNA hybridization studies have shown the species share between 12 and 69% relatedness [Brenner et al., 1991a].

Differentiation between the *Afipia* species has been achieved using ribotyping and multilocus enzyme analysis [Brenner et al., 1991a]. The species are also serologically distinct from one another, thus polyclonal antisera raised against each species can be used for specific identification when incorporated into immunofluorescence tests or other serological formats.

*The Genus* Bartonella

Unlike *Afipia*, the genus *Bartonella* has long been recognized. The genus was first proposed over 70 years ago as containing a single species, *B. bacilliformis*, the agent of Carrion's disease, an infection endemic to the Andean valleys of South America [Strong et al., 1915]. Although the genus remained unchanged for over 60 years, the past 5 years have seen numerous additions and alterations to *Bartonella* taxomony. In 1993, Brenner et al. proposed the unification of the genera *Rochalimaea* and *Bartonella*, and as taxonomic protocol states that the name of the elder genus be retained, the four former *Rochalimaea* species became *B. quintana, B. henselae, B. elizabethae* and *B. vinsonii*. In 1995, Birtles et al. proposed that the genera *Grahamella* and *Bartonella* also be combined, thus the two former *Grahamella* species became *B. talpae* and *B. peromysci*. Concurrently these authors proposed three new *Bartonella* species, namely *B. doshiae, B. grahamii* and *B. taylorii*. The genus gained an eleventh member in 1996 with the description of *B. clarridgeiae* [Lawson and Collins, 1996] and, additionally, a subspecies of *B. vinsonii*, named *B. vinsonii* subspecies *berkhoffii*, has been proposed [Kordick et al., 1996].

Following these changes, the general features of the *Bartonella* species are that they are Gram-negative, oxidase-negative, fastidious, aerobic rods. Two species, *B. bacilliformis* and *B. clarridgeiae*, have been shown to possess flagella. Isolates are best recovered on media containing 5% or more whole blood in the presence of 5% $CO_2$, although growth often remains scant. Optimal incubation temperatures are 30 °C for *B. bacilliformis* and 37 °C for all other species. Colonies can be polymorphic, but are typically small and off-white. All species are nonfermentative.

The major fatty acids observed are (18:1) and (18:0) octadecanoic acid and hexadecanoic acid (16:0). Some species possess more (17:0) and 16:1(7c) forms, but essentially no other fatty acids are present, distinguishing the *Bartonella* species from almost all other bacteria except *Brucella* and *Methylobacterium* species [Clarridge et al., 1995]. Estimations of the G+C content of *Bartonella* species range between 38.5 and 41%, and genome sizes have been calculated to be between 1,700 and 2,200 kb [Reschke et al., 1991; Roux and Raoult, 1995]. DNA relatedness between species ranges between 16 and 68% under optimal conditions [Brenner et al., 1993; Birtles et al., 1995].

In addition to the named *Bartonella* species, several reports have described numerous strains isolated from the blood of a wide variety of animals which are likely to represent new species [e.g. Birtles and Raoult, 1996]. Most of these isolates have been characterized by genotypic and serotypic methods, and although as yet unassigned to specific species, their existence serves to demonstrate that the true diversity of the genus is far from being recognized.

As the bartonellae remain all but inert in standard biochemical tests, and all are morphologically homologous, most schemes which have described the differentiation of species have been genotypic. Several methods based on restriction enzyme analysis (REA) of PCR-amplified genes or gene fragments have been developed, including those exploiting genetic variation in the 16S rRNA-encoding gene [Birtles, 1995], the citrate synthase (*gltA*) gene [Norman et al., 1995], or the 16S–23S intragenic spacer region [Roux and Raoult, 1995]. Base sequence determination of fragments of PCR-amplified 16S rRNA gene and *gltA* is also widely used to identify species [Sander et al., 1997; Regnery et al., 1996]. As *Bartonella*-specific PCRs based on both these genes have been described [Relman et al., 1990; Norman et al., 1995], the need to culture a *Bartonella* strain prior to its identification can now be circumvented, and this approach is particularly useful as bartonellae are notoriously fastidious organisms. Other PCR-based methods including repetitive element (ERIC)-PCR have also been described for distinguishing species [Rodriguez-Barradas et al., 1995].

Isolates can also be identifed by ribotyping [R.J. Birtles, unpubl. observation] and macrorestriction analysis using pulsed-field gel electrophoresis [Roux and Raoult, 1995]. In addition to these genotypic methods, serological differentiation is also reliable as the *Bartonella* species identified to date are serologically distinct from one another. Serovariation between strains of the same species has, however, been observed [Drancourt et al., 1996].

### *Afipia felis*

*Medical Relevance. A. felis* is without doubt an agent of CSD, although today its relative importance is debated. Although the infectious nature of CSD had long been recognized, it was not until 1983 that the presence of small pleomorphic, Gram-negative bacilli was demonstrated in lymph nodes of patients with the disease, a step achieved using the nonspecific Warthin-Starry silver stain [Wear et al., 1983]. Lymph node infections due to organisms of indistinguishable morphology were also observed by other groups [Cotter et al., 1986] and later, identical bacilli together with possible cell wall-defective forms were seen in skin and the conjunctiva [Margileth et al., 1984; Wear et al., 1985]. In 1988, English et al. reported the isolation of a bacterial agent from the lymph nodes of 10 of 19 patients who fulfilled at least three of the four classical criteria for CSD: (1) cat contact, with presence of a scratch or a primary dermal or eye lesion; (2) a positive skin test; (3) regional lymphadenopathy with normal results of laboratory studies for other causes of lymphadenopathy, and (4) characteristic histopathologic changes in a lymph node. The isolates were morphologically indistinguishable from the organisms observed previously. Serum samples were available for 7 patients and 3 of these demonstrated seroconversion to the cultured bacterium. Furthermore, rabbit antiserum raised against the isolate reacted with the vegetative bacilli earlier observed in lymph node, skin or conjunctiva of CSD patients. The isolates obtained by English et al. [1988] were subsequently assessed by polyphasic taxonomic criteria (see below), and on the basis of these results were assigned to a new species, *A. felis* [Brenner et al., 1991a].

Subsequent to this study, recovery of *A. felis* from CSD patients was not achieved again until 1996 when Giladi et al. obtained an isolate from pus aspirated from a lymph node of a patient with typical CSD. However, evidence for a pathogenic role for *A. felis* has also resulted from other approaches; Alkan et al. [1995] attempted to detect *A. felis* DNA in fixed lymph node sections with histological features of CSD using dot-blot hybridization with species-specific PCR-generated probes. *A. felis* was detected in three sections whereas the other proported agent of CSD, *B. henselae*, was detected in five, and, unexpectedly, both organisms were detected in two. The remaining two sections tested negative with both probes. Against these two studies, most other workers have failed to detect *A. felis* in numerous surveys of CSD aetiology; Bergmans et al. [1995] found no evidence of *A. felis* during PCR-based detection of bacterial DNA in pus samples collected from over 200 CSD patients. Szelc-Kelly et al. [1995] measured serological responses in American CSD patients and in a contol group, and demonstrated that antibody levels against *A. felis* did not differ between the two. A similar finding was also reported in a serological study of French CSD patients [Amerein et al., 1996].

Drancourt et al. [1992] detected seroconversion to *A. felis* in a 25-year-old woman with acute meningoencephalitis, suggesting the species may have pathogenic potential outside of CSD.

*Microbiology.* The original isolates of English et al. [1988] were subjected to rigorous phenotypic assessment following their recovery after 2–9 days' incubation of inoculated brain-heart infusion biphasic media. Blood agar subcultures were achieved at 32 °C with colonies appearing grey-white, glistening, convex and opaque with entire edges. Microscopic examination revealed bacilli which were pleomorphic, Gram-negative, single or in short chains, Y-forms, clumps or filaments. Their size was estimated to be 0.2–0.5 by 0.2–2.5 μm. The isolates were nonhaemolytic, motile by means of a single polar flagellum, tested oxidase-positive, reduced nitrate to nitrite and produced urease. All other biochemical tests were negative. Subsequently, characterizations of four of the isolates, together with seven other isolates which shared some morphological and biochemical features with the CSD bacillus, were completed by polyphasic methods including cellular fatty acid analysis, estimation of G + C content and DNA:DNA homology, multilocus enzyme analysis, ribotyping, plasmid content and serology [Brenner et al., 1991a]. The four CSD bacilli could not be distinguished using these methods and thus were all assigned to a newly proposed species, named *A. felis.* The seven CSD-like organisms were clearly different from the four CSD isolates in several assessments and were thus assigned to the five different species discussed below. *A. felis* can be distinguished from the other *Afipia* species using both genotypic and phenotypic (see above) criteria. Genotypically, the species has a unique G + C content (62.5 mol%), together with a unique 16S rRNA sequence, fatty acid profile, ribotype and mutilocus enzyme type. It also shares less than 50% DNA relatedness with the other species.

*Epidemiology and Natural Cycle.* All isolates of *A. felis* obtained to date have been clinical; no evidence of infections in cats has been found. As one of the *Afipia* genospecies has been isolated from water, it is possible that *A. felis* too persists in the environment. If this were to be the case, cats may act only as mechanical vectors, picking up the organism from soil and perhaps inoculating humans with contaminated claws.

In vitro, armadillos have responded to subdermal inoculation with *A. felis* by production of skin lesions which closely resembled those observed during the early stages of CSD in humans. *A. felis* infections could also be sustained in other laboratory animals, including mice, rats, hamsters and guinea pigs, although none developed symptoms compatible with human CSD [English et al., 1988]. No attempts have been made to assess the homogeneity of the handful of isolates available.

*Antibiotic Susceptibility.* On original isolation one of the CSD bacilli was subjected to testing against a wide range of antimicrobial agents. The isolate was found to be resistant to penicillin G, ampicillin, erythromycin, tetracycline, chloramphenicol, clindamycin, cephalothin, cefazolin, cefamandole, cefoperazone and nitrofurantoin. It was clearly sensitive to cefoxitin, cefotaxime, gentamicin, amikacin, tobramycin, netilmicin and mezlocillin. More recently, Maurin et al. [1993] have reassessed the susceptibilities of *A. felis* in both axenic medium and in cells. In axenic medium the organism was susceptible to imipenem, aminoglycosides and rifampin whereas when grown in HeLa cells, it was only susceptible to amikacin and tobramycin. Thus, despite an intracellular location, *A. felis* can be reached by aminoglycosides, an in vitro finding which concurs with clinical data obtained in CSD patients [Bogue et al., 1989].

### *Afipia clevelandensis*

*Medical Relevance.* This species is at present represented by a single strain. In 1991, Hall et al. reported the isolation of a bacterium associated with CSD from the tibial biopsy of a patient hospitalized in the Cleveland Clinic Foundation, Cleveland, Ohio, with severe necrotizing pancreatitis. The patient, a 69-year-old male, had been previously healthy and had no history of either alcohol abuse or biliary disease. During his hospitalization, multiple surgical procedures were required to drain abscesses in the pancreas, retroperitonal areas, and the left flank, and he developed acute renal failure, and had repeated bouts of sepsis and pneumonia. Eventually he became ventilator-dependent and died 8 months after admission. During the fifth month of his hospitalization he was found to have oedematous lower extremities with petechial lesions and erythematous plaques, as well as isolated areas of ulceration and crusting. The biopsy from which the bacterium was isolated revealed histological stasis without polymorphonuclear cell infiltrates.

The patient had no signs or symptoms of CSD, and histopathology of the lesion demonstrated no inflammation. In conclusion, the investigators reported that 'it is not known what, if any, clinical significance this isolate had, but it might possibly represent the first instance of a nosocomial organism resembling the CSD bacillus'.

*Microbiology.* The isolates grew well on both chocolate blood agar at 35 °C and brain-heart infusion agar with blood and potato dextrose agar at 25 °C (although not at 5 or 42 °C), in the presence of 5% $CO_2$. Biochemically the organism was oxidase-positive, but remained inert in all other standard tests applied. It was however motile, by use of a single, polar flagellum. The strain was further characterized during the study which led to the proposal as *A. clevelandensis* [Brenner et al., 1991a]. It appeared to be the most fastidious of all the *Afipia* species being, uniquely, unable to produce acid from *D*-xylose, although, again uniquely, it did manage delayed, weak growth on MacConkey agar. Polyvalent rabbit antiserum raised against *A. clevelandensis* yielded strong homologous titres and also reacted more weakly with strains of *A. felis*, but not with representatives of any other *Afipia* species.

Recently, Drancourt et al. [1997] have demonstrated significant cross-reactivity between *A. clevelandensis* antigens and antibodies from patients with brucellosis or *Yersinia entercolitica* infection. Serosurvey of over 30,000 sera submitted for routine diagnosis of possible rickettsial infection demonstrated 1.5% to exhibit detectable antibody to *A. clevelandensis*; however, among 52 seropositive patients for whom clinical data were available, 42% had brucellosis and 15% had *Y. enterocolitica* O:9 infection. Western blotting identified two cross-reacting antigens which were of presumptive lipopolysaccharide nature.

*Epidemiology and Natural Cycle.* With only a single isolate in existence, speculation on the natural cycle of this *A. clevelandensis* is difficult. It appears the one case to date was acquired nosocomially, and thus the possibility of cat contact was discounted.

*Antibiotic Susceptibility. A. clevelandensis* has demonstrated marked resistance to a range of agents including amoxycillin-clavulanate, ampicillin, cefoperazone, ceftazidine, gentamycin, piperacillin, tetracycline and ticarcillin. The species was, however, clearly sensitive to ceftriaxone, cephalothin and imipenem [Brenner et al., 1991a].

### *Afipia broomeae*

*Medical Relevance.* Three strains of *A. broomeae* have been described and their characteristics compared [Brenner et al., 1991a]. All three were recovered from clinical material, although from markedly different settings. The first strain to be isolated was recovered from the sputum of a New Zealander, whereas the subsequent isolates came from the bone marrow of a patient in

Massachusetts and the synovial fluid of a patient with a wrist abscess in Kentucky. No further details of any of these patients have yet been published.

*Microbiology. A. broomeae* exhibits all the characteristics for the genus, being weakly catalase-positive and showing delayed, weak acid production from *D*-xylose.

*Epidemiology and Natural Cycle.* Intra-species diversity was demonstrated in their measured fatty acid contents, although differences were only minor. Multilocus enzyme typing, based on 30 metabolic enzymes, divided the three strains into two electrophoretic types, one for the New Zealand isolate and the second for those originating from the USA. Genotypic analysis confirmed this heterogeneity with ribotyping of both *Eco*RI and *Pst*I-*Bgl* II-digested genomic DNA demonstrating indistinguishable profiles for the US strains, but a distinct profile for that from New Zealand. Furthermore, DNA:DNA homology results demonstrated that the two US strains shared 98% relatedness, whereas the Kentucky and New Zealand strains shared only 77% relatedness [Brenner et al., 1991a]. It would clearly be foolhardy at this stage to suggest solely a geographic basis for this variation, although as such a low level of intra-species DNA relatedness exists, the US strains may in the future become considered as belonging to a distinct subspecies.

*Antibiotic Sensitivity.* Antimicrobial sensitivity testing demonstrates the species to be markedly resistant to cefoperazone, piperacillin and tetracycline, but sensitive to a range of other agents especially cefoxitin, ceftriaxone, cephalothin and imipenem. Some variation in susceptibility profiles to β-lactams and ciprofloxacin was observed among the three *A. broomeae* strains [Brenner et al., 1991a].

## The Three *Afipia* Genospecies

*Medical Relevance.* The three *Afipia* genospecies are undoubtedly distinct species which, although differentiated from other members of the genus using polyphasic taxonomic criteria, were not named as it was considered that they could not be biochemically differentiated with certainty from each other or from the named *Afipia* species [Brenner et al., 1991a]. Each of the three species is represented by a single isolate. Interestingly, one of the isolates, that of genospecies 3, is of environmental origin, being isolated from a water sample collected in Indiana. The other two are clinical isolates, with genospecies 1 being isolated from pleural fluid in a fatal case of pulmonary obstruction, and genospecies 2 being recovered from a bronchial wash of a pneumonia patient.

*Microbiology.* That the genospecies were considered biochemically indistinguishable at the time of their proposal is somewhat surprising as the authors actually report unique biochemical profiles for two of the three strains [Brenner et al., 1991a]. Genospecies 1 was, uniquely among the *Afipia* species, citrate-positive as well as showing delayed, weak acid production from *D*-mannitol. Similarly, genospecies 3 was unique in yielding a weak production of hydrogen sulphide.

*Antibiotic Susceptibility.* In general the antibiotic susceptibilities of genospecies 1 and 2 were found to be very similar, and both showed marked resistance against more agents than any of the other *Afipia* species. High levels of resistance were found against aminoglycosides, amoxycillin, ureidopenicillins, second- and third-generation cephalosporins, fluoroquinolones and tetracycline. The two species could perhaps be considered sensitive only to a combination of amoxycillin and clavulanate, although even in this instance an MIC of 8/16 was obtained for genospecies 1. As opposed to the two genospecies isolated from clinical material, the environmental isolate, genospecies 3, was sensitive to almost all antibiotics with the exception of some of the cephalosporins and tetracycline [Brenner et al., 1991a].

### *Bartonella bacilliformis*

*Medical Relevance.* The oldest member of the genus was first recognized in 1909, when Alberto Barton observed the presence of intraerythrocytic organisms in blood films prepared from patients with Carrion's disease. Carrion's disease got its name from a Peruvian medical student who valiently died whilst demonstrating that its two manifestations were indeed part of the same disease.

Classically the disease first manifests as an acute, very severe, anaemia. During this phase of illness, bacteria penetrate [Cuadra and Takano, 1969] and parasitize up to all of the erythrocytes, and it is their demise, which results either as a direct result of infection or due to phagocytosis of infected cells, which leads to the anaemia together with fever, heptosplenomegaly, generalized lymphadenopathy, pallor, rapid pulse and possible circulatory collapse. It is at this stage of the illness, termed Oroya fever, that most fatalities occur, resulting either directly by suffocation through lack of functional erythrocytes, or through secondary infections. Untreated Oroya fever will result in death in 40–85% of patients, one of the highest mortality rates of all infectious diseases [Ihler, 1996]. The disease then enters an intercalary period during which the blood is cleared of infection and erythrocyte levels return to normal. This process may take weeks or months, and patients may remain bacteraemic for prolonged periods.

Subsequent to Oroya fever, angiogenic skin lesions, termed verrugas, erupt all over the body as a result of proliferation of subdermal vascular endothelial cells, mediated by factors released by infecting *B. bacilliformis* [Garcia et al., 1990]. The lesions occur in numerous forms which may be of varying sizes, numbers and distribution, and which may be confined to the papillary dermis or infect all layers of the dermis or subcutaneous tissue. In general, lesions are friable and bleed easily, although older forms may be more robust. These lesions resemble those observed in cases of bacillary angiomatosis due to either *B. henselae* or *B. quintana*, and may also be confused with atypical forms of Kaposi's sarcoma [Webster et al., 1992]. Although often disfiguring, the verrugas are self-limiting, and over a period of months they gradually disappear.

*Microbiology.* During the height of anaemia, *B. bacilliformis* can be easily observed infecting erythrocytes in Giemsa-stained blood films, and bacteria can be recovered on blood-rich axenic media. Isolates grow best if incubated at 28–32 °C in a 5% $CO_2$ atmosphere, typically taking a week to become visible. Growth of primary isolates does not occur at 37 °C which might explain why *B. bacilliformis* preferentially infects the skin, although this is not compatible with their rapid multiplication in the bloodstream. No other diagnostic methods are routinely used, although serological assays and PCR-based detection methods have been described [Knobloch et al., 1985; Maas et al., 1992].

*B. bacilliformis* is a highly motile species, being propelled by multiple unipolar flagella. Bacterial motility is necessary for optimal binding of the bacterium to the erythrocyte surface, and treatment of *B. bacilliformis* with antiflagellar antibodies reduces binding considerably [Ihler, 1996].

As expected, *B. bacilliformis* remains inert in most standard physiological tests, and is nonfermentative for a wide range of sugars. The G+C content of the species has been calculated as being about 40%, whereas genome molecular mass estimations vary between $4 \times 10^8$ and $1.3 \times 10^9$ [Brenner et al., 1991b; Birtles et al., 1991]. Small subunit (16S) rRNA gene sequence comparison demonstrated that *B. bacilliformis* is the most distinct member of the genus, although it retains a specific relationship with the other *Bartonella* species [Birtles et al., 1995]. This observation concurs with DNA homology data, which again indicates the species to be an outlying member of the genus [Birtles et al., 1995].

*Epidemiology and Natural Cycle.* Although recognized hundreds of years ago and despite its severity, bartonellosis remains little studied, probably because the disease is almost entirely limited to the inter-Andean valleys of Peru, Ecuador and Columbia. The basis of the disease's distribution in Peru is that it generally matches that of *Lutzomyia verriformis* [Carceres, 1993] which is thought to be the principle vector of the bacterium [Townsend, 1913]. However, as the disease occurs in regions of the country where this species of sandfly is absent, and a recent outbreak continued despite destruction of the local sandfly population by spraying, other vectors or modes of transmission must exist [Gray et al., 1990]. Interestingly, prior to a recent outbreak, villagers reported increased flea bites, which suggests a mode of transmission similar to that which has been observed for *Bartonella* species infecting rodents [Gray et al., 1990].

An infection which presents in an indistinguishable way to verruga peruana has been observed in the lowland province of Manabi in southern Ecuador, an area where none of the 'highland' species of *Lutzomyia* exist. In a recent study, 11 index cases of cutaneous 'bartonellosis' were investigated, and serosurvey of their close contacts revealed 21% seropositivity. Comparison of a partial 16S rRNA gene sequence obtained by PCR-based amplification of DNA in a fixed verrugal biopsy indicated the infecting organism to be *Bartonella*-like, but clearly different from Peruvian *B. bacilliformis* strains [Amano et al., 1997]; isolates are yet to be obtained. Outside South America, bartonellosis is only encountered in travel-associated cases [Matteelli et al., 1994].

At present, man is thought to be the reservoir for the disease, and Herrer [1990] has demonstrated that up to 10% of individuals living in endemic areas had asymptomatic infections, albeit on a seasonal basis (infections disappeared during the 'dry' season). Conversely, in a recent survey by Cooper et al. [1996] in Zamora Chinchipe province in southern Ecuador, an endemic region, no evidence of current blood-borne infection with *B. bacilliformis* was seen among almost 250 schoolchildren. Other reservoirs may therefore exist, and such a proposition is supported by several other observations, including (1) animal infections have been induced in vitro, (2) anecdotal evidence suggests that animals develop verruga-like warts in endemic regions, (3) bartonellosis can be acquired in uninhabited regions, and (4) increases in the rodent population have been reported prior to outbreaks [Gray et al., 1991]. However, in the only study of its kind to date, a survey of the blood of endemic intradomicillary animals in the Huayllacallan valley in Ancash, Peru, whilst demonstrating the presence of other *Bartonella* species, have failed to detect *B. bacilliformis* [Birtles et al., 1998].

In endemic regions of Ecuador and Peru, members of the indigenous population are prone to relapses of verruga, but not anaemia. Indeed, most of the population may well acquire the disease whilst young, and therefore be offered some degree of immunity. The disease appears to be most severe when acquired by visitors to the region, and historically, the most dramatic outbreaks have been reported among immigrant workers. Interestingly, today, the clearing of forests in the north of Peru for agricultural exploitation is leading to a new influx of people into regions where bartonellosis is endemic, and many new cases are being encountered. Similarly, border disputes between Peru and

Ecuador have also led to cases among the military personnel deployed in the conflict [Leon and Leon, 1986].

Estimation of the prevalence of bartonellosis is difficult, but it is certain that the remoteness of the endemic region prevents many cases being referred to the health services. The most recent national estimate available is for 1992, when about 1,500 cases were registered. In general, the prevalence of the disease is cyclic with widespread epidemics occurring every 15–20 years. As the last of these occurred in the late 1970s, a large-scale outbreak may be imminent.

*Antibiotic Susceptibility.* Urteaga and Payne [1955] proposed the use of chloramphenicol in the treatment of Oroya fever, and during the most recently reported outbreak of bartonellosis, as reported by Gray et al. [1990], chloramphenicol was the only antibiotic used. The case fatality rate for untreated patients was 88%, but among at least 10 acutely ill patients who were treated, all survived and were healthy in a survey conducted at the end of the outbreak. Although many antibiotics are effective, chloramphenicol is most commonly used as it is also effective against salmonellae which are frequently the cause of secondary infections. Antibiotic efficacy against verruga peruana is less clear cut; rifampin and streptomycin may be useful. Over the last 10 years, Peruvian clinicians have observed chloramphenicol resistance among some *B. bacilliformis* strains [Dr. H. Guerra, Universidad Cayetano Heredia, Lima, Peru, unpubl. observations].

### *Bartonella quintana*

*Medical Relevance. B. quintana* infection, manifesting as trench fever, was first encountered during World War I among allied and axis troops. Detailed descriptions of trench fever have been made [Byam et al., 1919]. Typically the incubation period for the disease is about 3 weeks, after which clinical manifestations ranging from mild infection to severe illness develop. The most frequently encountered presentation among World War I troops was a febrile illness of acute onset and of a 5-day periodic nature, often accompanied by severe headache and pain in the lower legs. The headache may indicate meningitis, especially when occipital and associated with stiffness of the neck. Although recurrent, each succeeding attack is usually less severe than its predecessor. Only in severe cases will a patient become weaker and leg pains more persistent. The tongue may become furred and conjunctival congestion as well as slow pulse may also be observed. Areas of tenderness occur around painful muscles, tendons, bones or joints, and the spleen becomes palpable. Major polymorphonuclear leukocytosis often accompanies the fever, and anaemia may occur in chronically ill patients. Nevertheless, despite chronic infection, fatalities among trench fever patients have not been recorded.

Trench fever was re-encountered during World War II, although not on such a widespread scale, and after the cessation of hostilities in 1945, only the odd sporadic case was reported [Vinson, 1966]. However, over the past 8 years there has been a re-emergence of *B. quintana* infections, predominantly encountered among the homeless and alcoholic populations of modern cities or those with AIDS.

In the most complete study of *B. quintana* infections among the former of these groups, an 'outbreak' of 10 cases of culture-confirmed bacteraemia in Seattle, Washington, was reported by Spach et al. [1995]. No consistent symptoms were recorded in this study other than fever and weight loss. The bacteraemia persisted for more than 10 days in 4 patients and for more than 8 weeks in 1 who refused antibiotic therapy. One patient died from concurrent *Streptococcus pneumoniae* bacteraemia. Prolonged *B. quintana* bacteraemia, similar to those observed above, was often reported among wartime trench fever patients [Byam et al., 1919].

A more profound manifestation of *B. quintana* infection among the urban deprived is endocarditis. One of the 10 patients in the above study had aortic valve vegetations, and Drancourt et al. [1995] concurrently reported the syndrome in 3 French homeless men. All patients required valve replacement surgery. All were blood culture-positive for *B. quintana* and possessed high titres of anti-*B. quintana* antibodies. A recent study by Raoult et al. [1996] described 22 cases of culture-negative native valve endocarditis caused by *Bartonella* species diagnosed using a combination of antibody estimations, culture and PCR-based detection methods. *B. quintana* was diagnosed as the cause of 5 of these cases, whereas 13 were not attributed to a specific species as the serological assays used for diagosis were not able to accurately differentiate between the different members of the genus. All patients fulfilled the criteria for endocarditis proposed by Durack et al. [1994].

*B. quintana* has also been demonstrated in a number of cases of bacillary angiomatosis (BA), a vascular proliferative disease which was first recognized in AIDS patients in 1983 by Stohler et al. Although most cases reported to date have been in HIV-seropositive individuals, some infections have been encountered in organ transplant patients and among the immunocompetent [Cockerell et al., 1990].

BA presents most often as skin lesions, which bleed profusely when punctured, and enlarged lymph nodes, usually corresponding to the regional drainage of skin lesions [Tappero et al., 1993]. The form, location and distribution of lesions can vary immensely, thus they can be superficial, dermal or subcutaneous, ranging in colour from blood-red to deep purple. Subdermal lesions may be mobile or fixed to underlying structures. Lesions can begin as papules then gradually increase in size to form larger nodules. BA can also effect the bone marrow, spleen, liver and the mucosal surfaces of the mouth, anus, conjunctiva or the gut [Koehler et al., 1988, 1992]. The clinical differential diagnosis of BA includes pyogenic granuloma, haemangioma, various subcutaneous tumours, and atypical Kaposi sarcoma; however, the demonstration of the presence of bacteria in histologic biopsy specimens should allow BA to be clearly distinguished. The skin lesions of BA are indistinguishable from those associated with bartonellosis, and it is likely that the two are formed by similar pathogenic processes.

Initial microbiological investigation of BA demonstrated it to be caused by *B. henselae* [Relman et al., 1990]; however, identification of the aetiological agent in an increasing number of cases led to the recognition of the role of *B. quintana* in the syndrome [Koehler et al., 1992; Maurin et al., 1994]. There appears to be no specific manifestations associated with either species.

In addition to trench fever, endocarditis and BA, *B. quintana* has been demonstrated to induce a number of other clinical manifestations. The species has been isolated from a woman with chronic cervical and mediastinal adenopathy [Raoult et al., 1994], and more recently from a woman with Goujerot-Sjögren disease who had been undergoing long-term renal dialysis [Maurin and Raoult, 1996]. Very recently, Holmberg et al. [1997] have reported a *Bartonella* infection in a 60-year-old with myocarditis who succumbed to sudden death, although as yet the causative species has not been confirmed.

*Microbiology.* Despite being first observed infecting trench fever patients during Wold War I, it was not until 1961 that Vinson and Fuller finally isolated *B. quintana* from blood drawn from a patient with experimentally induced trench fever. Lice infected with *B. quintana* were fed daily on the volunteer for about 6 weeks until he experienced a typical clinical course of the disease. Isolates were obtained on blood-rich media inoculated with blood following 12 days of incubation at 34 °C in a moist, $CO_2$-rich (5%) atmosphere and were of typical *Bartonella*-like appearance, being convex, transparent, mucoid, and with smooth edges. Postinfection, but not preinfection, sera collected from the volunteer reacted strongly with the isolate in an indirect immunofluorescence test. Vinson et al. [1969] subsequently fulfilled Koch's postulates by inducing trench fever in another volunteer following inoculation with the bacteria propagated on blood agar, then re-isolating the organism from the volunteer's blood on blood agar and in lice.

Following axenic culture, *B. quintana* could be subjected to rigorous characterization. Tyeryar et al. [1973] calculated the G+C content to be 39%. Weisburg et al. [1989] determined the 16S rRNA gene sequence of *B. quintana* and by comparison with those of other bacteria, inferred its phylogenetic position to be close to *Brucella abortus*. This provided the first clear evidence that, against the general opinion of the time, the species was not specifically related to the *Rickettsiaceae*. In keeping with other *Bartonella* species, *B. quintana* is inert in most standard physiological tests, although it has been reported to be weakly oxidase-positive [Brenner et al., 1993]. Assay for preformed peptidases demonstrated the species could be distinguished from all other species except *B. vinsonii* [Birtles et al., 1995]. DNA relatedness was found to be high (20–70%) with other *Bartonella* species, but low ($<20\%$) with *Rickettsia prowazekii* [Brenner et al., 1993].

Huang [1967] assessed the metabolic requirements of *B. quintana* and reported that the species can utilize succinate, pyruvate and glutamine or glutamate, but not glucose, as sources of energy. Growth is enhanced by increasing amounts of $CO_2$ and by fetal calf serum, and is hemin-dependent. *B. quintana* also requires sodium bicarbonate as a carbon source [Myers et al., 1972; Weiss and Dasch, 1984].

Current approaches to the microbiological diagnosis of *B. quintana* infections include culture, antibody estimation and PCR-based methods. The optimum conditions required for the recovery of isolates from clinical materials are disputed. Some studies used direct plating onto axenic media [Maurin et al., 1994; Drancourt et al., 1995; Spach et al., 1995] whereas others used co-cultivation in cell cultures [Koehler et al., 1992; Raoult et al., 1994].

Axenic culture conditions generally require blood-rich media and $CO_2$-rich, humid incubation conditions. Primary incubation times should be very prolonged, at least 45 days. Pretreatment of blood specimens by lysis centrifugation may enhance recovery [Welch et al., 1992]. Detection of *Bartonella* species in conventional blood cultures remains difficult as the organisms produce little or no $CO_2$ or visible growth, thus Larson et al. [1994] proposed a procedure by which bacteria are detected using an acridine orange dye staining procedure. Koehler et al. [1992] were the first to use co-cultivation methods, recovering *B. quintana* from BA patients via a bovine endothelial cell line. Similar cell lines were used by other groups to obtain isolates when direct plating failed [Drancourt et al., 1995; Raoult et al., 1994].

Among BA patients, most of whom are immunodeficient, significant antibody response to infection is often not mounted. Conversely, serological diagnosis is of most use among endocarditis patients who typically yield exceedingly high anti-*Bartonella* titres. In their review of 33 cases of *Bartonella*-induced endocarditis, Raoult et al. [1996] obtained serological data on all bar 4 patients. Of these 29, 28 yielded titres of $>1,600$ against *B. henselae*, and of $>400$ against *B. quintana*, confirming the usefulness of this diagnostic method, but demonstrating its limitation – differentiation between *Bartonella* species is not possible. Cross-reactivity between anti-*Bartonella* antibodies and other antigens, most importantly *Chlamydia* species, has been observed and led to misdiagnosis of cases of *Bartonella* endocarditis; 9 of the patients in the above series had previously been thought to have chlamydial endocarditis.

PCR-based detection methods have proven particularly useful for diagnosis of these fastidious organisms. The 16S rRNA gene and the *gltA* have been two regions of the genome on which efforts to produce PCRs specific for the *Bartonella* genus have concentrated [Relman et al., 1990; Norman et al., 1995], although Anderson et al. [1994] have also targeted a heat-shock gene fragment. The identity of amplified fragments has usually been confirmed by REA, hybridization with internal probes, or base sequence determination, as, as yet, no reliable species-specific PCRs have been evaluated.

*Epidemiology and Natural Cycle.* Subsequent to the Seattle 'outbreak' discussed above, Jackson et al. [1996] carried out a *B. quintana* serosurvey among the city's homeless and/or alcoholic population by testing sera collected from attendees of a downtown community clinic. Titres considered indicative of infection were detected in 39 of 192 compared to 4 of 199 blood donors, suggesting the prevalence of *B. quintana* infection was surprisingly high. Among the clinic patients, alcohol abuse was the only factor found to be independently associated with diagnostic titres. However, of the seropositive patients, 62% also yielded high titres against *B. henselae* indicating cross-reaction between the two species. Raoult et al. [1996] also collated epidemiological findings of 11 patients with *B. quintana* endocarditis, finding 8 were homeless, 7 were alcoholic and only 2 had had valvulopathy previously.

As with *B. bacilliformis*, man is presently the only recognized host for *B. quintana*. Infection is thought to be transmitted exclusively by the human body louse (*Pediculus humanis*), and survey of these ectoparasites in Burundi indicated about 15% to be infected with the bacterium [D. Raoult, unpubl. observations]. Early work by Wolbach et al. [1922] demonstrated the species multiplied extracellularly in the gut of the louse, in which it produced neither apparent pathology nor death.

Outbreaks of lice are induced by poor social and hygiene conditions and are thus usually associated with wars or natural disasters. Under such conditions, widespread *B. quintana* infection is likely, but as trench fever is usually a mild illness, its clinical diagnosis is difficult and therefore its prevalence is probably underestimated. Although it is feasible that inner-city homeless and alcoholics acquire infection from infesting lice, such a cycle seems far less likely for *B. quintana* infections in HIV-positive individuals. Although their immunodeficient state compromises them to infection, the HIV-positive patients with *B. quintana*-induced BA have not been louse-infested, nor have they led lifestyles compatible with ectoparasitic infestation.

Comparison of *B. quintana* isolates revealed some heterogeneity. Welch et al. [1992] used fatty acid analysis to distinguish between two strains, and later Roux and Raoult [1995] used macrorestriction analysis (MRA) to demonstrate genetic relationships among seven isolates. Although, in general, profile patterns were well conserved suggesting intraspecies homology, *Eag*I and *Sma*I were useful in differentiating the strains, and numerical analysis of profiles allowed dendrographic representation of their genetic relatedness. Although no correlation between the *B. quintana* genotypes and either their geographic distribution or clinical data from infected individuals was found, the usefulness of MRA for epidemiological typing of the species was demonstrated. Such an approach would be useful, for example, in determining the relationship of the Seattle outbreak strains. In the same study the 16S/23S intragenic spacer region of each of the seven isolates was also determined and compared. Two subgroups were found among the seven strains, although the sequence of each differed by less than 0.5%. This approach does not, therefore, appear to be as sensitive a method as MRA for the epidemiological study of *B. quintana* [Roux and Raoult, 1995].

*Antibiotic Susceptibility.* As most cases of trench fever occurred prior to the antibiotic era, very few records of treatment exist; Vinson et al. [1969] report of successful treatment with chloramphenicol being one of the few available. Data on more recently recognized *B. quintana* infections are more forthcoming. For the treatment of BA, nafcillin, dicloxacillin and cephalexin A regimens have been reported to be ineffective, findings which are consistent with results of in vitro susceptibility testing. Clinical data supported the use of amoxicillin, aminoglycosides, trimethoprim-sulphamethoxazole and doxycycline, although again regimen failures have been reported [Maurin and Raoult, 1996]. Information regarding the effective treatment of *B. quintana* endocarditis is more scarce as so few cases have been reported. In the series of 22 patients reported by Raoult et al. [1996], 15 received aminoglycoside therapy of whom 6 died and 9 recovered. Treatment of bacteraemia has also been described; 5 of the patients described by Spach et al. [1995] were treated for 7 days with ceftriaxone followed either by erythromycin or azithromycin for 3 weeks. Follow-up was possible on only 3 patients, in all of whom bacteraemia resolved. The poor efficacy of β-lactams in treatment does not reflect the susceptibility of bartonellae to these drugs in vitro [Myers et al., 1984], however, such an observation may be due to the intracellular location of infecting bacteria.

### *Bartonella elizabethae*

*Medical Relevance.* Only one confirmed isolate of *B. elizabethae* has been reported [Daly et al., 1993]. This strain was isolated from the blood of a patient with endocarditis. The patient had been unwell for 2 months prior to hospitalization for surgery with a history of fatigue, malaise, shortness of breath, and a 9-kg weight loss. Perhaps of relevance is that he had sustained lacerations on his left hand 2 weeks prior to onset of symptoms, however, he had no history of drug use, exposure to pets or other animals, or a chronic underlying clinical condition. On admission the patient was febrile, had multiple infected teeth and a diastolic murmur of aortic regurgitation. An echocardiogram revealed large vegetations on the aortic valve, and on subsequent valve replacement the tricuspid valve was found to be vegetated on all three cuspids. Gram staining of this vegetation revealed abundant minute coccobacillary organisms.

*Microbiology.* Direct culture of blood samples did not yield any isolates, but subculture of a sample from the aerobic bottle, done approximately 1 week after inoculation, grew small dry colonies after about 14 days of incubation at 35 °C in a 5–10% $CO_2$-enriched atmosphere. Biochemical assessment of the isolate was initially fruitless as it remained inert in all standard tests. Later, the strain, F9251, underwent complete characterization, during which it was found: (1) to be susceptible to all antibiotics tested; (2) to have a G + C content of 41.0 mol%; (3) to share between 32 and 67% DNA relatedness with the other *Bartonella* species recognized at the time; (4) to have a 16S rRNA gene sequence which was very similar to, but distinguishable from, those of the other *Bartonellae* (98.4–99.6% similarity), and (5) to possess a cellular fatty acid profile typical for the *Bartonella*. In phenotypic terms, F9251 could be differentiated from the other *Bartonella* species as it demonstrated hemolysis, albeit weak, on rabbit blood, and, along with *B. henselae*, did not demonstrate weak oxidase activity using the Kovacs procedure. On the basis of these findings, F9251 was proposed as the type strain of the new species *B. elizabethae* [Daly et al., 1993].

*Epidemiology and Natural Cycle. B. elizabethae* has only once been encountered in a clinical setting and, as discussed above, no epidemiological factors which could be specifically associated with the infection. However, Birtles et al. [1996] isolated a *Bartonella* from a rat in Peru which had a citrate synthase gene (*gltA*) sequence indistinguishable from that of F9251. *GltA*, rather than 16S rRNA gene, sequences were compared as it has been demonstrated that interspecies differences are about 12 times greater in the former than the latter, thus species can be more confidently differentiated from one another. However, despite sharing the same *gltA* sequence, a small degree of genetic variation between F9251 and the Peruvian isolate was found, so the precise relationship between the two strains is not clear. Regnery et al. [1996] and Ellis et al. [1997] also preliminarily reported the isolation of *B. elizabethae* from North American rodents although details of how they confirmed identity of their isolates have not yet been presented. Despite this, these three studies do provide some evidence to suggest that *B. elizabethae*, like *B. vinsonii* and three other *Bartonella* species discussed later in this chapter, naturally infects small mammals which therefore act as its reservoir. If this is confirmed, it is also likely that as with other rodent-borne bartonellae, *B. elizabethae* is transmitted between hosts by ectoparasite vectors. Whether this mode of transmission can also lead to human infections remains to be assessed.

*Antibiotic Susceptibility.* The patient with *B. elizabethae* endocarditis did not respond to nafcillin or gentamicin treatment, but symptoms resolved after cardiac valve replacement and a regimen of vancomycin and imipenem therapy was continued for 6 weeks, and oral trimethoprim-sulphamethoxazole was administered for a further 5 weeks [Daly et al., 1993].

### *Bartonella clarridgeiae*

*Medical Relevance.* Kordick et al. [1997] very recently reported a case of CSD caused by *B. clarridgeiae*. The patient was a veterinarian who, a few weeks after adopting a kitten, developed headache, fever and left axillary node lymphadenopathy. Although initial blood cultures from the patient and the cat were sterile, repeat cultures from the cat yielded *B. clarridgeiae*. Sera from the patient were reactive against the cat isolate (titre 1/1,024), but not against *B. henselae, B. quintana* or *B. elizabethae*. Sera from the cat were reactive at high titres to both *B. henselae* and *B. clarridgeiae*, and at a lower titre to *B. quintana*.

This is the only report of *B. clarridgeiae* involvement in CSD to date, however, as 16% or more of patients with clinically defined CSD are seronegative for *B. henselae* [Dalton et al., 1995; Bergmans et al., 1997b], it is possible that some of these cases may have been due to *B. clarridgeiae* and failure to obtain a diagnosis resulted from the use of the incorrect antigen in serological assays.

*Microbiology. B. clarridgeiae* was proposed in 1996 following characterization of a *Bartonella*-like organism isolated from the blood of a domestic cat. Although the colony morphology and biochemical reactions of the isolate were found to be similar to those of the recognized *Bartonella* species, the presence of flagella and a characteristic 16S rRNA sequence, together with earlier evidence based on citrate synthase gene sequence and cellular fatty acid analysis, were cited in support of it representing a new species [Lawson and Collins, 1996].

The isolate was first encountered during investigation into a case of *B. henselae* bacteraemia [Clarridge et al., 1995]. The patient had a cat which was suspected as being the source of infection, thus a blood sample was taken from the animal. *Bartonella* were recovered from the sample by first inoculating a paediatric Isolator tube, then plated the contents of the tube onto blood-rich media. The resulting colonies were originally differentiated from those of other *Bartonella* species as they were indurated yet did not embed in the agar. Microscopic analysis revealed they also possessed flagella, which other species except *B. bacilliformis* lack. The biochemical profile of the isolate was assessed using the RapID ANA II panel, and, as expected, it was inert except for the production of peptidases. The isolate shared the same profile as *B. henselae* and *B. quintana*, cleaving only leucyl-glycine, glycine, proline, phenylalanine, arginine and serine.

Lawson and Collins [1996] further characterized the isolate using electron microscopy to confirm the presence of flagella, and 16S rRNA sequence analysis to yield a unique sequence which demonstrated 97.4–98.5% similarity to those of the other *Bartonella* species. On the basis of these findings, the isolate was proposed as a new species, despite the difference in 16S rRNA sequence not being sufficient to fulfill the 97% cut-off criterion proposed for species delineation. This is an interesting taxonomic precedent, justified on the grounds that (1) the levels of sequence divergence between *B. clarridgeiae* and other *Bartonella* species are substantially higher than observed values between other *Bartonella* species known to be genotypically distinct using DNA:DNA pairing, and (2) *B. clarridgeiae* forms a distinct evolutionary line within phylogenetic reconstructions for the *Bartonella* genus.

*Epidemiology and Natural Cycle. B. clarridgeiae* has now been isolated from a number of apparently healthy cats in the USA and Europe. In a recent survey in France, Heller et al. [1997] reported that 53% of 94 stray cats sampled yielded a *Bartonella* isolate, and of these 30% (15 cats) yielded *B. clarridgeiae*. In this study primary isolates of *B. clarridgeiae* were only recovered from bloods treated using paediatric Isolator tubes and inoculated into BACTEC medium; strains could not be recovered by direct inoculation of blood-rich agars with the Isolator tube contents. A further study by the same group [Gurfield et al., 1997] demonstrated that 5 of 436 domestic cats in France were coinfected with *B. henselae* and *B. clarridgeiae*. In a concurrent study, Bergmans et al. [1997a] detected presumptive *B. clarridgeiae* in 9 of 113 (8%) bloods collected from cats living in four shelters in different regions of The Netherlands. Blood samples were treated by lysis centrifugation, pellets were resuspended in NZ broth, then plated onto blood-rich agar. Again, co-infection with *B. henselae* was demonstrated in 5 cats. Furthermore, *B. clarridgeiae* DNA was detected in fleas collected from 1 bacteraemic cat, suggesting these ectoparasites may have a role in the transmission of the species.

*Antibiotic Susceptibility.* The in vitro antibiotic suceptibility of *B. clarridgeiae* has not been assessed. The one human case to date recovered following a 2-week regimen of doxycycline (500 mg every 12 h).

### *Bartonella vinsonii*

*Veterinary Relevance.* Veterinary interest in *B. vinsonii* has followed recent evidence implicating the species in endocarditis. In 1995, Breitschwerdt et al. described a case of vegetative valvular endocarditis involving aortic and to a lesser extent, mitral valves in a 3-year old Labrador retriever. The dog had been unwell for about 5 months, initially appearing lethargic, intermittently inappetent and with shifting leg lameness, then suffering increasing weight loss and the appearance of numerous intradermal haemorrhages on the neck and trunk. Despite the administration of tetracycline and prednisone, the dog continued to show signs of listlessness and epistaxis. Electrocardiograms confirmed the presence of isolated, infrequent ventricular extrasystoles and revealed a large vegetative lesion involving aotic valve and a smaller vegetative lesion on the anterior mitral valve leaflet. The dog had anaemia and thrombocytopenia, together with mild hypoalbuminaemia, azotaemia and hypokalaemia. Blood cultured by the lysis centrifugation technique grew a fastidious Gram-negative bacterium.

Treatment for presumed bacterial endocarditis accompanied by congestive heart failure consisted of enrofloxacin, doxycycline, clavulanate-potentiated amoxicillin, furosemide, digoxin and enalapril. However, due to a lack of substantial clinical improvement and intractable epitaxis, the owners elected euthanasia 17 days later. Post-mortem examination confirmed partially mineralized vegetations up to 1.25 cm in diameter replacing all three valvulae of the tricuspid aortic valve and a few smaller nodules on the mitral valve. Petechiae and ecchymoses were scattered throughout the brain, lungs and kidneys, and focally there were a few regions of marked haemorrhage and haematomas within the cerebellum, lungs and nasal cavity. Warthin-Starry silver staining of the aortic valve lesion revealed the presence of a dense bacterial vegetation, the organisms being of a morphology compatible with them being bartonellae.

Subsequent analysis of the bacterial isolate obtained confirmed it to be a *Bartonella* species. On the basis of 16S rRNA gene sequence comparison and DNA:DNA homology data the strain was assigned to the species *B. vinsonii*, although it was considered to demonstrate sufficient phenotypic and genotypic differences from the type strain of the species to warrant being classified as a new subspecies, thus it was proposed under the name *B. vinsonii* subspecies *berkhoffii*. To date this case is the only one of its kind to be reported; the same group has reported obtaining a number of additional isolates, but their source has not yet been disclosed [Pappalardo et al., 1997].

*Microbiology.* Prior to the case described above, *B. vinsonii* was represented by a sole isolate which orginated from the blood of a vole captured on Grosse Isle in the St. Lawrence Seaway, Canada, in 1940 [Baker, 1946]. At this time the island was being used as a war disease control station, however 100 years earlier it had been a quarantine island for immigrants prior to their admittance into Canada. During the 1840s a massive outbreak of typhus occurred among Irish immigrants, and many had died during quarantine and were buried on the island. James Baker, a member of a detachment of the US Army Veterinary Corps which was stationed on the island during World War II, researched this outbreak and suspected that the typhus rickettsiae may persist in the island's fauna. During survey of captured voles for the presence of the rickettsiae, Baker encountered a microorganism which he considered as possibly being the agent he searched for, particularly as he could only recover it in egg yolk sacs.

In 1978, Weiss et al. demonstrated Baker had been mistaken – the organism he had isolated was not a *Rickettsiae* and could be cultured axenically on blood-rich media. Initial characterization of the isolate demonstrated it to share an enzyme reactivity pattern with the then named *R. quintana*, and to have an identical G+C content (39%). Furthermore, serological studies demonstrated strong cross-reactivity between antiserum raised against the vole agent and *R. quintana*. The conclusion of this analysis was therefore that the vole isolate was a strain of *R. quintana*, however, a more thorough comparative study followed and led to a different opinion. This study, which used additional polyphasic characterization methods including DNA:DNA homogy studies, led to Weiss and Dasch [1984] amending their earlier identification, and proposing Baker's isolate to be a new species, *Rochalimaea vinsonii*. As described above for *B. quintana, R. vinsonii* was renamed *Bartonella vinsonii* in 1993 following demonstration of close evolutionary links between the members of the two genera [Brenner et al., 1993].

As described above, recent interest in *B. vinsonii* has followed the isolation of new strains of the species. Although the species has been demonstrated as the cause of endocarditis in one animal, it has also been recovered from an apparently healthy dog [Breitschwerdt et al., 1995]. The primary cultures of both isolates were obtained on blood-rich axenic media, although bloods were processed using lysis centrifugation methods prior to plating (direct plating of bloods onto agar did not yield isolates). Bacterial colonies appeared on primary isolate plates after their prolonged incubation at 35 °C in a 5–10% $CO_2$-enriched atmosphere. Microscopic examination of the isolates revealed their *Bartonella*-like morphology, and they remained inert in all standard biochemical tests. Cellular fatty acid analysis confirmed that the two isolates had profiles that in general were similar to that of the *B. vinsonii*-type strain, and those of the other *Bartonella* species. The 16S rRNA gene sequences of the strains were determined and on comparison were found to be almost indistinguishable from one another (99.8% similarity), and from the *B. vinsonii* type strain (99.4–99.6%). Very high levels of similarity were also found with the other *Bartonella* species (98.0–99.3%). The 16S rRNA gene sequence of both dog isolates included a 12 base pair insert in one of the highly variable regions of the gene; this feature had not previously been observed for either *B. vinsonii* or the other *Bartonella* species. DNA:DNA homology studies demonstrated that although the isolates were specifically related to the *B. vinsonii* type strain (72–82% relatedness under optimum conditions), they were markedly more closely related to one another (91%), thus they were proposed as members of a new *berkhoffii* subspecies.

*Epidemiology and Natural Cycle.* Pappalardo et al. [1997] very recently completed the evaluation of the risk factors associated with exposure and seroreactivity to *B. vinsonii* subspecies *berkhoffii* in a study of 69 case and 138 control dogs. Dogs testing seropositive to the organism were found to be 8.5 times more likely to live outdoors than to be kept predominantly indoors. Similarly, dogs which were allowed to roam free were 4.8 times more likely to be seropositive than those kept in a yard or leashed. Living in a rural area was also a factor which led to marked increase in risk of infection. Moreover, seropositive dogs were 5.6 times more likely to have a history of heavy flea exposure and were 14 times more likely to have a history of heavy tick exposure, suggesting, not unexpectedly, that ectoparasites act as vectors for the bacterium.

### *Bartonella doshiae, B. grahamii* and *B. taylorii*

*Veterinary Relevance.* These three species were isolated from the blood of apparently healthly small woodland mammals trapped in the UK. Microscopic observation of blood films made from infected animals demonstrated, in some cases, a significant number of infected erythrocytes, and under such circumstances it is difficult to believe that infection does not bear some cost on the host. Some work demonstrated that blood-borne infections are enhanced by immunosuppression due to splenectomy or concurrent infection with other pathogenic agents [Cox and Wedderburn, 1972], and that interaction between different forms of blood parasites occurs [Tyzzer, 1941]. However, to date there has been no evidence to suggest these species induce any specific illness on their hosts. As *B. elizabethae*, a species known to be pathogenic to humans, has also now been isolated from apparently healthy rodents, it is feasible that outside their nature hosts, all *Bartonella* species are potentially pathogenic. A lack of contact between infected rodents, their ectoparasites and humans, rather than a lack of virulence among these species, may limit infections in man.

*Microbiology.* In 1994, Birtles et al. surveyed '*Grahamella*' species infecting the blood of a population of small rodents trapped in Shropshire, UK, consisting predominantly of *Clethrionomys glareolus*, *Apodemus* species, and *Sorex auranus.* Isolates with a characteristic *Bartonella*-like appearance were obtained following incubation of blood-rich axenic media inoculated with blood pellets for up to 14 days at 37 °C in a $CO_2$-rich (5%) atmosphere. Characterization of the isolates revealed the presence of three species, all previously unencountered. The genus *Grahamella* had long been recognized as a repository for intraerythrocytic rod-shaped bacteria observed infecting a wide range of hosts. Very few of these organisms were grown let alone characterized, and their speciation was derived solely from the species of their host, thus *G. gallinarum* were associated with chicken erythrocytes, *G. canis* with dog erythrocytes, etc. In a review of Weinman and Kreier [1977], a list of over 35 species was so named. The shortcomings of these species descriptions led to exclusion of the genus from the official list of bacterial names published in 1980 [Skerman et al., 1980], however, Ristic and Kreier revived the genus together with the type species, *G. talpae* (from moles) and *G. peromysci* (from deer mice) in 1984.

The work by Birtles et al. [1994] not only identified new *Grahamella* species, but also confirmed their close relationship to *Bartonella* species, and demonstrated that the bacteria were not host-specific. Subsequently, a unification of the genera *Grahamella* and *Bartonella* was proposed, and the three new species were assigned as *B. grahamii*, *B. taylorii* and *B. doshiae* [Birtles et al., 1995]. Taxonomic protocol dictated that the species *G. talpae* and *G. peromysci* be also transferred into the *Bartonella* genus, despite there no longer being strains of either held in any culture collections.

The three species have been well characterized using polyphasic taxonomic methods. In keeping with other *Bartonella* species they were found to be generally unreactive in physiological tests, although preformed peptidase activity was detected, and could be used to distinguish between *B. doshiae* and the other two species [Birtles et al., 1995]. *B. taylorii* could be distinguished from the other species as it was not able to hydrolyse tributyrin. The three species were demonstrated to share between 40 and 51% DNA relatedness with one another and between 16 and 64% relatedness with the other *Bartonella* species, confirming them to be closely related but distinct. This finding has been confirmed by 16S rRNA gene and *gltA* sequence comparisons [Birtles et al.,

1995; Birtles and Raoult, 1996]. REA of PCR-amplified DNA fragments has been demonstrated to be useful for differentiating between the three species and other *Bartonella* strains; this approach has exploited sequence variation in both the 16S rRNA gene [Birtles, 1995] and the 16S/23S intragenic spacer region [Birtles et al., 1997].

*Epidemiology and Natural Cycle.* With a prevalence of infection of at least 40%, rodents are likely to be the natural reservoirs of *B. grahamii* and *B. taylorii*. To date, *B. doshiae* has only been isolated on one occasion, so speculation on its natural cycle is difficult. Krampitz [1962] demonstrated that '*Grahamella*' infections could be transmitted in vitro between infected and uninfected rodents by fleas. When fleas were absent, infection was not transmitted even if animals were kept in close contact, thus these ectoparasites are capable vectors. Turner [1986] demonstrated seasonal variations in the prevalence of '*Grahamella*' among UK small rodents, supporting the role of arthropods in their transmission; however, the ability of other ectoparasites such as mites or ticks to transmit infection has not been assessed. The natural cycle of bacteria within fleas has also not been determined, thus it is not known if they act as more than mere mechanical vectors of infected blood.

Birtles et al. [1997] presented preliminary data on intraspecies variation among bartonellae isolated from an isolated population of *Psammomys obesus* in Tunisia. REA of PCR-amplified 16S/23S intragenic spacer regions was used to demonstate the presence of clear heterogeneity among the most predominant species of *Bartonella* encountered. Similar observations have been made among strains of *B. grahamii* from UK rodents [R.J. Birtles, unpubl. observations], but the basis of this phenomenon is not yet apparent.

### Other Unnamed *Bartonella* Strains

Recent surveys of small mammal populations in Europe, Africa and North and South America have encountered *Bartonella* strains which are likely to be representatives of new species or subspecies. Ball [1995] encountered several isolates of a strain, now designated N40, whilst surveying intraerythrocytic bartonellae in small rodents in Staffordshire, UK, which has been shown to be genotypically and serologically distinct from other species. Birtles et al. [1998] isolated several new strains during a fruitless search for an animal reservoir for *B. bacilliformis* in Peru. Regnery et al. [1996] reported a diversity of strains infecting rodents captured in different regions of the USA, including one closely related to *B. elizabethae* and one closely related to *B. clarridgeiae*. Ellis et al. [1997] assessed *Bartonella* isolates obtained from *Rattus rattus* and

*Rattus norvegicus* captured in five North American states and in Bolivia and Paraguay using comparison of partial *gltA* sequences. All isolates clustered together, sharing a specific evolutionary relatedness with *B. elizabethae* and *B. grahamii*, with similarity values ranging from identity to 93%. These isolates also shared a specific relationship with the two rat isolates obtained by Birtles et al. [1998] in Peru, and, as proposed by both groups, these observations support a hypothesis that these strains are of Old World origin and were not present in the New World pre-Columbus. Jones et al. [1997] used the same method of comparative analysis to divide bartonellae isolated from North American rodents into seven different groupings. Some, but not all groups appeared to be host-specific, while others were found within specific geographical boundaries. Birtles et al. [1997] isolated and characterized two new strains of *Bartonella* from *Psammomys obesus* trapped in the Tunisian Sahara as well as detecting the presence of a third novel strain by PCR. *Bartonella*-like organisms have been observed parasitizing the erythrocytes of a wide range of animals throughout the world, and although rodents are the hosts which are most frequently implicated, it is likely that this is solely because it is this group of animals which is investigated most often. Infections have also been reported in other mammals such as cattle, bats, dogs, wolves and monkeys as well as in amphibians, turtles and fish [Weinman and Kreier, 1977].

All these studies serve to demonstrate the enormous diversity and potential ubiquitous incidence of *Bartonella* species, and it is clear that our knowledge of the range of the genus is presently woefully limited. In general, the bartonellae remain a group of bacteria for which we understand little. Clearly efforts to date have concentrated in assessing the pathogenic role of these organisms in humans, but as our knowledge of their diversity increases, we will also need to consider their ecological role on a broader scale.

## References


Alkan S, Morgan MB, Sandin RL, Moscinski LC, Ross CW: Dual role for *Afipia felis* and *Rochalimaea henselae* in cat scratch disease. Lancet 1995;345:385.

Amano Y, Rumbea J, Knobloch J, Olsen J, Kron M: Bartonellosis in Ecuador: Serosurvey and current status of cutaneous verrucous disease. Am J Trop Med Hyg 1997;57:174–179.

Amerein MP, De Briel D, Jaulhac B, Meyer P, Monteil H, Piemont Y: Diagnostic value of the indirect immunofluorescence assay in cat scratch disease with *Bartonella henselae* and *Afipia felis* antigens. Clin Diagn Lab Immunol 1996;3:200–204.

Anderson B, Sims K, Regnery R, Robinson L, Schmidt MJ, Goral S, Hager C, Edwards K: Detection of *Rochalimaea henselae* DNA in specimens from cat scratch disease patients by PCR. J Clin Microbiol 1994;32:942–948.

Baker JA: A rickettsial infection in Canadian voles. J Exp Med 1946;84:37–50.

Ball ML: MSc thesis, Liverpool School of Tropical Medicine, University of Liverpool, 1994.

Barton AL: Description de elementos endoglobulares en los enfermos de fiebre de verruga. Cron Med Lima 1909;26:7.

Bergmans AMC, Groothedde JW, Schellekens JFP, Van Embden JD, Ossewaarde JM, Schouls LM: Etiology of cat scratch disease: Comparison of polymerase chain reaction detection of *Bartonella* (formerly *Rochalimaea*) and *Afipia felis* DNA with serology and skin tests. J Infect Dis 1995;171: 916–923.

Bergmans AMC, De Jong CMA, Van Amerongen G, Schot CS, Schouls LM: Prevalence of *Bartonella* species in domestic cats in The Netherlands. J Clin Microbiol 1997a;35:2256–2261.

Bergmans AMC, Peeters MF, Schellekens JFP, Vos MC, Sabbe LJM, Ossewaarde JM, Verbakel H, Hooft HJ, Schouls LM: Pitfalls and fallacies of cat scratch disease serology: Evaluation of *Bartonella henselae*-based indirect fluorescence assay and enzyme-linked immunoassay. J Clin Microbiol 1997b; 35:1931–1937.

Birtles RJ: Differentiation of *Bartonella* species using restriction endonuclease analysis of PCR-amplified 16S rRNA genes. FEMS Microbiol Lett 1995;129:261–266.

Birtles RJ, Canales J, Alvarez E, Ventosilla P, Guerra H, Llanos-Cuentas, A, Raoult D, Doshi N, Harrison TG: Survey of *Bartonella* species infecting intra-domicillary animals in the Huayllacallan valley Ancash. Peru, a region of endemic for human bartonellosis. Am J Trop Med Hyg 1998; in press.

Birtles RJ, Fichet-Calvet E, Raoult D, Ashford RW: Detection and genotypic differentiation of *Bartonella* species infecting a Tunisian *Psammomys obesus* population. 13th Sesqui-Annual Meeting of the American Society for Rickettsiology, Seven Springs, Pa, Sept 1997, abstr 34.

Birtles RJ, Harrison TG, Fry NK, Saunders NA, Taylor AG: Taxonomic considerations of *Bartonella bacilliformis* based on phylogenetic and phenotypic characteristics. FEMS Microbiol Letts 1991; 83:187–192.

Birtles RJ, Harrison TG, Saunders NA, Molyneux DH: Proposals to unify the genera *Grahamella* and *Bartonella*, with descriptions of *Bartonella talpae* comb nov, *Bartonella peromysci* comb nov, and three new species, *Bartonella grahamii* sp nov, *Bartonella taylorii* sp nov, and *Bartonella doshiae* sp nov. Int J Syst Bacteriol 1995;45:1–8.

Birtles RJ, Raoult D: Comparison of citrate synthase gene (*gltA*) sequences for phylogenetic analysis of *Bartonella* species. Int J Syst Bacteriol 1996;46:891–897.

Bogue CW, Wise JD, Gray GF, Edwards KM: Antibiotic therapy for cat scratch disease. JAMA 1989; 262:813–816.

Breitschwerdt EB, Kordick DL, Malarkey DE, Keene B, Hadfield TL, Wilson K: Endocarditis in a dog due to infection with a novel *Bartonella* subspecies. J Clin Microbiol 1995;33:154–160.

Brenner DJ, Hollis DG, Moss CW, English CK, Hall GS, Vincent J, Radosevic J, Birkness KA, Bibb WF, Quinn FD, Swaminathan B, Weaver RE, Reeves MW, O'Connor SP, Hayes PS, Tenover FC, Steigerwalt AG, Perkins BA, Daneshvar MI, Hill BC, Washington JA, Woods TC, Hunter SB, Hadfield TL, Ajello GW, Kaufmann AF, Wear DJ, Wenger JD: Proposal of *Afipia* gen nov, with *Afipia felis* sp nov (formerly cat scratch disease bacillus), *Afipia clevelandensis* (formerly the Cleveland Clinic Foundation Strain), *Afipia broomeae* sp nov, and three unnamed genospecies. J Clin Microbiol 1991a;29:2450–2460.

Brenner DJ, O'Connor SP, Hollis DG, Weaver RE, Steigerwalt AG: Molecular characterisation and proposal of a neotype strain for *Bartonella bacilliformis.* J Clin Microbiol 1991b;29:1299–1302.

Brenner DJ, O'Connor SP, Winkler HH, Steigerwalt AG: Proposals to unify the genera *Bartonella* and *Rochalimaea*, with descriptions of *Bartonella quintana* comb nov, *Bartonella vinsonii* comb nov, *Bartonella henselae* comb nov, and *Bartonella elizabethae* comb nov, and to remove the family *Bartonellaceae* from the order *Rickettsiales.* Int J Syst Bacteriol 1993;43:777–786.

Byam W, Carroll JH, Churchill JH, Dimond L, Sorapure VE, Wilson RM, Lloyd LL: Trench fever: A louse-borne disease. London, Oxford University Press, 1919.

Caceres AG: Distribucion geographica de *Lutzomyia verrucarum* (Townsend, 1913) (*Diptera, Psychodidae, Phlebotominae*), vector de la bartonellosis humana en el Peru. Rev Inst Med Trop São Paulo 1993; 35:485–490.

Clarridge JE III, Raich TJ, Pirwani D, Simon B, Tsai L, Rodriguez-Barradas MC, Regnery R, Zollo A, Jones DC, Rambo C: Strategy to detect and identify *Bartonella* species in routine clinical laboratory yields *Bartonella henselae* from human immunodeficiency virus-positive patient and unique *Bartonella* strain from his cat. J Clin Microbiol 1995;33:2107–2113.

Cockerell CJ, Bergstresser PR, Myrie-Williams C, Tierno PM: Bacillary epithelioid angiomatosis occurring in an immunocompetent individual. Arch Dermatol 1990;126:787–790.
Cooper P, Guderian R, Paredes W, Daniels R, Perera D, Espinel M, Valdez M, Griffin G: Bartonellosis in Zamora Chinchipe province in Ecuador. Trans R Soc Trop Med Hyg 1996;90:241–243.
Cotter B, Maurer R, Hedinger C: Cat scratch disease: Evidence for a bacterial etiology: A retrospective analysis using Warthin-Starry strain. Virchows Arch A 1986;410:103–106.
Cox FEG, Wedderburn N: Enhancement and prolongation of *Babesia microti* infections in mice infected with oncogenic viruses. J Gen Microbiol 1972;72:79–85.
Cuandra M, Takano J: The relationship of *Bartonella bacilliformis* to the red blood cell as revealed by electron microscopy. Blood 1969;33:708–716.
Dalton MJ, Robinson LE, Cooper J, Regnery RL, Olsen JG, Childs JE: Use of *Bartonella* antigens for serologic diagnosis of cat scratch disease at a national referral center. Arch Intern Med 1995;155: 1670–1676.
Daly JS, Worthington MG, Brenner DJ, Moss CM, Hollis DG, Weyant RS, Steigerwalt AG, Weaver RE, Daneshvar MI, O'Connor SP: *Bartonella elizabethae* sp nov isolated from a patient with endocarditis. J Clin Microbiol 1993;31:872–881.
Drancourt M, Birtles RJ, Chaumentin G, Vandendenesch F, Etienne J: A new serogroup of *Bartonella henselae* causes endocarditis and cat scratch disease. Lancet 1996;347:441–443.
Drancourt M, Brouqui P, Raoult D: *Afipia clevelandensis* antibodies and cross-reactivity with *Brucella* spp and *Yersinia enterocolitica* O:9. Clin Diag Lab Immunol 1997;4:748–752.
Drancourt M, Donnet A, Pelletier J, Raoult D: Acute meningoencephalitis associated with seroconversion to *Afipia felis*. Lancet 1992;340:558.
Drancourt M, Mainardi JL, Brouqui P, Vandenesch F, Carta A, Lehnert F, Etienne J, Goldstein F, Acar J, Raoult D: *Bartonella (Rochalimaea) quintana* endocarditis in three homeless men. N Engl J Med 1995;332:419–423.
Durack DT, Lukes AS, Bright DK: New criteria for diagnosis of infective endocarditis: Utilization of specific echocardiographic findings. Am J Med 1994;96:200–209.
Ellis B, Regnery R, Marston E, Jones D, Olsen J, Glass GE, Childs JE: Recovery and characterisation of *Bartonella* from the genus *Rattus*. 13th Sesqui-Annual Meeting of the American Society for Rickettsiology, Seven Springs, Pa, Sept 1997, abstr 21.
English CK, Wear DJ, Margileth AM, Lissner CR, Walsh GP: Cat scratch disease. Isolation and culture of the bacterial agent. JAMA 1988;259:1347–1352.
Garcia FU, Wojta J, Broadley KN, Davidson JM, Hoover RL: *Bartonella bacilliformis* stimulates endothelal cells in vitro and is angiogenic in vivo. Am J Pathol 1990;136:1125–1135.
Gray GC, Angulo Johnson A, Thornton SA, Alexander-Smith W, Knobloch J, Kelley PW, Obregon Escudero L, Arones Huayda M, Wignall FS: An epidemic of Oroya fever in the Peruvian Andes. Am J Trop Med Hyg 1990;42:215–221.
Gurfield AN, Boulouis H-J, Chomel BB, Heller R, Kasten RW, Yamamoto K, Piemont Y: Coinfection with *Bartonella clarridgeiae* and *Bartonella henselae* and with different *Bartonella henselae* strains in domestic cats. J Clin Microbiol 1997;35:2120–2123.
Hall GS, Pratt-Rippin K, Washington JA: Isolation of agent associated with cat scratch disease bacillus from pretibial biopsy. Diagn Microbiol Infect Dis 1991;34:511–513.
Heller R, Artois M, Xemar V, De Briel D, Gehin H, Jaulhac B, Monteil H, Piemont Y: Prevalence of *Bartonella henselae* and *Bartonella clarridgeiae* in stray cats. J Clin Microbiol 1997;35:1327–1331.
Herrer A: Epidemiologia de la verruga peruana. Lima, Pribaceb, 1990.
Holmberg M, Wesslen L, Hjelm E, Pahlson C, Lindquist O, Friman G, Regnery RL: *Bartonella* spp in a 60 year-old Swedish male with myocarditis who succumbed to sudden death. 13th Sesqui-Annual Meeting of the American Society for Rickettsiology, Seven Springs, Pa, Sept 1997, abstr 31.
Huang KY: Metabolic activities of the trench fever rickettsia, *Rickattsia quintana*. J Bacteriol 1967;93: 853–859.
Ihler GM: *Bartonella bacilliformis*: Dangerous pathogen slowly emerging from a deep background. FEMS Microbiol Lett 1996;144:1–11.

Jackson LA, Spach DH, Kippen DA, Sugg NK, Regnery RL, Sayers MH, Stamm WE: Seroprevalence to *Bartonella quintana* among patients at a community clinic in downtown Seattle. J Infect Dis 1996;173:1023–1026.

Jones D, Kosoy M, Marston E, Regnery D, Regnery R: A phylogenetic analysis of recently isolated *Bartonella* species using *gltA*. 13th Sesqui-Annual Meeting of the American Society for Rickettsiology, Seven Springs, Pa, Sept 1997, abstr 15.

Knobloch J, Solano L, Alvarez O, Delgado E: Antibodies to *Bartonella bacilliformis* as detected by fluorescence antibody test, indirect haemagglutination and ELISA. Trop Med Parasitol 1985;16:183–185.

Koehler JE, LeBoit PE, Egbert BM, Berger TG: Cutaneous vascular lesions and disseminated cat scratch disease in patients with the acquired immunodeficiency syndrome (AIDS) and AIDS-related complex. Ann Intern Med 1988;109:449–455.

Koehler JE, Quinn FD, Berger TG, LeBoit PE, Tappero JW: Isolation of *Rochalimaea* species from cutaneous and osseous lesions of bacillary angiomatosis. N Engl J Med 1992;327:1625–1631.

Kordick DL, Hilyard EJ, Hadfield TL, Wilson KH, Steigerwalt AG, Brenner DJ, Breitschwerdt EB: *Bartonella clarridgeiae*, a newly recognised zoonotic pathogen causing inoculation papules, fever, and lymphadenopathy (cat scratch disease). J Clin Microbiol 1997;35:1813–1818.

Kordick DL, Swaminathan B, Greene CE, Wilson KH, Whitney AN, O'Connor S, Hollis DG, Matar GM, Steigerwalt AG, Malcolm GB, Hayes PG, Hadfield TL, Breitschwerdt EB, Brenner DJ: *Bartonella vinsonii* subsp *berkhoffii* subsp nov, isolated from dogs; *Bartonella vinsonii* subsp *vinsonii*, and emended description of *Bartonella vinsonii*. Int J Syst Bacteriol 1996;46:704–709.

Krampitz HE: Weitere Untersuchungen an *Grahamella* Brumpt 1911. Z Tropenmed Parasitol 1962;13: 34–53.

Larson AM, Dougherty MJ, Nowowiejski DJ, Welch DF, Matar GM, Swaminathan B, Coyle MB: Detection of *Bartonella (Rochalimaea) quintana* by routine acridine orange staining of broth blood cultures. J Clin Microbiol 1994;32:1492–1496.

Lawson PA, Collins MD: Description of *Bartonella clarridgeiae* sp nov isolated from the cat of a patient with *Bartonella henselae* septicemia. Med Microbiol Lett 1996;5:64–73.

Leon LA, Leon R: Bartonellosis o enfermedad de Carrion en la Republica del Ecuador. Enfermededes Nativas No 1. Instituto de Investigaciones, Facultad de Ciencias Ledicas, Universidad Central del Ecuador, Quito, Ecuador 1986.

Maas M, Schreiber M, Knobloch J: Detection of *Bartonella bacilliformis* in cultures, blood and formulin-preserved skin biopsies by use of polymerase chain reaction. Trop Med Parasitol 1992;43:191–194.

Margileth AM, Wear DJ, Hadfield TL: Cat scratch disease: Bacteria in skin at the primary inoculation site. JAMA 1984;252:928–931.

Matteelli A, Castelli F, Spinetti A, Bonetti F, Graifenberghi S, Carosi G: Verruga peruana in an Italian traveller from Peru. Am J Trop Med Hyg 1994;50:143–144.

Maurin M, Lepocher H, Mallet D, Raoult D: Antibiotic susceptibilities of *Afipia felis* in axenic medium and in cells. Antimicrob Agents Chemother 1993;37:1410–1413.

Maurin M, Raoult D: *Bartonella (Rochalimaea) quintana* infections. Clin Microbiol Rev 1996;9:273–292.

Maurin M, Roux V, Stein A, Ferrier F, Viraben R, Raoult D: Isolation and characterisation by immunofluorescence, sodium dodecyl sulphate polyacrylamide gel electrophoresis, Western blot, restriction fragment length polymorphism-PCR, 16S rRNA gene sequencing, and pulsed-field gel electrophoresis of *Rochalimaea quintana* from a patient with bacillary angiomatosis. J Clin Microbiol 1994; 32:1166–1171.

Myers WF, Grossman DM, Wisseman CL: Antibiotic susceptibility patterns in *Rochalimaea quintana*, the agent of trench fever. Antimicrob Agents Chemother 1984;25:690–693.

Myers WF, Osterman JV, Wisseman CL: Nutritional studies of *Rickettsia quintana*. J Bacteriol 1972;109: 89–95.

Norman AF, Regnery RL, Jameson P, Greene C, Krause DC: Differentiation of *Bartonella*-like isolates by PCR-restriction fragment length polymorphism in the citrate synthase gene. J Clin Microbiol 1995;33:1797–1803.

Pappalardo BL, Correa MT, York CC, Peat CY, Breitschwerdt EB: Epidemiologic evaluation of the risk factors associated with exposure and seroreactivity to *Bartonella vinsonii* in dogs. Am J Vet Res 1997;58:467–471.

Raoult D, Drancourt M, Carta A, Gastaut JA: *Bartonella (Rochalimaea) quintana* isolation in patient with chronic adenopathy, lymphopenia, and a cat. Lancet 1994;343:977.

Raoult D, Fournier PE, Drancourt M, Marrie TJ, Etienne J, Cosserat J, Cacoub P, Poinsignon Y, Leclercq P, Sefton AM: Diagnosis of 22 new cases of *Bartonella* endocarditis. Ann Intern Med 1996;125: 646–652.

Regnery R, Jones D, Regnery D: Genotypic analysis of *Bartonella* genus isolates. 12th Sesqui-Annual Meeting of the American Society for Rickettsiology, Monterey, Calif, March 1996, abstr 49.

Relman DA, Loutit JS, Schmidt TM, Falkow S, Tompkins LS: The agent of bacillary angiomatosis. An approach to the identification of uncultured pathogens. N Engl J Med 1990;323:1573–1580.

Reschke DK, Frazier ME, Mallavia LP: Transformation and genomic restriction mapping of *Rochalimaea* species. Acta Virol 1991;35:519–525.

Ristic M, Kreier JP: Family II. *Bartonellaceae* Gieszczykiewicz (sic) 1939, 25AL; in Kreig NR, Holt JG (eds): Bergey's Manual of Systematic Bacteriology. Baltimore, Williams & Wilkins, 1984, vol 1, pp 717–718.

Rodriguez-Barradas MC, Hamill RJ, Houston ED, Georghiou PR, Clarridge JE, Regnery RE, Koehler JE: Genomic fingerprinting of *Bartonella* species by repetitive element PCR for distinguishing species and isolates. J Clin Microbiol 1995;33:1089–1093.

Roux V, Raoult D: Inter- and intra-species identification of *Bartonella (Rochalimaea)* species. J Clin Microbiol 1995;33:1573–1579.

Sander A, Bühler C, Pelz K, Von Cramm E, Bredt W: Detection and identification of two *Bartonella henselae* variants in domestic cats in Germany. J Clin Microbiol 1997;35:584–587.

Skerman VBD, McGowan V, Sneath PHA: Approved lists of bacterial names. Int J Syst Bacteriol 1980; 30:225–420.

Spach DH, Kanter AS, Dougherty MJ, Larson AM, Coyle MB, Brenner DJ, Swaminathan B, Matar GM, Welch DF, Root RK, Stamm WE: *Bartonella (Rochalimaea) quintana* bacteraemia in inner-city patients with chronic alcoholism. N Engl J Med 1995;332:424–428.

Stohler MH, Bonfiglo TA, Steigbigel RT, Pereira M: An atypical subcutaneous infection associated with acquired immunodeficiency syndrome. Am J Clin Pathol 1983;80:714–718.

Strong RP, Tyzzer EE, Sellards AW: Oroya fever, second report. JAMA 1915;64:806–808.

Szelc-Kelly CM, Goral S, Perez-Perez GI, Perkins BA, Regnery RL, Edwards KM: Serologic responses to *Bartonella* and *Afipia* antigens in patients with cat scratch disease. Pediatrics 1995;96: 1137–1142.

Tappero JW, Koehler JE, Berger TG, Cockerell CJ, Lee TH, Busch MP, Stites DP, Mohle-Boetani J, Reingold AL, LeBoit PE: Bacillary angiomatosis and bacillary splenitis in immunocompetent adults. Ann Intern Med 1993;118:363–365.

Townsend CHT: The transmission of verruga by phlebotomus. JAMA 1913;61:1717–1718.

Turner CMR: Seasonal and age distributions of *Babesia, Hepatozoon, Trypanosoma* and *Grahamella* species in *Clethrionomys glareolus* and *Apodemus sylvaticus* populations. Parasitology 1986;93:279–289.

Tyeryar FJ, Weiss E, Millar DB, Bozeman FM, Ormsbee RA: DNA base composition of rickettsiae. Science 1973;180:415–417.

Tyzzer EE: Interference in mixed infections of *Bartonella* and *Eperythrozoon* in mice. Am J Pathol 1941; 17:141–148.

Urteaga BO, Payne EH: Treatment of the acute febrile phase of Carrion's disease with chloramphenicol. Am J Trop Med Hyg 1955;4:507–511.

Vinson JW: In vitro cultivation of the rickettsial agent of trench fever. Bull WHO 1966;35:155–164.

Vinson JW, Fuller HS: Studies on trench fever. I. Propagation of *Rickettsia*-like organisms from a patient's blood. Pathol Microbiol 1961;24(suppl):152–166.

Vinson JW, Varela G, Molina-Pasquel C: Trench fever. III. Induction of clinical disease in volunteers inoculated with *Rickettsia quintana* propagated on blood agar. Am J Trop Med Hyg 1969;18: 713–722.

Wear DJ, Malaty RH, Zimmerman LF: Cat scratch disease bacilli in the conjunctiva of patients with Parinaud's oculoglandular syndrome. Ophthalmology 1985;92:1282–1287.

Wear DJ, Margileth AM, Hadfield TL, Fischer GW, Schlagel CJ, King FM: Cat scratch disease: A bacterial infection. Science 1983;221:1403–1405.

Webster GF, Cockerell CJ, Friedman-Klein AE: The clinical spectrum of bacillary angiomatosis. Br J Dermatol 1992;126:535–541.

Weinman D, Kreier JP: *Bartonella* and *Grahamella*; in Kreier JP (ed): Parasitic Protozoa. London, Academic Press, 1977, pp 197–233.

Weiss E, Dasch GA: Differential characteristics of strains of *Rochalimaea vinsonii* sp nov, the Canadian vole agent. Int J Syst Bacteriol 1984;32:305–314.

Weiss E, Dasch GA, Woodman DR, Williams JC: The vole agent identified as a strain of the trench fever *Rickettsia, Rochalimaea quintana*. Infect Immun 1978;19:1013–1020.

Welch DF, Pickett DA, Slater LN, Steigerwalt AG, Brenner DJ: *Rochalimaea henselae* sp nov, a cause of septicemia, bacillary angiomatosis and parenchymal bacillary peliosis. J Clin Microbiol 1992;30: 275–280.

Willems A, Collins MD: Evidence for a close genealogical relationship between *Afipia felis* (the casual organism of cat scratch disease), *Bradyrhizobium japonicum* and *Blastobacter denitrificans*. FEMS Microbiol Lett 1992;96:241–246.

Wolbach SB, Todd JL, Palfrey FW: The Etiology and Pathology of Typhus. Cambridge, Harvard University Press, 1922.

R.J. Birtles, Unité des Rickettsies, CNRS UPRESA 6020, Faculté de Médecine,
27, boulevard Jean-Moulin, F–13385 Marseille (France)
Tel. (+33) 4 91 32 43 75, Fax (+33) 4 91 83 03 90, E-Mail bartonella@medecine.univ-mrs.fr

Schmidt A (ed): *Bartonella* and *Afipia* Species Emphasizing *Bartonella henselae*.
Contrib Microbiol. Basel, Karger, 1998, vol 1, pp 32–62

# Cat-Scratch Disease and an Overview of Other *Bartonella henselae*-Related Infections

*Pierre-Edouard Fournier, Didier Raoult*

Unité des Rickettsies, CNRS UPRESA 6020, Faculté de Médecine,
Université de la Méditerranée, Marseille, France

## Introduction

It has long been recognized that cat-scratch disease (CSD) is a worlwide zoonosis. Athough it has been attributed to several species of bacteria or viruses, this disease was first related to *Afipia felis* (*A. felis*), and then to the emerging pathogen *Bartonella henselae* (*B. henselae*), which seems to be the main etiological agent. However, the exact role of *A. felis* remains an open question. The most striking pathological feature of *B. henselae*, as well as the other members of the genus *Bartonella*, is their apparent ability to produce angioproliferative lesions, specifically among immunocompromised patients such as those infected with HIV. Domestic cats are the reservoir of *B. henselae* and thus most related infections are probably acquired from infected cats, either directly by cat scratch or bite, or indirectly via cat fleas. CSD is a usually benign and self-limiting lymphadenitis, but severe forms have been described in young children and immunocompromised patients: encephalitis, meningitis, myelitis, granulomatous hepatitis, endocarditis, and osteomyelitis. Two recently described HIV-associated infections, bacillary angiomatosis (BA) and bacillary peliosis hepatitis have been attributed to *B. henselae* on the basis of 16S rRNA gene amplification. Diagnosis of CSD mainly relies upon clinical and epidemiological features, but can be confirmed using microbiological or histological methods. Serology is the easiest way to confirm the diagnosis. Cultivation of *B. henselae* is difficult, as these bacteria are extremely fastidious. Polymerase chain reaction (PCR)-based or immunological methods for the detection of *Bartonella* species in infected tissues have proven useful. Although bartonellae are susceptible to most antibiotics, only aminoglycosides display in vitro bactericidal activity against both, *B. henselae* and *A. felis.*

## Historical Aspects

The first report of CSD was made by Parinaud et al. [1] in 1889 when he observed a patient with conjunctivitis and regional lymphadenopathy following contacts with cats. CSD was first recognized as a clinical entity in the 1930s by Debré, in Paris, and Foshay, in Cincinnati, who examined several patients with suppurative adenitis following cat scratches on the hand or arm on the same side. By using pus from infected adenopathies, Foshay produced an intradermal skin test and observed positive reactions in his patients. In 1946, Rose, in New York, performed an intradermal skin test on a fellow physician, Hanger, suffering from an epitrochlear adenopathy following scratches from his cat. As antigen, he used pus from Hanger's node. He obtained an intense tuberculin-like response. In honor of these two physicians, the skin test was called Hanger-Rose skin test [2]. During the 1940s, Debré [4] used material provided by Foshay for the skin tests he performed on his patients. In 1950, Debré et al. [4], studying the occurrence of suppurative adenitis following cat scratches in children, described for the first time the clinical presentation of the disease, which they called 'maladie des griffes du chat'. At the same time, Presme and Marchand [5] observed an association between cat ownership and CSD in child with Parinaud's oculoglandular syndrome. From that moment, numerous studies and reports of CSD cases were published, some of which comprising large series, such as Warwick [6], in 1967, who described 160 cases, and Carithers [7] who reported 1,200 cases in 1985.

Many microorganisms have been suspected as the etiologic agent of CSD. In 1913, Verhoeff [8] examined stained sections of nodes from patients with Parinaud's syndrome, observed filamentous organisms and labeled the disease as mycotic. Several authors [9–12] suspected chlamydiae to be the causative agents, based on complement fixation serology results. Others [13–19] presented data consistent with a viral infection, especially a hemagglutinin activity in the pus from CSD adenopathies. Other arguments in favor of a virus were the absence of growth of the organism on usual bacteriologic media and the poor efficacy of antibiotics. Acid-fast bacteria have also been suspected [20], as well as 'leptothrix' [8, 21] and *Rothia*-like organisms [22]. A major advance in the discovery of the CSD agent was made by Wear et al. [23] in 1983 and Margileth et al. [24] in 1984. They examined lymph nodes, skin at the inoculation site and conjunctiva from patients with CSD after Warthin-Starry silver impregnation stain and observed small argyrophilic pleomorphic bacilli which proved to be Gram-negative with the modified Brown-Hopp's tissue Gram stain and reacted positively when immunoperoxidase stained using sera from patients with CSD. The presence of such microorganisms was confirmed by Hadfield et al. [25] in 1985 by electron microscopy. In 1988, English et al. [26] isolated and cultured a bacterium in vitro from CSD adenopathies. This microorganism, a pleomorphic Gram-negative bacillus, was similar to that described by Wear et al. [23]. Isolates were obtained from 10 patients, one was further characterized [27], included into a new genus, *Afipia*, and called *A. felis* [28]. However, other investigators published studies that challenged the identity of the agent of CSD. In 1990, Relman et al. [29] PCR-amplified DNA from bacilli into biopsies from BA lesions in AIDS patients. This bacterium was close to *Rochalimaea quintana* (*R. quintana*) [30], the well-known agent of trench fever [31]. At the same moment, Slater et al. [32], and then Regnery et al. [33], isolated a bacterium closely related to *R. quintana* in the blood of febrile and bacteremic immunocompromised patients. The 16S rRNA analysis demonstrated that this strain was identical to that amplified in BA lesions [29]. The bacterium was characterized and named *Rochalimaea henselae* (*R. henselae*) [34]. The same microorgansim was also cultivated from BA lesions [35]. Therefore, apparently distinct syndromes encountered in immunocompromised patients were related to a single agent. More evidence of the role of *R. henselae* in CSD was brought by Regnery et al. [36] who isolated *R. henselae* from the blood of an asymptomatic cat, thus supporting that domestic cats were the reservoir of *R. henselae*. Moreover, the same authors [37] and Zangwill et al. [38] developed an indirect immunofluorescence assay using *R. henselae* as antigen and demonstrated that 88 and 84%, respectively, of patients with a clinical CSD had antibodies whereas none had antibodies to *A. felis* [39]. *R. henselae*, but not *A. felis*, was also PCR-amplified from skin test antigens [40]. The first isolation of *R. henselae* from CSD adenopathies was made by Dolan et al. [41] in 1993. The bacterium was then amplified and isolated from cat fleas, suggesting a potential role in *R. henselae* infections [42]. In 1993, members of the genus *Rochalimaea* have been included in the genus *Bartonella* [43]. Few more recent studies have emphasized the role of *B. henselae* as causative agent of CSD and have failed to demonstrate more evidence for *A. felis* [44–46].

Therefore, *B. henselae* is now considered as the primary agent of CSD. However, in a minority of cases of typical clinical CSD, no evidence of *B. henselae* infection can be found, possibly indicating that, although less frequently, other etiologic agents including *A. felis* may be responsible for the disease [47]. Moreover, recently, a new species, *Bartonella clarridgeiae*, has been isolated from a domestic cat [48] and then found together with *B. henselae* in coinfected cats [49]. This species was also isolated from the blood of a cat whose proprietary had developed a febrile lymphadenopathy after a bite [50]. Therefore, *B. clarridgeiae* species may be responsible for certain CSD cases.

## Bacteriology

*B. henselae* presents as short (0.6 × 1.0 μm), pleomorphic, Gram-negative, oxidase-negative rods [51, 52]. They are fastidious, aerobic, and do not produce acid from carbohydrates. They are motile due to the presence of pili. Their G+C content is 41% [43] and their genome size is 2.0 Mb [53]. A 14-kb linear extrachromosomal DNA element [54] has been found in *B. henselae* and *Bartonella bacilliformis*, and may correspond to a bacteriophage-like particle [55]. The role of this particle in pathophysiology of *B. henselae* infections remains unknown. Antigenic variations in *B. henselae* have recently been described [56]. Moreover, recent data indicate the existence of two *B. henselae* genotypes [57]. Although extracellular, the intraerythrocytic presence of *B. henselae* in cat erythrocytes has also been recently observed [58]. These bacteria highly depend on hemin for their growth [59]. They grow in axenic medium, either on blood-enriched agar (rabbit blood or horse blood are more effective than sheep blood) in the presence of 5% $CO_2$ or in broth [60, 61]. The optimal growth temperature is 37 °C. Growth is slow. On blood agar, primary isolates are obtained typically after 12–14 days, although prolonged incubation periods of up to 45 days have been reported to be necessary [33, 34, 51, 62]. First subcultures of an isolate are also difficult to obtain, with colony formation again taking 10–15 days. Repeated subculture, however, reduces this time to only 3–5 days, although significantly affects colonial morphology. Colonies are gray-white, opaque, rough, adherent, pitting the agar on primary isolation, and become smooth and less adherent after several passages. First described as *R. henselae, B. henselae* was included in the genus *Bartonella* in 1993 [43]. Prior to these recent taxonomic changes, *B. bacilliformis* was the only member of the genus. Following taxonomic studies [43, 63], the genus *Bartonella* presently includes 12 validated species, 5 of which have been described as human pathogens. The genera which currently comprise the *Bartonella* were previously classified in the order *Rickettsiales*. However, modern phylogenetic methods demonstrated the evolutionary diversity within the order [64]. Currently, *Bartonella* species lie within the $\alpha_2$ subdivision of the *Proteobacteria* and *Rickettsia* species in the $\alpha_1$ subdivision.

## Pathogenesis

*B. henselae* is capable of intracellular growth. It has been demonstrated to localize intracellularly [38] when cocultivated with Vero cells, to grow into human epithelial cells [65] and into cat erythrocytes [58]. The interactions between *B. henselae* and eukaryotic cells is suggested by the improved recovery of this microorgansim from clinical material when cell lysis procedures or cell culture systems are used [35, 66–68]. Type IV-like pili have been observed by electron microscopy and are supposed to be important factors in cell attachment and virulence [65, 69]. They may also play a role in adherence to agar. *B. henselae* strongly adheres to blood agar plates when first isolated from clinical specimens [32–34], but this property can be lost after subculture. This phenotypic variation from adherent to nonadherent is similar to the rough-smooth shift observed in enterobacteriaceae and may be related to a differential expression of pili [69]. Another argument in favor of interaction between cells and *B. henselae* was brought by Anderson et al. [70] who characterized an HtrA-like encoding gene. Such a protein protects intracellular bacteria from oxidative destruction.

Concerning the human immune response, *B. henselae* interacts with the immune system, which may play a role in its pathogenesis. It activates the alternative pathway of the complement [71], induces the expression of specific antigens on the surface of tissue macrophages [72], adheres to lymphocytes [73] and reduces the oxidative function of polymorphonuclear leukocytes [74]. This last property was confirmed by Rodriguez-Barradas et al. [71] who demonstrated that polymorphonuclear leukocytes were less inhibited in the presence of opsonized bacteria. The lesions induced by *B. henselae* highly depend upon the host immune status. In immunocompetent hosts, *B. henselae* induces lymphoid hyperplasia in affected lymph nodes, resulting in the formation of granulomas and, later, suppuration. The most striking pathogenic feature of *B. henselae* is its ability to induce the formation of proliferative vascular tumors in immunocompromised hosts. Koehler et al. [35] reported that when *B. henselae* is inoculated onto bovine endothelial cells, the cell monolayers remain intact and viable for longer periods than do uninfected monolayers. The cells do, however, undergo morphological changes described as similar to those seen in endothelial cells exposed to angiogenic factors. Conley et al. [75] and Palmari et al. [76] have shown that *B. henselae* stimulates the migration and proliferation of human umbilical vein endothelial cells in vitro. In humans, the neovascularization begins in small blood vessels and is responsible for the lesions of BA and peliosis hepatitis. This angiogenesis phenomenon has also been reported with *Bartonella quintana* (BA and peliosis hepatitis) [77] and *B. bacilliformis* (verruga peruana) [78]. The role of *B. henselae* in human lesions has been emphasized by the regression of lesions when antimicrobial agents are administered [77]. *Bartonella* species are the only known bacteria with the ability to stimulate endothelial cell proliferation in humans.

Although the immune status of the patients seems to be a major determinant of the manifestations of *B. henselae* infections, a variation in the virulence among strains has also been suggested by the occurrence of a cluster of cases of encephalitis associated with CSD in immunocompetent patients [79, 80].

## Epidemiology

CSD has been reported worldwide [81–83]. It is likely that this disease is the most common *Bartonella* infection. Only few studies have been performed so far to estimate the incidence rate of CSD. Jackson et al. [84], studying epidemiological databases, have estimated that approximately 24,000 cases occur yearly in the United States, and calculated an incidence of 9.3/10,000 ambulatory patients, per year. Depending on studies, seroprevalence in the population ranges from 3.6 to 6%, and is higher in intravenous drug users [38, 85, 86]. However, since it is a usually benign and self-limiting disease, its real prevalence is probably underestimated. Although CSD has been reported at all ages, a large majority of cases (around 80% in most studies) occur in patients 18 years or younger, especially males, between ages 2 and 14 years [7, 38, 84, 87, 88]. This can be explained by the fact that children are more likely to be in contact with kittens. However, in other studies, the disease in equally common among adults and children, but less likely to be recognized in the former [7, 89, 90]. CSD is one of the most common causes of chronic lymphadenopathy in children. The incidence is seasonal, most cases being encountered in August through October in temperate areas [7, 90]. The prevalence also varies with the geographic location [84].

Many studies have demonstrated the role of cats in transmission of the causative agent of CSD [38, 42, 45, 83, 91–96]. Cats may infect humans either directly through scratches, bites, of licks; or indirectly via an arthropod vector. Zangwill et al. [38] were amongst the first to show an epidemiological association between patients with CSD, the ownership of a cat, especially a kitten 12 months or younger, scratches or bites by a kitten, and cat fleas. *B. henselae* infections are common among the cat population [36, 42, 45, 80, 91, 93, 94, 97–99]. Regnery et al. [36] first reported bacteremia in cats. They can present with bacteremia that can last 2 or more months [36, 94]. Relapsing bacteremia has also been described [100]. Chomel et al. [92] demonstrated that cats, especially stray cats younger than 1 year of age, were more likely to have a high-grade bacteremia and to be infested with fleas. However, most of the infected cats appeared healthy [42]. Prevalence of bacteremia among cats was found to be 22% in The Netherlands [101] and 9.1% in Japan [102]. Moreover, Gurfield et al. [49] demonstrated that 0.5% of their studied cats were coinfected with two distinct *B. henselae* strains. Jameson et al. [93] reported that prevalence of antibodies to *B. henselae* was higher in areas with warm humid climates, which also have a higher incidence and degree of cat flea infestation. The overall seroprevalence was 28% in the United States, 35% in Australia [103], 24% in Zimbabwe and 21% in South Africa [104]. Similar results were found by other authors [83, 99, 105, 106]. Dalton et al. [107] have demonstrated that the highest seroprevalence in humans parallels that of cats [93]. Childs et al. [99] observed that peak seroconversion occurs in kittens 3–6 months old. Prevalence of antibodies to *B. henselae* has also been studied in wild cats [108]. 30% of the 114 tested animals were positive, most of which had fleas or ear mites. Recently, the newly described species *B. clarridgeiae* was demonstrated as a human cat-related pathogen [50]. A French report revealed that 1.1% of the 436 studied cats were coinfected with both *B. henselae* and *B. clarridgeiae* [49]. Therefore, cats, and more generally felids are a reservoir for *B. henselae*. Thus, *B. henselae* infections of humans can be considered zoonoses.

Cat fleas (*Ctenocephalides felis*) have been suspected to play a role as a vector of *B. henselae* in human infections [42, 109, 110]. The presence of the bacterium in these fleas has been demonstrated [36, 91, 111, 112]. More recently, Chomel et al. [113] demonstrated that *B. henselae* could be transmitted to pathogen-free kittens by infested fleas, whereas flea-free bacteremic kittens do not transmit this bacterium to pathogen-free cats. Higgins et al. [114] have found similar results. However, although epidemiological studies have identified ownership of flea-infested cats as being a predisposing factor in CSD and BA [38, 95], no evidence of any direct transmission by fleas to humans could be demonstrated and thus, the precise role of fleas in the transmission of infection to humans remains uncertain.

However, although contact with kittens and cats can be documented in a majority of cases, in a small percentage of CSD patients, no history of animal contact is reported [90, 115, 116].

## Clinical Manifestations of *B. henselae* Infections

Various *B. henselae* infections are currently described. Their presentation and severity highly depend upon the immune status of the patient. CSD is the most common manifestation of *B. henselae* infection in immunocompetent hosts, whereas immunocompromised patients are more likely to have systemic disease.

*Cat-Scratch Disease*

First described in 1950 [4], CSD most often presents as a benign, self-limiting, lymphadenopathy in nodes draining the site of the cat scratch in children and young adults [2, 6, 7, 84, 87–90, 96, 115, 117–122]. A history of scratch, bite, lick or contact with a cat, often a kitten, is reported by most patients. After a 3- to 10-day incubation period, a nontender erythematous papule or pustule, measuring 0.5–1 cm in diameter, develops at the site of inoculation in 50% of cases [24, 38, 90, 123]. Regression of the lesion occurs after a few days to 8 weeks. One to 2 weeks after the primary cutaneous lesion, one, more often than several, regional lymph nodes draining the area enlarge over a 2- to 3-week period. The location of the lymphadenopathy depends on the site of inoculation. In most patients, the upper extremities are involved, with nodes being axillar more than epitrochlear [7, 122]. The cervical and submandibulary regions represent the second most common location, followed by the inguinal, popliteal, preauricular, clavicular, mesenteric and retroperitoneal areas. The adenopathies can reach a size of a few centimeters, are freely movable, tender and overlaid by an erythematous skin area, especially during the first 2 weeks of enlargement, or nontender, and persist for a few weeks before recovery. The usual duration of the disease is 2–6 months. The enlarged lymph nodes may seldom persist for up to 24 months. Lymphadenopathy represents the most common clinical manifestation of CSD and is found in more than 80% of cases [7, 124]. In up to 50% cases, patients may present with a mild fever $\leq$39 °C, anorexia, malaise, arthralgia, myalgia, headache, sore throat, or abdominal, neck, back or extremity pain [7, 125]. While most cases are mild and regress spontaneously, some are totally asymptomatic and others are severe. Of the 24,000 cases reported yearly in the United States, only 2,000 resulted in a hospital admission [84]. They may last several months and/or proceed to fluctuation and then suppuration in about 10% of cases. Similar clinical symptoms were described in the patient infected with *B. clarridgeiae* [50].

Also designated as atypical CSD, the other clinical manifestations of CSD include Parinaud's oculoglandular syndrome, hepatitis, hepatic and splenic abscesses, involvement of the central nervous system, and pulmonary, ophthalmic or musculoskeletal manifestations. Parinaud's oculoglandular syndrome, first described in 1889 [1], is characterized by unilateral conjunctivitis with adjacent preauricular lymphadenopathy [126]. The evidence of *B. henselae* as the etiologic agent of Parinaud's syndrome has been brought by Wear et al. [127] who observed in 1985 typical CSD bacilli in conjunctival lesions using the Warthin-Starry silver stain. More recently, Le et al. [128] PCR-amplified *B. henselae* DNA from conjunctival lesions of Parinaud's syndrome. It occurs in up to 17% of CSD cases. Contamination is more likely to result from rubbing the eye with the fingers after a contact with a cat, than by direct inoculation. The important swelling of the involved eye stands in contrast with the absence of pain and discharge. The evolution is usually spontaneously favorable, with the regression of the lesions in 2–4 months. Rare cases of temporary blindness have been reported [124]. Hepatic and splenic abscesses usually present as a prolonged fever of unknown origin with abdominal pain [129–133]. Rizkallah et al. [132] were amongst the first to describe a hepatic involvement due to *B. henselae*. In their study, 4 immunocompetent children presented with adenopathies, prolonged fever and abdominal pain. They reported a history of a cat scratch. Ultrasonography showed multiple hepatic and/or splenic hypoechoic lesions, which were confirmed by computed tomography (CT) scan. Results of liver function tests were found to be normal, but leukocyte count and erythrocyte sedimentation rate were moderately elevated. Other studies have described similar findings [129–131, 133–135]. Microscopic examination of microabscess biopsies shows necrotizing granuloma, and occasionally bacilli after Warthin-Starry staining. The lesions may spontaneously resolve over 2–3 months. Granulomatous hepatitis has also been described, in patients with prolonged fever but without any lymphadenopathy [136].

Neurologic manifestations occur in about 2% of cases of CSD. Several syndromes have been described: encephalopathy, seizures, Leber's neuroretinitis, myelitis, radiculitis, polyneuritis, paraplegia and cerebral arteritis [122]. First described by Stevens [137], encephalopathy is the most frequent neurological manifestation of CSD. Children 7–12 years old are more likely to develop such a complication. It occurs a few days to 2 months after onset of lymphadenopathy [80, 138–140]. The onset is sudden [7]. Clinical symptoms may include fever, convulsions, status epilepticus, headache, malaise, behavior changes, lethargy, coma, respiratory depression, hemiplegia, aphasia, ataxia, cranial nerve palsy and hearing loss [80, 138, 141–143]. Patients fully recover within 2 weeks to 1 year. Cerebrospinal fluid may either be normal or show pleocytosis and elevated protein concentration. Antibodies to *B. henselae* can usually be detected in the spinal fluid. Although electroencephalogram shows nonspecific diffuse slowing or focal abnormalities, cranial CT scan is usually normal. However, an intracranial mass, in the middle fossa, has also been reported in a 10-year-old girl who presented with prolonged fever, headache, hemiparesthesia of the face and abdominal pain related to hepatic nodules [144]. Cranial or peripheral nerve involvement are the second most common neurological manifestation of CSD. Amongst these, Leber's neuroretinitis, also called Leber's idiopathic stellate retinopathy, Leber's idiopathic stellate maculopathy or Leber's idiopathic stellate neuroretinitis, is the most commonly encountered. It was first described in 1916 [145] and related to CSD in the 1970s [146, 147]. It occurs both in children and adults and is characterized by a painless, most often unilateral, loss of vision with a central scotoma, stellate macular exudates and optic disc edema. Clinical symptoms result from exudates which leak from capillaries and extend into the macular area. Complete recovery generally occurs spontaneously after 1–3 months [145, 148–154].

The prevalence of osteomyelitis in CSD is 0.3% of cases. It usually results from the extension from an adjacent lymphadenopathy. Any bone may be involved [90, 155–159]. It presents as a febrile disease with pain at the infected site. The patients generally recover within 4–12 months. In 1994, Bernini et al. [160] reported a case of paravertebral abscess, necessitating a drainage for the treatment. Pulmonary manifestations occur in 0.2% of CSD cases [122]. They include pneumonia, sometimes severe and requiring intubation and ventilatory support, and exudative pleural effusion [122, 161, 162].

Although CSD is usually benign and self-limited in immunocompetent hosts, *B. henselae* may also be responsible for life-threatening generalized infections in immunocompromised patients, especially those who are HIV-infected.

*Bacillary Angiomatosis*

In 1983, Stoler et al. [163] observed atypical subcutaneous lesions in HIV patients. On pathological examination of cutaneous biopsies, vascular proliferation was noted, and the disease was considered to be infectious because, after Warthin-Starry silver staining, bacilli were observed within the lesions. Moreover, they resolved on antibiotic treatment [164]. Relman et al. [29] were the first to amplify *B. henselae* DNA from such lesions. Since then, *B. quintana* has also been described as a causative agent of BA [35, 165].

In 1996, Mohle-Boetani et al. [166] differentiated several clinical presentations of BA, the most frequent being the cutaneous form, in 50% of cases, followed by abdominal pain in 20% of cases, and fever and adenopathy in another 20%. Primary skin lesions correspond to papules, which gradually increase in size to form nodules. A characteristic feature is that these lesions may bleed profusely when punctured. Cutaneous lesions may be solitary or multiple, they may be superficial, dermal, or subcutaneous, and are usually tender. Superficial lesions may be reddish or uncolored [77, 167–169]. Deep lesions are usually uncolored and either motile of fixed to underlying structures, including bones. BA may also present as a malleolar ulcer [170]. Oral, respiratory, conjunctival, anal and gastrointestinal mucosa have also been involved [164, 168, 171]. The presence of regional adenopathies in the drainage territory of skin lesions has been extensively reported [29, 35, 172]. Other localizations of BA have been described, such as lymph nodes, spleen, bones, bone marrow, heart, muscles, brain and liver [35, 109, 167, 172–183]. However, abdominal nodes together with hepatic and splenic enlargement have also been reported as the sole lesions of BA [172, 184, 185]. Fever, chills, malaise, headache or weight loss may also be encountered. BA may rarely resolve spontaneously [164].

A history of cat contact is reported in many cases [167]. Furthermore, although mostly described among HIV-infected patients [163, 164, 179, 186], especially those who suffer from leukopenia and CD4+ cell counts of <100 per $mm^3$, BA has also been encountered in other immunocompromised patients, such as those undergoing immunosuppressive therapy [162, 183, 187, 188] or chronic alcoholics [66, 189], and even in immunocompetent patients [68, 109, 190, 191].

*Peliosis Hepatitis*

Peliosis hepatitis (PH) has been considered as a visceral manifestation of BA [34, 176, 192, 193]. It is a vascular proliferation resulting in cystic blood-filled spaces in the liver. It was first reported in patients suffering from diseases such as tuberculosis and advanced cancers, and in association with the use of drugs such as anabolic steroids [34, 95, 172, 194, 195]. PH may be associated with BA lesions or may occur as an isolated condition in HIV-infected individuals [34, 172, 196, 197]. The same lesions may also involve the spleen. Patients with PH may present with fever, abdominal pain, nausea, vomiting and diarrhea. Hepatosplenomegaly is generally present. On CT scan, PH lesions are hypodense and scattered throughout the hepatic and/or splenic parenchyma.

*Bacteremia*

Bacteremia due to *B. henselae* was first reported in 1990 [32]. Bacteria were isolated after prolonged incubation of blood cultures in patients without any focus of *B. henselae* infection. Since then, bacteremia has been reported in HIV-infected patients, transplant recipients, and immunocompetent individuals [32, 34, 68]. Bacteremia may also present as a relapsing fever [68].

*Endocarditis*

*Bartonella* endocarditis has rarely been described in the literature. So far, few cases of proved *B. henselae* endocarditis have been reported [56, 198–201]. Since usual blood culture systems do not allow the growth of these bacteria and since the clinical presentation is aspecific, it is likely that their incidence is underestimated. We have reported recently 22 cases of *Bartonella* endocarditis, 4 of which were due to *B. henselae* [199]. From our data and data from reference centers in three different countries, we could estimate the *Bartonella* species accounted for 3–4% of all cases of endocarditis. Our 4 patients had native valves. We could demonstrate specific epidemiological factors associated with *B. henselae* endocarditis when compared to other *Bartonella* endocarditis cases. *B. henselae* endocarditis most often occurred in patients with known valvulopathy, in contact with cats whereas *B. quintana* endocarditis was most often observed in homeless, chronic alcoholic patients, without previous known valvulopathy.

In the absence of a treatment, the outcome of *B. henselae* endocarditis may rarely be fatal or more often lead to extensive valve lesions necessitating valvular replacement. Therefore, *Bartonella* should systematically be suspected when diagnosing patients with endocarditis, especially if regular blood cultures remain sterile despite the absence of antibiotic therapy.

*Rare Manifestations of* B. henselae *Infections*

Rare manifestations of *B. henselae* infections include aseptic meningitis, encephalopathy with dementia in HIV-infected people, erythema nodosum, erythema multiforme, erythema annulare, maculopapular eruption, thrombocytopenia, reactive arthritis, systemic illness with septic shock, thyroiditis, urethritis, breast tumor, uveitis, and lymphedema, especially in immunocompromised patients [6, 7, 38, 149, 202–207].

## Laboratory Diagnosis

Historically, the diagnosis of CSD relied upon four lose criteria: (1) a history of cat contact and the presence of a primary lesion; (2) development of lymphadenopathy approximately 2 weeks after the primary inoculation, with the exclusion of other causes of lymphadenopathy; (3) a positive CSD skin test result; (4) histopathologic findings on lymph node biopsy specimens showing a granulomatous process with stellate necrosis and pleomorphic bacilli visualized by Warthin-Starry silver staining. However, recent improvements in the isolation of *B. henselae* and PCR procedures have allowed the diagnosis of an increased number of cases. Currently, the diagnosis of CSD should be considered in any patient with unique or regional lymphadenitis, acute or chronic, especially with a history of a cat scratch or bite. The diagnosis of *B. henselae* infection should also be systematically evocated in case of a blood culture-negative endocarditis, or in front of an immunocompromised patient with fever of unknown origin or cutaneous lesions consistent with BA.

*Cat-Scratch Skin Test*

Although considered to be reliable to confirm the diagnosis of CSD [208], the skin test is no longer recommended because of its lack of specificity and sensitivity when compared to PCR and serology [44], and because no test is commercially available. Positive skin tests have been reported in up to 36% of family contacts whereas false-negative tests were observed in about 5% of cases [2].

*Histology*

Biopsy of lymph nodes should be reserved to atypical cases. Pathologic findings depend on the stage of infection. Early in the course of the disease, the findings may include lymphoid hyperplasia comprising arteriolar proliferation, reticulum cell hyperplasia and widening of arteriolar walls [209]. At later stages, nonspecific granulomas appear, some of which are centered with necrosis. Later, necrosis forms microabscesses and then abscesses. The demonstration of CSD bacilli in adenopathy biopsies may be obtained with the Warthin-Starry silver stain. The bacteria are more easily found in the walls of vessels in nonnecrotic areas of vascular inflammation [209].

The diagnosis of BA should be confirmed by histological examination of skin biopsies. In contrast to CSD, BA biopsies reveal the presence of specific lesions. In hematoxylin and eosin-stained sections, BA is characterized by lobular capillary proliferation [77], the lobules being rounded aggregates of capillaries. The stroma surrounding the lobules is edematous in early lesions, becoming fibrotic in later stages. The endothelial cells of BA may protrude into vascular lumina, which may become occluded. Nuclear atypia of endothelial cells may be seen. Amphophilic granular aggregates are highly indicative of BA. Such aggregates are revealed to be masses of bacteria using Warthin-Starry silver staining, electron microscopy, or immunofluorescence. Neutrophils frequently cluster around these aggregates of bacteria. Clinical differential diagnosis of BA includes pyogenic granuloma, hemangioma, various subcutaneous tumors and atypical Kaposi's sarcoma, although demonstration of the presence of bateria in histologic specimens of skin biopsies clearly distinguishes BA from these other conditions. Differentiation of cutaneous BA from the skin lesions of Carrion's disease (verruga peruana) may not be possible in endemic areas. Microscopic observation of the lesions characteristic of *B. henselae*-induced BA reveals tumor-like capillary lobules [77], which are rounded aggregates of capillaries with rapidly proliferating endothelial cells [77].

In PH, histologic examination of hematoxylin and eosin-stained liver biopsies reveals dilated, cystic blood-filled spaces in the fibromyxoid stroma containing inflammatory cells, dilated capillaries, and clumps of granular purple material which are revealed as masses of bacteria by Warthin-Starry silver staining [172]. Lesions with histological appearance similar to those of PH have also been reported in the spleen of HIV-infected patients with BA [34, 109], the less specific term 'parenchymal peliosis' has been proposed.

In endocarditis cases, histologic preparations of valvular biopsies reveals massive vegetations on the valve surface, with extensive destruction of the underlying valve tissue, and the presence of numerous bacteria on Warthin-Starry staining.

*Culture*

The two most widely used methods are either direct plating onto solid media [62, 66, 189, 210] or cocultivation in cell cultures [35, 66, 67, 189], although even groups using the same methods describe differing levels of success [34, 62, 66, 67, 210]. Cell culture systems have been previously reported to be more sensitive and allow more rapid growth of bartonellae than the blood agar technique. This was verified in our experience, some isolates being obtained only in cell cultures. Also, subculture of bartonellae grown in cell culture systems onto blood agar was often difficult to obtain. In a few cases, however, only the blood agar technique allowed isolation of the bacteria. A combination of both methods is probably most useful for optimizing recovery of *B. henselae*.

*Blood Agar-Based Culture.* On 10% fresh rabbit blood-enriched agar and BCYE, *B. henselae* is best cultivated in a humid, $CO_2$-enriched (5%) atmosphere [31, 33, 211]. Primary isolation from the blood of infected patients may require up to 45 days' incubation before colonies become apparent. Horse and rabbit blood have been reported to be more effective supplements than sheep blood [34, 35]. Both the use of blood-enriched agar and the need for prolonged incubation of the plates provoke the possibility of contamination, especially from fungi. Adding amphotericin B in the culture medium may therefore be beneficial. However, due to the high level of in vitro susceptibility of bartonellae to most antibiotics, their inclusion in culture medium in order to prevent bacterial overgrowth would also impair growth of bartonellae themselves. The use of lysis centrifugation has been shown to enhance the recovery of *Bartonella* from blood [34], as well as freezing the samples. Detection of fastidious organisms such as *B. henselae* in conventional automated blood culture systems remains difficult as the organisms produce little or no $CO_2$ and yield little visible growth. Thus, systematic detection of bacteria in blood cultures by using an acridine orange dye-staining procedure has been proposed [210] as an approach to improving recovery of *B. henselae*.

*Cell Culture Systems. B. henselae* can be grown in vitro in a number of cell culture systems, including endothelial cells, L929, HeLa cells [35, 66, 212]. Endothelial cell cutlures, however, are considered the most effective and have been reported to support more efficiently bartonellae growth. Cocultivation of cutaneous biopsy material with a bovine endothelial cell line was used to isolate for the first time *B. quintana* from a BA patient [35]. In our laboratory, we routinely use HEL cells to isolate *Bartonella* species from clinical specimens [213].

*Identification*

*B. henselae* should be suspected when nonmotile, small, Gram-negative bacilli are recovered following prolonged incubation of inoculated blood-enriched media in a $CO_2$-enriched, humid environment at 30–37 °C. Several methods for confirming the identity of presumptive *B. henselae* have been described, ranging from the comparison of the biochemical reactivities of isolates [214] to more complex genotypic and phenotypic analyses. *B. henselae* is virtually inert in all standard biochemical assays, only few biochemical tests are positive: leucine arylamidase, esculin hydrolysis, hippurate hydrolysis, and acid production from lactose [59]. *Bartonella* species have been differentiated on the basis of the presence of different preformed aminopeptidases [43, 63]. Rabbit antisera raised against type strains of *B. henselae* appear not to significantly cross-react with nonhomologous antigens [63], and provide a useful method of identification.

A number of PCR-based differentiation methods have also been described, including repetitive element PCR [215] and various PCR-RFLP analyses exploiting variation within the RNA operon [27, 29, 33, 62, 64, 216–219], or the citrate synthase (*gltA*) gene [29, 33, 62, 66, 98, 220]. Determination of partial 16S rRNA or *gltA* sequences is also regularly reported. Macrorestriction analysis using pulse-field gel electrophoresis has been used to demonstrate intraspecies differences [53, 221].

*Serology*

Serology is the most widely used method for the diagnosis of CSD. Various tests have been developed. Currently, specific antibody detection and estimation are now used in the diagnosis of *B. henselae* infections, including the immunofluorescence antibody test (IFAT) and (ELISAs) [107, 222, 223]. It must be noted that in most HIV-infected patients, a group particularly prone to *B. henselae* infections, a significant antibody response to infection is not mounted. In contrast, up to 88% [37] of patients involved with CSD were found to present *B. henselae*-specific antibodies in their sera when using the IFA technique, and 95% when using ELISA [223]. The titer to which antibodies are detected, however, appears to depend on the strain used as antigen [56], on the method by which the antigen used in the assay is prepared, and even different batches of the same antigen preparation can yield different results [224]. In the study by Drancourt et al. [66], antigen prepared from plate-grown *Bartonella* species reacted with antisera to dilutions of 1:400 to 1:800, whereas titers of 6,400 to 12,800 were obtained when the same sera were tested against antigens prepared from organisms cocultivated with cell monolayers.

Genetic heterogeneity among *B. henselae* strains was observed during preliminary characterization of the species [29], and subsequently genotypic and phenotypic differences were observed among *B. benselae* isolates made from cat blood [42]. Drancourt et al. [56] characterized new *B. henselae* strains from French patients with endocarditis and CSD, and from English and Swiss cats, and demonstrated them to have antigenic differences from previously assessed isolates. Other phenotypic and genotypic differences were also noted, and it was proposed that these strains could be considered to belong to a separate serogroup of the species. Examination of 16S rRNA gene fragment sequences derived from *B. henselae*-infected tissues of Dutch CSD identified two distinct groups of strains; the respective 'signature sequences' of the 16S rRNA genes of the two groups matched those of the two serogroups proposed above [57]. It therefore appears that a widely distributed group of serovariant strains exists. Drancourt et al. [56] were also able to demonstrate significant reactivities in 18 of 113 apparently negative serum specimens when a strain of the new serogroup was incorporated as antigen into a diagnostic IFT. Antigenic variation among *B. henselae* strains may therefore explain inconsistent results in the serological diagnosis of CSD.

Since most *Bartonella*-related infections have only recently been described and the number of cases identified is still relatively low, the titer at which antibody levels become significant (i.e. the 'cut-off' value) for diagnosis of infection has yet to be determined. Over 12,000 sera from patients with suspected *Bartonella* infections have been tested in our laboratory for the presence of specific antibodies using IFAT and antigen from plate-grown organisms. IgG titers of $>100$ against *B. quintana* have been found in 70 of these sera, with titers of $>400$ in 31 of these 70. At present, we would consider an IgG titer of $>100$ as significant. Raoult et al. [225] demonstrated that such an IgG titer had a positive predictive value of 65%.

The specificity of antibody estimation tests has been questioned by several groups. Current serological tests may not reliably distinguish *B. henselae* antibody responses from *B. quintana* responses. Cross-reactivity between *Bartonella* species and other organisms, including *Coxiella burnetii* [226] and *Chlamydia* species [66], have also been reported. Emmons et al. [19] first demonstrated that antisera from CSD patients reacted with *Chlamydia trachomatis* antigens. This cross-reactivity was confirmed using immunoblotting. The susceptibility of the cross-reacting antigens to proteinase K indicated their protein nature. Very recently, we tested 8 sera from 8 patients previously diagnosed as chlamydial endocarditis upon serological data. All sera reacted strongly against both *Chlamydia* and *Bartonella* antigens. Adsorption procedures and Western blotting confirmed cross-reactions between *Bartonella* and *Chlamydia* antigens, and indicated that antibody reactivities were more compatible with antibody response observed in *Bartonella*-infected patients. All patients were considered to have been involved with *Bartonella* endocarditis rather than chlamydial endocarditis. La Scola and Raoult [227] have also reported that more than 50% of chronic Q-fever patients tested had antibodies which reacted with *B. henselae* antigen to a significant level. These reactions were confirmed by a cross-adsorption study and protein immunoblotting.

Clearly, the cross-reactivity between *Bartonella, Chlamydia* and *C. burnetii* is of diagnostic importance, as all are potential etiologic agents of endocarditis. However, given that the levels of specific antibodies observed in *Bartonella*-induced endocarditis are extremely high, low level cross-reaction with other antigens should not lead to misdiagnosis, provided serology for all suspected agents is performed.

Alternatively, antigenic variations in *B. henselae* strains, as recently detected [56], may explain the apparent lack of specific antigens in patients with typical clinical signs of CSD. Recent data indicate the existence of two *B. henselae* genotypes [57].

*PCR-Based Detection Methods*

The 16S rRNA gene [29, 33, 35, 67, 228], the 16S–23S intergenic spacer region [53, 221, 229, 230] and the citrate synthase gene [66] have been the DNA fragments on which efforts have been focused in attempts to develop specific PCR-based assays for the diagnosis of *Bartonella* infections. An alternative approach based on PCR amplification of a heat-shock gene fragment has also been described [231].

In 1990, Relman et al. [29] were the first to design *Bartonella*-specific PCR primers based on unique regions of the 16S rRNA gene. As described earlier, these primers were used to amplify a 280-bp fragment of *B. henselae* 16S rRNA gene from clinical material from three BA patients. The primers, p24E and p12B, have subsequently been used successfully in several different studies to amplify 16S rRNA gene from different *Bartonella* species [29, 33, 35, 67]. These primers are, however, not genus-specific, and also amplify 16S rRNA gene fragments from other members of the $\alpha_2$ subdivision of the *Proteobacteria*. The production of a suitably sized fragment using this PCR cannot therefore be considered as evidence for the presence of *Bartonella* DNA, and amplicons need to be further characterized, most effectively by sequencing or probing.

The amplification of citrate synthase gene (*gltA*) fragments, coupled with RFLP, was first described for the detection and identification of rickettsiae [232] and the scheme was later extended to the former *Rochalimaea* species. The primers used in the amplification are not *Bartonella*-specific, although RFLP of amplification products allows discrimination of *Bartonella* species from other bacteria.

Matar et al. [221, 230] and Roux et al. [53, 229] amplified the 16S–23S intergenic spacer region of *B. henselae, B. quintana, B. vinsonii* and *B. eliza-*

*bethae*. However, a discrepancy existed betweeen the investigators. The amplified fragment was 1,600 bp long in the study of Matar et al. [221] whereas Roux and Raoult [229] obtained a 1,262-bp fragment. The amplification was followed by restriction fragment length polymorphism using various enzymes or by sequencing. The PCR based on this gene has demonstrated to be a reliable tool for the identification of *Bartonella* species, and also to amplify *B. henselae* from clinical specimens.

In 1994, Anderson et al. [231] described a PCR assay using degenerate primers that allowed amplification of a 414-bp fragment of DNA either from *B. quintana* or *B. henselae*. Internal oligonucleotides were used as hybridization probes and allowed rapid differentiation of these two species. Conversely, the 414-bp DNA fragment was not amplified in the PCR assay from *B. quintana* or *A. felis*. The technique was applied to 16 fresh node tissue and 9 node aspirates from patients involved with CSD [231]. The 414-bp fragment was amplified from 21/25 samples, and in all cases the 414-bp fragment hybridized with *B. henselae*-specific probe.

## Treatment

*In vitro Antibiotic Susceptibility*

Only few data [233] on the in vitro antibiotic susceptibility of *Bartonella* species were available since the 1990s, mainly because so few strains had been isolated. Recent development of *Bartonella*-specific cultures in routine laboratory practice allowed more frequent isolation of *B. henselae*. Both agar-based and cell culture methods have recently been reported for the sudy of the in vitro antibiotic susceptibility of *Bartonella* species Maurin et al. [234, 235] used horse blood-supplemented Columbia agar as the assay medium, and an incubation time at 37 °C of 5 days, and Wolfson et al. [236] used Etest antibiotic-impregnated strips to assess the antibiotic suceptibility of chocolate agar-grown *B. henselae*. On the other hand, Musso et al. [237] evaluated the bactericidal activity of antibiotics against *B. henselae* in cell cultures either using a murine macrophage-like cell line (ATCC TIB63) or a human endothelial cell line (ECV 304,9) [237], whereas Ives et al. [238] used Vero cells and an immunofluorescence-based detection method. Cocultivation of *B. henselae* species with eukaryotic cells did not change the bacteriostatic activity of antibiotics. However, only the aminoglycosides such as gentamicin, tobramycin, and amikacin were bactericidal on either axenic or cell-line cultured organisms. Although it should be emphasized that in vitro MIC determination for the fastidious species *B. henselae* must be considered cautiously, the results indicated that all isolates were highly susceptible to β-lactams, aminoglycosides, macrolides, including the newer compounds, tetracyclines, and rifampin. *Bartonella* species were less susceptible to penicillinase-resistant penicillins, first-generation cephalosporins and clindamycin, and were resistant to vancomycin. High variations were noted in the susceptibility to fluoroquinolone compounds. Interestingly, although *A. felis* is highly resistant to antibiotics in vitro, only the aminoglycosides display significant in vitro bacteriostatic and bactericidal activity both in axenic medium and in cell systems [239].

*Clinical Data on Antibiotic Therapy of* Bartonella *Infections*

Data on the efficacy of antibiotics in the treatment of the newly recognized *B. henselae*-induced infections, and mainly BA, are more widely available. A regimen of erythromycin (250–500 mg, 4 times/day) has been reported to be the most effective method of treating cutaneous BA [29, 32, 34, 172], although relapses may occur after antibiotic treatment withdrawal, particularly in HIV-infected patients on short (< 15 days) courses of treatment [32]. Failures have been reported for the treatment of BA when using nafcillin, dicloxacillin and cephalexin, and such data are consistent with in vitro results of antibiotic susceptibility. Clinical data suggest that amoxicillin [68], aminoglycosides [68, 172], doxycycline [33] and trimethoprim-sulfamethoxazole [32, 240] may be suitable for treatment, even though several patients on these regimens relapsed. A wide range of other antibiotics has been reported to successfully treat *Bartonella*-induced BA. Lesions resolved in 2 patients treated with ceftriaxone [32, 68]. Successful therapy of 3 cases of BA has also been reported using norfloxacin [32] and ciprofloxacin [32, 68]. Antimycobacterial drugs are also reported to be effective in eradicating BA, supposedly because of the rifampin component [172]. It should be emphasized that the duration of therapy may be more important than the choice of antibiotic, especially in the immunocompromised host. Fewer relapses have been noted in patients treated for more than a month.

Data on the requirements for the effective treatment of *B. henselae*-induced endocarditis are scarce, again because so few cases have yet been reported. Successful treatment has been reported with a complex regimen consisting of intravenous amoxycillin combined with gentamicin [66]; intravenous vancomycin with ofloxacin and netilmicin, followed by oral therapy with rifampin, ofloxacin and pristinamycin [66]; and intravenous ceftriaxone followed by long-term erythromycin [241]. Intravenous antibiotic therapy was continued for 6 weeks and oral trimethoprim-sulfamethoxazole was administered for a further 5 weeks. It should be noted that *Bartonella*-induced endocarditis usually results in extensive valve damage requiring replacement [66, 242].

CSD typically does not respond to antibiotic therapy. Only the aminoglycosides, mainly gentamicin, were reported as effective in patients suffering from suppurative complications [243, 244]. Few reports indicate that ciprofloxacin, rifampin, and sulfamethoxazole-trimethoprim may be active [134, 245, 246].

*Considerations on Antibiotic Therapy and Prophylactic Measures for* Bartonella *Infections*

The poor efficacy of the β-lactams in the treatment of *Bartonella*-induced illness and the frequency of relapses when antibiotic therapy is withdrawn despite high in vitro susceptibility of bartonellae to antibiotics are striking. As discussed earlier, several observations and experiments have indicated that *Bartonella* species are also found intracellularly in infected tissue [247]. On the other hand, recent in vitro experiments have shown that most antibiotics except the aminoglycosides do not display any bactericidal activity against bartonellae [237], and a bactericidal activity may be more important in vivo especially in immunocompromised patients or patients with chronic infections or endocarditis. Although the formulation of a standard antibiotic regimen for antibiotic treatment of *Bartonella*-related diseases remains hazardous, both the use of aminoglycosides and prolonged administration of the antibiotic therapy should be advocated.

As the cycle of the *Bartonella* species in nature remains unclear, likely predisposing epidemiological factors also remain uncertain and thus it remains difficult to establish valid recommendations for prevention of *Bartonella*-induced illnesses. Delousing procedures were recommended for prevention of trench fever, and may fit for prevention of bacteremia [189], and endocarditis [66] in homeless people. As for *B. henselae* infections, immunocompromised persons, including those infected with HIV, may avoid contact with cats.

## References


1 Parinaud H: Conjonctivite infectieuse transmise par les animaux. Ann Ocul 1889;101:252–253.
2 Moriarty RA, Margileth AM: Cat scratch disease. Infect Dis Clin North Am 1987;1:575–590.
3 Debré R, Job JC: La maladie des griffes du chat. Acta Pediatr Scand 1954;43:1–87.
4 Debré R, Lamy M, Jammet ML, Costil L, Mozziconacci P: La maladie des griffes du chat. Soc Méd Hôp Paris 1950;66:76–79.
5 Presme P, Marchand E: Un nouveau type de conjonctivite infectieuse probablement transmise par le chat. J Méd Bordeaux 1950;127:131.
6 Warwick WJ: The cat-scratch syndrome, many diseases or one disease? Prog Med Virol 1967;9: 256–301.
7 Carithers HA: Cat-scratch disease: An overview based on a study of 1,200 patients. Am J Dis Child 1985;139:1124–1133.
8 Verhoeff FH: Parinaud's conjunctivitis: A mycotic disease due to a hitherto undescribed filamentous organism. Arch Ophthalmol 1913;42:344–351.
9 Kalter SS, Prier JE, Prior JT: Recent studies on the diagnosis of cat scratch fever. Ann Intern Med 1955;42:562–573.

10 Gifford H: Skin test reactions to cat scratch disease among veterinarians. Arch Intern Med 1955; 95:828–833.

11 Gifford H: Cat scratch disease. Pediatr Clin North Am 1955;2:33–40.

12 Fowler RS, Bailey JD: Cat scratch disease in childhood. Can Med Assoc J 1961;84:1365–1368.

13 Mollaret P, Reilly J, Bastin R, Tournier P: La découverte du virus de la lymphoréticulose bénigne d'inoculation. I. Caractérisation sérologique et immunologique. Presse Méd 1951;59:681–682.

14 Dodd MC, Graber CD, Anderson G: Hemagglutination of rabbit erythrocytes by pus from cases of cat scratch fever. Proc Soc Exp Biol Med 1959;102:556–558.

15 Turner W, Bigley NJ, Dodd MC, Anderson G: Hemagglutinating viruses isolated from cat scratch disease. J Bacteriol 1960;80:430–435.

16 Kalter SS, Herberling RL: Cat scratch disease-virus particles in lymph nodes. Bibl Haematol 1970; 36:773–774.

17 Kalter SS, Kim CS, Herberling RL: Herpes-like virus particles associated with cat scratch disease. Nature 1969;224:190.

18 Blank H, Haines H: Viral diseases of the skin, 1975: A 25-year perspective. J Invest Dermatol 1976; 67:169–176.

19 Emmons RW, Riggs JL, Schachter J: Continuing search for the etiology of cat scratch disease. J Clin Microbiol 1976;4:112–114.

20 Boyd GL, Craig G: Etiology of cat-scratch fever. J Pediatr 1961;59:313–317.

21 Henry M: Leptotrichosis conjunctivae (Parinaud's conjunctivitis). Trans Pacific Coast Otoophthalmol Soc 1952;33:173–196.

22 Gerber MA, Sedgwick AK, MacAlister TJ, Gustafson KB, Ballow M, Tilton RC: The aetiological agent of cat scratch disease. Lancet 1985;i:1236–1239.

23 Wear DJ, Margileth AM, Hadfield TL, Fischer GW, Schlagel CJ, King FM: Cat scratch disease: A bacterial infection. Science 1983;221:1403–1405.

24 Margileth AM, Wear DJ, Hadfield TL, Schlagel CJ, Spigel T, Muhlbauer JE: Cat-scratch disease: Bacteria in skin at the primary inoculation site. JAMA 1984;252:928–931.

25 Hadfield TL, Malaty RH, Van Dellen A, Wear DJ, Margileth AM: Electron microscopy of the bacillus causing cat-scratch disease. J Infect Dis 1985;152:643–645.

26 English CK, Wear DJ, Margileth AM, Lissner CR, Walsh GP: Cat-scratch disease: Isolation and culture of the bacterial agent. JAMA 1988;259:1347–1351.

27 O'Connor SP, Dorsch M, Steigerwalt AG, Brenner DJ, Stackebrandt E: 16S rRNA sequences of *Bartonella bacilliformis* and cat scratch disease bacillus reveal phylogenetic relationships with the alpha-2 subgroup of the class proteobacteria. J Clin Microbiol 1991;29:2144–2150.

28 Brenner DJ, Hollis DG, Moss CW, English CK, Hall GS, Vincent J, Radosevic J, Birkness KA, Bibb WF, Quinn FD, Swaminathan B, Weaver RE, Reeves MW, O'Connor SP, Hayes PS, Tenover FC, Steigerwalt AG, Perkins BA, Daneshvar MI, Hill BC, Washington JA, Woods TC, Hunter SB, Hadfield TL, Ajello GW, Kaufmann AF, Wear DJ, Wenger JD: Proposal of *Afipia* gen nov, with *Afipia felis* sp nov (formerly the cat scratch disease bacillus), *Afipia clevelandensis* sp nov (formerly the Cleveland Clinic Foundation strain), *Afipia broomeae* sp nov, and three unnamed genospecies. J Clin Microbiol 1991;29:2450–2460.

29 Relman DA, Loutit JS, Schmidt TM, Fallow S, Tompkins LS: The agent of bacillary angiomatosis: An approach to the identification of uncultured pathogens. N Engl J Med 1990;323:1573–1580.

30 Birtles RJ, Harrison TG, Taylor AG: The causative agent of bacillary angiomatosis (letter). N Engl J Med 1991;325:1447.

31 Vinson JW: In vitro cultivation of the rickettsial agent of trench fever. Bull WHO 1966;35:155–164.

32 Slater LN, Welch DF, Hensel D, Coody DW: A newly recognized fastidious gram-negative pathogen as a cause of fever and bacteremia. N Engl J Med 1990;323:1587–1593.

33 Regnery RL, Anderson BE, Clarridge JE, Rodriguez-Barradas MC, Jones DC, Carr JH: Characterization of a novel *Rochalimaea* species, *R. henselae* sp nov, isolated from blood of a febrile, human immunodeficiency virus-positive patient. J Clin Microbiol 1992;30:265–274.

34 Welch DF, Pickett DA, Slater LN, Steigerwalt AG, Brenner DJ: *Rochalimaea henselae* sp nov, a cause of septicemia, bacillary angiomatosis, and parenchymal bacillary peliosis. J Clin Microbiol 1992;30:275–280.

35 Koehler JE, Quinn FD, Berger TG, Leboit PE, Tappero JW: Isolation of *Rochalimaea* species from cutaneous and osseous lesions of bacillary angiomatosis. N Engl J Med 1992;327:1625–1631.
36 Regnery RL, Martin M, Olson JG: Naturally occurring '*Rochalimaea henselae*' infection in domestic cat. Lancet 1992;340:557.
37 Regnery RL, Olson TG, Perkins BA, Bibb W: Serological response to *Rochalimaea henselae* antigen in suspected cat-scratch disease. Lancet 1992;339:1443–1445.
38 Zangwill KM, Hamilton DH, Perkins BA, Regnery RL, Plikaytis BD, Hadler JL, Cartter ML, Wenger JD: Cat scratch disease in Connecticut – Epidemiology, risk factors, and evaluation of a new diagnostic test. N Engl J Med 1993;329:8–13.
39 Perkins BA, Swaminathan B, Jackson LA, Brenner DJ, Wenger JD, Regnery RL, Wear DJ: Case 22–1992. Pathogenesis of cat scratch disease. N Engl J Med 1992;327:1599–1601.
40 Anderson B, Kelly C, Threlkel R, Edwards K: Detection of *Rochalimaea henselae* in cat-scratch disease skin test antigens. J Infect Dis 1993;168:1034–1036.
41 Dolan MJ, Wong MT, Regnery RL, Jorgensen JH, Garcia M, Peters J, Drehner D: Syndrome of *Rochalimaea henselae* adenitis suggesting cat scratch disease. Ann Intern Med 1993;118:331–336.
42 Koehler JE, Glaser CA, Tapero JW: *Rochalimaea henselae* infection: A new zoonosis with the domestic cat as a reservoir. JAMA 1994;271:531–535.
43 Brenner DJ, O'Connor S, Winkler HH, Steigerwalt AG: Proposals to unify the genera *Bartonella* and *Rochalimaea*, with descriptions of *Bartonella quintana* comb nov, *Bartonella vinsonii* comb nov, and to remove the family *Bartonellaceae* from the order *Rickettsiales*. Int J Syst Bacteriol 1993;43: 777–786.
44 Bergmans AMC, Groothedde JW, Schellekens JFP, Van Embden JDA, Ossewaarde JM, Schouls LM: Etiology of cat scratch disease: Comparison of polymerase chain reaction detection of *Bartonella* (formerly *Rochalimaea*) and *Afipia felis* DNA with serology and skin tests. J Infect Dis 1995;171: 916–923.
45 Demers DM, Bass JW, Vincent JM, Person DA, Noyes DK, Staege CM, Samlaska CP, Lockwood NH, Regnery RL, Anderson BE: Cat-scratch disease in Hawaii: Etiology and seroepidemiology. J Pediatr 1995;127:23–26.
46 Szelckelly CM, Goral S, Perezperez GI, Perkins BA, Regnery RL, Edwards KM: Serologic responses to *Bartonella* and *Afipia* antigens in patients with cat scratch disease. Pediatrics 1995;96: 1137–1142.
47 Alkan S, Morgan M, Sandin R, Moscinski L, Ross C: Dual role for *Afipia felis* and *Rochalimaea henselae* in cat-scratch disease. Lancet 1995;345:385.
48 Lawson PA, Collins MD: Description of *Bartonella clarridgeiae* sp nov isolated from the cat of a patient with *Bartonella henselae* septicemia. Med Microbiol Lett 1996;5:64–73.
49 Gurfield AN, Boulouis HJ, Chomel BB, Heller R, Kasten RW, Yamamoto K, Piemont Y: Coinfection with *Bartonella clarridgeiae* and *Bartonella henselae* and with different *Bartonella henselae* strains in domestic cats. J Clin Microbiol 1997;35:2120–2123.
50 Kordick DL, Hilyard EJ, Hadfield TL, Wilson KH, Steigerwalt AG, Brenner DJ, Breitschwerdt EB: *Bartonella clarridgeiae*, a newly recognized zoonotic pathogen causing inoculation papules, fever, and lymphadenopathy (cat scratch disease). J Clin Microbiol 1997;35:1813–1818.
51 Welch DF, Slater LN: *Bartonella*; in Murray PR, Baron EJ, Pfaller MA, Tenover FC, Yolken RH (eds): Manual of Clinical Microbiology. Washington, ASM Press, 1995, pp 690–695.
52 Slater LN, Welch DF, Mandell GL, Bennett JE, Dolin R (eds): Principles and Practice of Infectious Diseases, ed 4. Edinburgh, Churchill Livingstone, 1995, p 170; *Rochalimaea* species (recently renamed *Bartonella*), pp 1741–1747.
53 Roux V, Raoult D: Inter- and intraspecies identification of *Bartonella* (*Rochalimaea*) species. J Clin Microbiol 1995;33:1573–1579.
54 Anderson BE, Goldsmith CS, Johnson AJ, Padmalayam I, Baumstark BR: Bacteriophage-like particle of *Rochalimaea henselae*. Mol Microbiol 1994;13:67–73.
55 Umemori E, Sasaki Y, Amano K, Amano Y: A phage in *Bartonella bacilliformis*. Microbiol Immunol 1992;36:731–736.
56 Drancourt M, Birtles RJ, Chaumentin G, Vandenesch F, Etienne J, Raoult D: A new serotype of *Bartonella henselae* causes endocarditis and cat-scratch disease. Lancet 1996;347:441–443.

57 Bergmans AMC, Schellekens JFP, Vanembden JDA, Schouls LM: Predominance of two *Bartonella henselae* variants among cat-scratch disease patients in The Netherlands. J Clin Microbiol 1996; 34:254–260.
58 Kordick DL, Breitschwerdt EB: Intraerythrocytic presence of *Bartonella henselae*. J Clin Microbiol 1995;33:1655–1656.
59 Drancourt M, Raoult D: Routine identification of *Rochalimaea* species. Eur J Clin Microbiol Infect Dis 1993;12:710–713.
60 Mason RA: Propagation and growth cycle of *Rickettsia quintana* in a new liquid medium. J Bacteriol 1970;103:184–190.
61 Wong MT, Thornton DC, Kennedy RC, Dolan MJ: A chemically defined liquid medium that supports primary isolation of *Rochalimaea* (*Bartonella*) *henselae* from blood and tissue specimens. J Clin Microbiol 1995;33:742–744.
62 Maurin M, Roux V, Stein A, Ferrier F, Viraben R, Raoult D: Isolation and characterization by immunofluorescence, SDS-PAGE, Western blot, RFLP-PCR, 16S rRNA gene sequencing and pulsed-field gel electrophoresis of *Rochalimaea quintana* from a French patient with bacillary angiomatosis. J Clin Microbiol 1994;33:1166–1171.
63 Birtles RJ, Harrison TG, Saunders NA, Molyneux DH: Proposals to unify the genera *Grahamella* and *Bartonella*, with descriptions of *Bartonella talpae* comb nov, *Bartonella peromysci* comb nov, and three new species, *Bartonella grahamii* sp nov, *Bartonella taylorii* sp nov, and *Bartonella doshiae* sp nov. Int J Syst Bacteriol 1995;45:1–8.
64 Weisburg WG, Dobson ME, Samuel JE, Dasch GA, Mallavia LP, Baca O, Mandelco L, Sechrest JE, Weiss E, Woese CR: Phylogenetic diversity of the rickettsiae. J Bacteriol 1989;171:4202–4206.
65 Batterman HJ, Peek JA, Loutit JS, Falkow S, Tompkins LS: *Bartonella henselae* and *Bartonella quintana* adherence to and entry into cultured human epithelial cells. Infect Immunity 1995;63: 4553–4556.
66 Drancourt M, Mainardi JL, Brouqui P, Vandenesch F, Carta A, Lehnert F, Etienne J, Goldstein F, Acar JF, Raoult D: *Bartonella* (*Rochalimaea*) *quintana* endocarditis in three homeless men. N Engl J Med 1995;332:419–423.
67 Raoult D, Drancourt M, Carta A, Gastaut JA: *Bartonella* (*Rochalimaea*) *quintana* isolation in patient with chronic adenopathy, lymphopenia, and a cat. Lancet 1994;343:977.
68 Lucey D, Dolan MJ, Moss CW, Garcia M, Hollis DG, Weigner S: Relapsing illness due to *Rochalimaea henselae* in immunocompetent hosts: Implication for therapy and new epidemiological associations. Clin Infect Dis 1992;14:683–688.
69 Anderson BE, Newman MA: *Bartonella* spp as emerging human pathogens. Clin Microbiol Rev 1997;10:203–219.
70 Anderson B, Jones D, Burgess A: Cloning, expression and sequence analysis of the *Bartonella henselae* gene encoding the HtrA stress-response protein. Gene 1996;178:35–38.
71 Rodriguez-Barradas MC, Bandres JC, Hamill RJ, Trial J, Clarridge JEI, Baughn RE, Rossen RD: In vitro evaluation of the role of humoral immunity against *Bartonella henselae*. Infect Immunity 1995;63:2367–2370.
72 O'Laughlin S, Braverman M, Smith-Jeffries M, Buckley P: Macrophages (histiocytes) in various reactive and inflammatory conditions express different antigenic phenotypes. Hum Pathol 1992;23: 1410–1418.
73 Pece S, Maffione AB, Petruzzelli R, Greco B, Giuliani G, Partipilo MR, Amarri S, Schettini F, Jirillo E, Fumarola D: *Rochalimaea henselae* organisms possess an elevated capacity of binding to peripheral blood lymphocytes from patients with cat scratch disease. Microbios 1995;77:95–100.
74 Fumarola DS, Pece S, Fumarola R, Petruzzelli R, Greco B, Giuliani G, Maffione AB, Jirillo E: Downregulation of human polymorphonuclear cell activities exerted by microorganisms belonging to the alpha-2 subgroup of *Proteobacteria* (*Afipia felis* and *Rochalimaea henselae*). Immunopharmacol Immunotoxicol 1994;16:449–461.
75 Conley T, Slater L, Hamilton K: *Rochalimaea* species stimulate human endothelial cell proliferation and migration in vitro. J Lab Clin Med 1994;124:521–528.

76 Palmari J, Teysseire N, Dussert C, Raoult D: Image cytometry and topographical analysis of proliferation of endothelial cells in vitro during *Bartonella* (*Rochalimaea*) infection. Anal Cell Pathol 1996;11:13–30.
77 Leboit PE, Berger TG, Egbert BM, Beckstead JH, Yen BTS, Stoler MH: Bacillary angiomatosis. The histopathology and differential diagnosis of a pseudoneoplastic infection in patients with human immunodeficiency virus disease. Am J Surg Pathol 1989;13:909–920.
78 Arias-Stella J, Lieberman PH, Erlandson RA: Histology, immunochemistry, and ultrastructure of the verruga in Carrion's disease. Am J Surg Pathol 1986;10:595–610.
79 Centers for Disease Control and Prevention: Encephalitis associated with cat scratch disease. Broward and Palm Beach counties, Florida 1994. MMWR 1994;43:915–916.
80 Noah DL, Bresee JS, Gorensek MJ, Rooney JA, Cresanta JL, Regnery RL, Wong J, Del Toro J, Olson JG, Childs JE: Cluster of five children with acute encephalopathy associated with cat-scratch disease in south Florida. Pediatr Infect Dis J 1995;14:866–869.
81 Waldvogel K, Regnery RL, Anderson BE, Caduff R, Caduff J, Nadal D: Disseminated cat-scratch disease: Detection of *Rochalimaea henselae* in affected tissue. Eur J Pediatr 1994;153:23–27.
82 Flexman JP, Lavis NJ, Kay ID, Watson M, Metcalf C, Pearman JW: *Bartonella henselae* is a causative agent of cat scratch disease in Australia. J Infect 1995;31:241–245.
83 Ueno H, Muramatsu Y, Chomel BB, Hohdatsu T, Koyama H, Morita C: Seroepidemiological survey of *Bartonella* (*Rochalimaea*) *henseale* in domestic cats in Japan. Microbiol Immunol 1995; 39:339–341.
84 Jackson LA, Perkins BA, Wenger JD: Cat scratch disease in the United States: An analysis of three national databases. Am J Public Health 1993;83:1707–1711.
85 Noah DL, Kramer CM, Verbsky MP, Rooney JA, Smith KA, Childs JE: Survey of veterinary professionals and other veterinary conference attendees for antibody to *Bartonella henselae* and *B. quintana*. J Am Vet Med Assoc 1997;210:342–344.
86 Comer JA, Flynn C, Regnery RL, Vlahov D, Childs JE: Antibodies to *Bartonella* species in inner-city intravenous drug users in Baltimore, Md. Arch Intern Med 1996;156:2491–2495.
87 Klein JD: Cat scratch disease. Pediatr Rev 1994;15:348–353.
88 Margileth AM: Dermatological manifestations and update of cat scratch disease. Pediatr Dermatol 1988;5:1–9.
89 Margileth AM: Cat scratch disease: Nonbacterial regional lymphadenitis. The study of 145 patients and a review of the literature. Pediatrics 1968;42:803–818.
90 Carithers HA, Carithers CM, Edwards RO: Cat scratch disease: Its natural history. JAMA 1969; 207:312–316.
91 Childs JE, Rooney JA, Cooper JL, Olson JG, Regnery RL: Epidemiologic observations on infection with *Rochalimaea* species in cats living in Baltimore. J Am Vet Med Assoc 1994;11:1775–1778.
92 Chomel BB, Abbott RC, Kasten RW, Floydhawkins KA, Kass PH, Glaser CA, Pedersen NC, Koehler JE: *Bartonella henselae* prevalence in domestic cats in California. Risk factors and association between bacteremia and antibody titers. J Clin Microbiol 1995;33:2445–2450.
93 Jameson P, Greene C, Regnery R, Dryden M, Marks A, Brown J, Cooper J, Glaus B, Greene R: Prevalence of *Bartonella henselae* antibodies in pet cats throughout regions of North America. J Infect 1995;172:1145–1149.
94 Kordick DL, Wilson KH, Sexton DJ, Hadfield TL, Berkhoff HA, Breitschwerdt EB: Prolonged *Bartonella* bacteremia in cats associated with cat-scratch disease patients. J Clin Microbiol 1995; 33:3245–3251.
95 Tappero JW, Mohle-Boetani JC, Koehler JE, Swaminathan B, Berger TG, Leboit PE, Smith LL, Wenger JD, Pinner RW, Kemper CA, Reingold AL: The epidemiology of bacillary angiomatosis and bacillary peliosis. JAMA 1993;269:770–775.
96 Groves MG, Harrington KS: *Rochalimaea henselae* infections: Newly recognized zoonoses transmitted by domestic cats. J Am Vet Med Assoc 1994;204:267–271.
97 Magnarelli LA, Stafford KC, Mather TN, Yeh MT, Horn KD, Dumler JS: Hemocytic *Rickettsia*-like organisms in ticks: Serologic reactivity with antisera to *Ehrlichiae* and detection of DNA of agent of human granulocytic ehrlichiosis by PCR. J Clin Microbiol 1995;33:2710–2714.

98 Norman AF, Regnery RL, Jameson P, Greene C, Krause DC: Differentiation of *Bartonella*-like isolates at the species level by PCR-restriction fragment length polymorphism in the citrate synthase gene. J Clin Microbiol 1995;33:1797–1803.
99 Childs JE, Olson JG, Cohen WN, Wolf A, Fakile Y, Rooncy JA, Bacellar F, Regnery RL: Prevalence of antibodies to *Rochalimaea* species (cat scratch disease agents) in cats. Vet Rec 1995;136:519–520.
100 Kordick DL, Breitschwerdt EB: Relapsing bacteremia after blood transmission of *Bartonella henselae* to cats. Am J Vet Res 1997;58:492–497.
101 Bergmans AMC, de Jong CMA, Van Amerongen G, Schot CS, Schouls LM: Prevalence of *Bartonella* species in domestic cats in the Netherlands. J Clin Microbiol 1997;35:2256–2261.
102 Maruyama S, Nogami S, Inoue I, Namba S, Asanome K, Katsube Y: Isolation of *Bartonella henselae* from domestic cats in Japan. J Vet Med Sci 1996;58:81–83.
103 Branley J, Wolfson C, Waters P, Gottlieb T, Bradbury R: Prevalence of *Bartonella henselae* bacteremia, the causative agent of cat scratch disease, in an Australian cat population. Pathology 1996; 28:262–265.
104 Kelly PJ, Matthewman LA, Hayter D, Downey S, Wray K, Bryson NR, Raoult D: *Bartonella* (*Rochalimaea*) *henselae* in Southern Africa – Evidence for infections in domestic cats and implications for veterinarians. J S Afr Vet Assoc 1996;67:182–187.
105 Allerberger F, Schonbauer M, Zangerle R, Dierich M: Prevalence of antibody to *Rochalimaea henselae* among Austrian cats. Eur J Pediatr 1995;154:165.
106 Chomel BB, Gurfield AN, Boulouis HJ, Kasten RW, Piemont Y: Réservoir félin de l'agent de la maladie des griffes du chat, *Bartonella henselae*, en région parisienne: Résultats préliminaires. Rec Med Vet 1995;171:841–845.
107 Dalton MJ, Robinson LE, Cooper J, Regnery RL, Olson JG, Childs JE: Use of *Bartonella* antigens for serologic diagnosis of cat-scratch disease at a National Referral Center. Arch Intern Med 1995; 155:1670–1676.
108 Yamamoto K, Chomel B, Lowenstine L, Phillips L, Blackwell J, Kasten R, Pedersen N: Prevalence of *Bartonella henselae* antibodies in captive wild felids, California, and association with ectoparasite infestation. Epidémiol Santé Anim 1997;31:2.
109 Tappero JW, Koehler JE, Berger TG, Cockerell CJ, Lee TH, Busch MP, Stites DP, Mohle-Boetani JC, Reingold AL, Leboit PE: Bacillary angiomatosis and bacillary splenitis in immunocompetent adults. Ann Intern Med 1993;118:363–365.
110 Tompkins LS: *Rochalimaea* infections: Are they zoonoses? JAMA 1994;271:553–554.
111 Kirkpatrick CE, Whiteley HE: Argyrophilic, intracellular bacteria in the lymph node of a cat: Cat-scratch disease bacilli? J Infect Dis 1987;156:690–691.
112 Kirkpatrick CE, Glickman LT: Cat-scratch disease and the role of the domestic cat: Vector, reservoir, and victim? Med Hypotheses 1989;28:145–149.
113 Chomel BB, Kasten RW, Floyd-Hawkins K, Chi B, Yamamoto K, Roberts-Wilson J, Nikos Gurfield A, Abbott RC, Pedersen NC, Koehler JE: Experimental transmission of *Bartonella henselae* by the cat flea. J Clin Microbiol 1996;34:1952–1956.
114 Higgins JA, Radulovic S, Jaworski DC, Azad AF: Acquisition of the cat scratch disease agent *Bartonella henselae* by cat fleas (*Siphonaptera: Pulicidae*). J Med Entymol 1996;33:490–495.
115 Daniels WB, MacMurray FG: Cat scratch disease. Report of one hundred sixty cases. JAMA 1954; 154:1247–1251.
116 Spaulding WB, Hennessy JN: Cat scratch disease. A study of eighty-three cases. Am J Med 1960; 28:504–509.
117 Schwartzman WA: Infections due to *Rochalimaea*: The expanding clinical spectrum. Clin Infect Dis 1992;15:893–902.
118 Margileth AM: Cat scratch disease and nontuberculous mycobacterial disease: Diagnostic usefulness of PPD-Batty, PPD-T and cat scratch skin test antigens. Ann Allerg 1992;68:149–154.
119 Margileth AM, Hayden GF: Cat scratch disease. From feline affection to human infection. N Engl J Med 1993;329:53–54.
120 Shinall EA: Cat scratch disease: A review of the literature. Pediatr Dermatol 1990;7:11–18.
121 Chen SCA, Gilbert GL: Cat scratch disease: Past and present (a review). J Pediatr Child Health 1994;30:467–469.

122 Margileth AM: Cat scratch disease. Adv Pediatr Infect Dis 1993;8:1–21.
123 Margileth AM: Sorting out the causes of lymphadenopathy. Contemp Pediatr 1995;12:23–40.
124 Margileth AM: Antibiotic therapy for cat scratch disease: Clinical study of therapeutic outcome in 268 patients and a review of the literature. Pediatr Infect Dis J 1992;11:474–478.
125 Margileth AM, Hadfield TL: A new look at old cat scratch disease. Contemp Pediatr 1990;7:26–50.
126 Carithers HA: Oculoglandular disease of Parinaud. Am J Dis Child 1978;132:1195–1200.
127 Wear DJ, Malaty RH, Zimmerman LE, Hadfield TL, Margileth AM: Cat scratch disease bacilli in the con-junctival of patients with Parinaud's oculoglandular syndrome. Ophthalmology 1985;92:1282–1287.
128 Le HH, Palay DA, Anderson BE, Steinberg JP: Conjunctival swab to diagnose ocular cat scratch disease. Am J Ophthalmol 1994;118:249–250.
129 Delahoussaye PM, Osborne BM: Cat-scratch disease presenting as abdominal visceral granulomas. J Infect Dis 1990;161:71–78.
130 Lenoir AA, Storch GA, Deschryver-Kecskemeti K, Shackelford GD, Rothbaum RJ, Wear DJ, Rosemblum JL: Granulomatous hepatitis associated with cat scratch disease. Lancet 1988;1:1132–1135.
131 Malatack JJ, Altman HA, Nard JA, Wiener ES, Urbach AH, McGregor RS: Cat scratch disease without adenopathy. J Pediatr 1989;114:104.
132 Rizkallah MF, Meyer L, Ayoub EM: Hepatic and splenic abscesses in cat-scratch disease. Pediatr Infect Dis J 1988;7:191–195.
133 Golden SE: Hepatosplenic cat scratch disease associated with elevated anti-*Rochalimaea* antibody titers. Pediatr Infect Dis J 1993;12:868–871.
134 Bogue CW, Wise JD, Gray GF, Edwards KM: Antibiotic therapy for cat-scratch disease. JAMA 1989;262:813–816.
135 Dangman BC, Albanese BA, Kacica MA, Lepow ML, Wallach MT: Cat scratch disease in two children presenting with fever of unknown origin: Imaging features and association with a new causative agent, *Rochalimaea henselae*. Pediatrics 1995;95:767–771.
136 Malatack JJ, Jaffe R: Granulomatous hepatitis in three children due to cat-scratch disease without peripheral adenopathy. Am J Dis Child 1993;147:949–953.
137 Stevens H: Cat-scratch fever encephalitis. Am J Dis Child 1952;84:218–222.
138 Carithers HA, Margileth AM: Cat scratch disease. Acute encephalopathy and other neurologic manifestations. Am J Dis Child 1991;145:98–101.
139 Lewis LW, Tucker SH: Central nervous system involvement in cat-scratch disease. Pediatrics 1986; 77:714–721.
140 Centers for Disease Control and Prevention: Encephalitis associated with cat scratch disease. Broward and Palm Beach Counties, Florida 1994. MMWR 1994;43:915–916.
141 Hadley S, Albrecht AM, Tarsy D: Cat scratch encephalopathy: A cause of status epilepticus and coma in a healthy young adult. Neurology 1995;45:196.
142 Lewis DW, Tucker SH: Central nervous system involvement in cat scratch disease. Pediatrics 1986; 77:714–721.
143 Marra CM: Neurologic complications of *Bartonella henselae* infection. Curr Opin Neurol 1995;8:164–169.
144 Oran B, Ceri A, Yilmaz H: Fever, abdominal pain and intracranial mass. Pediatr Infect Dis J 1995; 14:725–728.
145 François J, Verriets G, DeLayey JJ: Leber's idiopathic stellate retinopathy. Am J Ophthalmol 1982; 93:96–101.
146 Sweeny VP, Drance SM: Optic neuritis and compressive neuropathy associated with cat scratch disease. Can Med Assoc J 1970;103:1380–1381.
147 Gass JDM: Diseases of the optic nerve that may stimulate macular disease. Trans Am Acad Ophthalmol 1977;83:763–770.
148 Newsom RW, Martin TJ, Wasilauskas B: Cat-scratch disease diagnosed serologically using an enzyme immunoassay in a patient with neuroretinitis. Arch Ophthalmol 1996;114:493–494.
149 Wong MT, Dolan MJ, Lattuada CP, Regnery RL, Garcia ML, Mokulis EC, Labarre RC, Ascher DP, Delmar JA, Kelly JW, Leigh DR, McRae AC, Reed JB, Smith RE, Melcher GP: Neuroretinitis, aseptic meningitis, and lymphadenitis associated with *Bartonella* (*Rochalimaea*) *henselae* infection in immunocompetent patients and patients infected with human immunodeficiency virus type 1. Clin Infect Dis 1995;21:352–360.

150 Golnik KC, Marotto ME, Fanous MM, Heiter D, King LP, Halpern JI, Holley PHJ: Ophthalmic manifestations of *Rochalimaea* species. Am J Ophthalmol 1994;118:145–151.
151 Dreyer RF, Hopen G, Gass JDM, Smith JL: Leber's idiopathic stellate neuroretinitis. Arch Ophthalmol 1984;102:1140–1145.
152 Weiss AH, Beck RW: Neutoretinitis in childhood. J Pediatr Ophthalmol Strab 1989;26:198–203.
153 Ulrich GG, Waecker NJ, Meister SJ, Peterson TJ, Hooper DG: Cat scratch disease associated with neuroretinitis in a 6-year-old girl. Ophthalmology 1992;99:246–249.
154 McCrary B, Cockerham W, Pierce P: Neuroretinitis in cat scratch disease associated with macular star. Pediatr Infect Dis J 1994;13:838–839.
155 Adams WC, Hindman SM: Cat scratch disease associated with an osteolytic lesion. J Pediatr 1954; 44:665–669.
156 Collipp PJ, Koch R: Cat scratch fever associated with an osteolytic lesion. N Engl J Med 1959; 260:278–280.
157 Shauon AB, Marchessault JH, McDonald P: Cat scratch disease associated with a vertebral osteolytic lesion. Pediatr Infect Dis J 1989;8:51–52.
158 Carithers HA: Cat scratch disease associated with an osteolytic lesion. Am J Dis Child 1983;137: 968–970.
159 Muszynski MJ, Eppes S, Riley HD: Granulomatous osteolytic lesion of the skull associated with cat scratch disease. Pediatr Infect Dis J 1987;6:199–201.
160 Bernini PM, Gorczyca JT, Modlin JF: Cat scratch disease presenting as a paravertebral abscess. A case report. J Bone Joint Surg Am 1994;76:1858–1863.
161 Koranyi K: Fever, back pain and pleural effusion in a four-year old boy. Pediatr Infect Dis J 1993; 13:657–672.
162 Caniza MA, Granger DL, Wilson KH, Washington MK, Kordick DL, Frush DP, Blitchington RB: *Bartonella henselae*: Etiology of pulmonary nodules in a patient with depressed cell-mediated immunity. Clin Infect Dis 1995;20:1505–1511.
163 Stoler MH, Bonfiglio TA, Steigbigel MT, Pereira M: An atypical subcutaneous infection associated with acquired immune deficiency syndrome. Am J Clin Pathol 1983;80:714–718.
164 Cockerell CJ, Whitlow MA, Webster GF, Friedman-Kien AE: Epithelioid angiomatosis: A distinct vascular disorder in patients with the acquired immunodeficiency syndrome or AIDS-related complex. Lancet 1987;ii:654–656.
165 Maurin M, Birtles RJ, Raoult D: Current knowledge of *Bartonella* species. Eur J Clin Microbiol Infect Dis 1997;16:487–506.
166 Mohle-Boetani JC, Koehler JE, Berger TG, Leboit PE, Kemper CA, Reingold AL, Plikaytis BD, Wenger JD, Tappero JW: Bacillary angiomatosis and bacillary peliosis in patients infected with human immunodeficiency virus: Clinical characteristics in a case-control study. Clin Infect Dis 1996;22:794–800.
167 Kemper CA, Lombard CM, Deresinski SC, Tompkins LS: Visceral bacillary epithelioid angiomatosis possible manifestations of disseminated cat scratch disease in the immunocompromised host: A report of two cases. Am J Med 1990;89:216–222.
168 Szaniawski WK, Don PC, Bitterman SR, Schachner JR: Epithelioid angiomatosis in patients with AIDS: A report of seven cases and review of the literature. J Am Acad Dermatol 1990;23: 41–48.
169 Schwartz RA, Nychay SG, Janniger CK, Lambert WC: Bacillary angiomatosis: Presentation of six patients, some with unusual features. Br J Dermatol 1997;136:60–65.
170 Carrascosa JM, Ribera M, Bielsa I, Raventos A, Vaquero M, Ferrandiz C: Bacillary angiomatosis presenting as a malleolar ulcer. Arch Dermatol 1995;131:963–964.
171 Levell NJ, Bewley AP, Chopra S, Churchill D, French P, Miller R, Gikes JJH: Bacillary angiomatosis with cutaneous and oral lesions in an HIV-infected patient from the UK. Br J Dermatol 1995;132: 113–115.
172 Perkocha LA, Geaghan SM, Yen BTS, Nishimumra SL, Chan SP, Garcia-Kennedy R, Honda G, Stoloff AC, Klein HZ, Goldman RL, Van Meter S, Ferrell LD, LeBoit PE: Clinical and pathological features of bacillary peliosis hepatis in association with human immunodeficiency virus infection. N Engl J Med 1990;323:1581–1586.

173 Adal KA, Cockerell CJ, Petri WAJ: Cat scratch disease, bacillary angiomatosis, and other infections due to *Rochalimaea*. N Engl J Med 1994;330:1509–1515.
174 Baron AL, Steinbach LS, Leboit PE, Mills CM, Gee JH, Berger TG: Osteolytic lesions and bacillary angiomatosis in HIV infection: Radiologic differentiation from AIDS-related Kaposi sarcoma. Radiology 1990;177:77–81.
175 Leboit PE, Berger TG, Egbert BM, Benedict Yen TS, Stoler MH, Bonfiglio TA, Strauchen JA, English CK, Wear DJ: Epithelioid haemangioma-like vascular proliferation in AIDS: Manifestation of cat scratch disease bacillus infection? Lancet 1988;1:960–966.
176 Koehler JE, Tappero JW: Bacillary angiomatosis and bacillary peliosis in patients infected with human immunodeficiency virus. Clin Infect Dis 1993;17:612–624.
177 Black JR, Herrington DA, Hadfield TL, Wear DJ, Margileth AM, Shigekawa B: Life-threatening cat-scratch disease in an immunocompromised host. Arch Intern Med 1986;146:394–396.
178 Koehler JE, Leboit PE, Egbert BM, Berger TG: Cutaneous vascular lesions and disseminated cat-scratch disease in patients with the acquired immunodeficiency syndrome (AIDS) and AIDS-related complex. Ann Intern Med 1988;109:449–455.
179 Cockerell CJ, Leboit PE: Bacillary angiomatosis: A newly characterized, pseudoneoplastic, infectious, cutaneous vascular disorder. J Am Acad Dermatol 1990;22:501–512.
180 Koehler JE, Cederberg L: Intra-abdominal mass associated with gastrointestinal hemorrhage: A new manifestation of bacillary angiomatosis. Gastroenterology 1995;109:2011–2014.
181 Fagan WA, Skinner SM, Ondo A, Williams JT, Anthony K, De Villez RL, Pulitzer DR: Bacillary angiomatosis of the skin and bone marrow in a patient with HIV infection. J Am Acad Dermatol 1995;32:510–512.
182 Milam MW, Balerdi MJ, Toney JF, Foulis PR, Milam CP, Behnke RH: Epithelioid angiomatosis secondary to disseminated cat scratch disease involving the bone marrow and skin in a patient with acquired immune deficiency syndrome: A case report. Am J Med 1990;88:180–183.
183 Bruckert F, de Kerviler E, Zagdanski AM, Molina JM, Casin I, Guermazi A, Bedrossian J, Frija J: Sternal abscess due to *Bartonella* (*Rochalimaea*) *henselae* in a renal transplant patient. Skeletal Radiol 1997;26:431–433.
184 Haught WH, Steinbach J, Zander DS, Wingo CS: Bacillary angiomatosis with massive visceral lymphadenopathy. Am J Med Sci 1993;306:236–240.
185 Shinella RA, Alba Greco M: Bacillary angiomatosis presenting as a soft-tissue tumor without skin involvement. Hum Pathol 1990;21:567–569.
186 Regnery RL, Childs JE, Koehler JE: Infections associated with *Bartonella* species in persons infected with human immunodeficiency virus. Clin Infect Dis 1995;21:S94–S98.
187 Apalsch AM, Nour B, Jaffe R: Systemic cat scratch disease in a pediatric liver transplant recipient and review of the literature. Pediatr Infect Dis J 1993;12:769–774.
188 Myers SA, Prose NS, Garcia JA, Wilson KH, Dunsmore KP, Kamino H: Bacillary angiomatosis in a child undergoing chemotherapy. J Pediatr 1992;121:574–578.
189 Spach DH, Kanter AS, Dougherty MJ, Larson AM, Coyle MB, Brenner DJ, Swaminathan B, Matar GM, Welch DF, Root RK, Stamm WE: *Bartonella* (*Rochalimaea*) *quintana* bacteremia in inner-city patients with chronic alcoholsim. N Engl J Med 1995;332:424–428.
190 Paul MA, Fleischer AB, Wieselthier JS, White WL: Bacillary angiomatosis in an immunocompetent child: The first reported case. Pediatr Dermatol 1994;11:338–341.
191 Lee WR, Chawla JC, Reid R: Bacillary angiomatosis of the conjunctiva. Am J Ophthalmol 1994;118:152–157.
192 Slater LN, Welch DF, Min KW: *Rochalimaea henselae* causes bacillary angiomatosis and peliosis hepatis. Arch Intern Med 1992;152:602–606.
193 Alkan S, Orenstein JM: Bacillary peliosis hepatis (letter; comment). N Engl J Med 1991;324:1513–1514.
194 Czapar CA, Weldon-Linne M, Moore DM, Rhone DP: Peliosis hepatitis in the acquired immunodeficiency syndrome. Arch Pathol Lab Med 1986;110:611–613.
195 Young JM: Peliosis hepatitis: Report of two cases. Am Rev Tuberc 1953;67:385–390.
196 Leong SS, Cazen RA, Yu GS, LeFevre L, Carson JW: Abdominal visceral peliosis associated with bacillary angiomatosis. Arch Pathol Lab Med 1992;116:866–871.

197 Steeper TA, Rosenstein H, Weiser J, Inampudi S, Snover DC: Bacillary epithelioid angiomatosis involving the liver, spleen, and skin in an AIDS patient with concurrent Kaposi's sarcoma. Am J Clin Pathol 1992;97:713–718.
198 Breathnach AS, Hoare JM, Eykyn SJ: Culture-negative endocarditis: Contribution of *Bartonella* infections. Heart 1997;77:474–476.
199 Raoult D, Fournier PE, Drancourt M, Marrie TJ, Etienne J, Cosserat J, Cacoub P, Poinsignon Y, Leclercq P, Sefton A: Diagnosis of 22 new cases of *Bartonella* endocarditis. Ann Intern Med 1996; 125:646–652.
200 Hadfield TL, Warren R, Kass M, Brun E, Levy C: Endocarditis caused by *Rochalimaea henselae*. Hum Pathol 1993;24:1140–1141.
201 Holmes AH, Greenough TC, Balady GJ, Regnery RL, Anderson BE, Okeane JC, Fonger JD, McCrone EL: *Bartonella henselae* endocarditis in an immunocompetent adult. Clin Infect Dis 1995; 21:1004–1007.
202 Spach DH, Panther LA, Thorning DR, Dunn JE, Plorde JJ, Miller RA: Intracerebral bacillary angiomatosis in a patient infected with human immunodeficiecny virus. Ann Med Intern 1992;116: 740–742.
203 Schwartzman WA, Patnaik M, Angulo FJ, Visscher BR, Miller EN, Peter JB: *Bartonella* (*Rochalimaea*) antibodies, dementia, and cat ownership among men infected with human immunodeficiency virus. Clin Infect Dis 1995;21:954–959.
204 Revol A, Vinhetto A, Jourvet A, Airmard G, Trillet M: Encephalitis in cat scratch disease with persistent dementia. J Neurol Neurosurg Psychol 1992;55:133–135.
205 Margileth AM, Wear DJ, English CK: Systemic cat scratch disease: Report of 23 patients with prolonged or recurrent severe bacterial infection. J Infect Dis 1987;155:390–404.
206 Arnold MM, McKenna F: Reactive arthritis in a patient with cat scratch disease. Postgrad Med J 1994;70:147.
207 Soheilian M, Markomichelakis N, Foster CS: Intermediate uveitis and retinal vasculitis as manifestations of cat scratch disease. Am J Ophthalmol 1996;122:582–584.
208 Kalter SS, Rodriguez AR, Heberling RL: Cat-scratch disease skin-test antigen preparation. Lancet 1977;ii:606–607.
209 Lamps LW, Gray GF, Scott MA: The histologic spectrum of hepatic cat scratch disease – A series of six cases with confirmed *Bartonella henselae* infection. Am J Surg Pathol 1996;20:1253–1259.
210 Larson AM, Dougherty MJ, Nowowiejski DJ, Welch DF, Matar GM, Swaminathan B, Coyle MB: Detection of *Bartonella* (*Rochalimaea*) *quintana* by routine acridine orange staining of broth blood cultures. J Clin Microbiol 1994;32:1492–1496.
211 Myers WF, Cutler LD, Wisseman CL Jr: Role of erythrocytes and serum in the nutrition of *Rickettsia quintana*. J Bacteriol 1969;97:663–666.
212 Zbinden R, Höchli M, Nadal D: Intracellular location of *Bartonella henselae* cocultivated with vero cells and used for an indirect fluorescent-antibody test. Clin Diagn Lab Immunol 1995;2:693–695.
213 Drancourt M, Reboul-Paris D, Enea M, Raoult D: The diagnosis of cat-scratch disease; in Kazar J, Toman R (eds): *Rickettsiae* and Rickettsial Diseases. Bratislava, Veda, 1996, pp 628–640.
214 Drancourt M, Raoult D: Proposed tests for the routine identification of *Rochalimaea* species. Eur J Clin Microbiol Infect Dis 1993;12:710–713.
215 Rodriguez-Barradas MC, Hamill RJ, Houston ED, Georgiou PR, Clarridge JE, Regnery RL, Koehler JE: Genomic fingerprinting of *Bartonella* species by repetitive element PCR for distinguishing species and isolates. J Clin Microbiol 1995;33:1089–1093.
216 Relman DA, Falkow S, Leboit PE, Perkocha LA, Min KW, Welch DF, Slater LN: The organism causing bacillary angiomatosis, peliosis hepatitis, and fever and bacteremia in immunocompromised patients. N Engl J Med 1991;324:1514.
217 Relman DA, Lepp PW, Sadler KN, Schmidt TM: Phylogenetic relationships among the agent of bacillary angiomatis, *Bartonella bacilliformis*, and other alphaproteobacteria. Mol Microbiol 1992; 6:1801–1807.
218 Birtles RJ: Differentiation of *Bartonella* species using restriction endonuclease analysis of PCR-amplified 16S rRNA genes. FEMS Microbiol Lett 1995;129:261–266.

219 Birtles RJ, Harrison TG, Fry NK, Saunders NA, Taylor AG: Taxonomic considerations of *Bartonella bacilliformis* based on phylogenetic and phenotypic characteristics. FEMS Microbiol Lett 1991;83: 187–192.
220 Joblet C, Roux C, Drancourt M, Gouvernet J, Raoult D: Identification of *Bartonella* (*Rochalimaea*) species among fastidious Gram-negative bacteria based on the partial sequence of the citrate-synthase gene. J Clin Microbiol 1995;33:1879–1883.
221 Matar GM, Swaminathan B, Hunter SB, Slater LN, Welch DF: Polymerase chain reaction-based restriction fragment length polymorphism analysis of a fragment of the ribosomal operon from *Rochalimaea* species for subtyping. J Clin Microbiol 1993;31:1730–1734.
222 Patnaik M, Peter JB: Cat-scratch disease, *Bartonella henselae*, and the usefulness of routine serological testing for *Afipia felis*. Clin Infect Dis 1995;21:1064.
223 Barka NE, Hadfield T, Patnaik M, Schartzman WA, Peter JB: EIA for detection of *Rochalimaea henselae*-reactive IgG, IgM and IgA antibodies in patients with suspected cat-scratch disease. J Infect Dis 1993;167:1503–1504.
224 Amerein MP, De Briel D, Jaulhac B, Meyer P, Monteil H, Piemont Y: Diagnostic value of the indirect immunofluorescence assay in cat scratch disease with *Bartonella henselae* and *Afipia felis* antigens. Clin Diagn Lab Immunol 1996;3:200–204.
225 Raoult D, Tissot-Dupont H, Enea Mutillod M: Positive predictive value of *Rochalimaea henselae* antibodies in the diagnostic of cat scratch disease. Clin Infect Dis 1994;19:335.
226 Cooper MD, Hollingdale MR, Vinson JW, Costa J: A passive hemagglutination test for diagnosis of trench fever due to *Rochalimaea quintana*. J Infect Dis 1976;134:605–609.
227 La Scola B, Raoult D: Serological cross-reactions between *Bartonella quintana, Bartonella henselae*, and *Coxiella burnetii*. J Clin Microbiol 1996;34:2270–2274.
228 Jalava J, Kotilainen P, Nikkari S, Skurnik M, Vanttinen E, Lehtonen OP, Eerola E, Toivanen P: Use of the polymerase chain reaction and DNA sequencing for detection of *Bartonella quintana* in the aortic valve of a patient with culture-negative infective endocarditis. Clin Infect Dis 1995;21: 891–896.
229 Roux V, Raoult D: The 16S-23S rRNA integenic spacer region of *Bartonella* (*Rochalimaea*) species is longer than usually described in other bacteria. Gene 1995;156:107–111.
230 Matar GM: Inter- and intraspecies identification of *Bartonella* species by PCR-restriction fragment length polymorphism analysis of a fragment of the ribosomal operon. J Clin Microbiol 1995;33: 3370.
231 Anderson B, Sims K, Regnery R: Detection of the *Rochalimaea henselae* DNA in specimens from cat-scratch disease patients by polymerase chain reaction. J Clin Microbiol 1994;32:942–948.
232 Regnery RL, Spruill CL, Plikaytis BD: Genotypic identification of rickettsiae and estimation of intraspecies sequence divergence for portions of two rickettsial genes. J Bacteriol 1991;173:1576–1589.
233 Myers WF, Grossman DM, Wisseman CL Jr: Antibiotic susceptibility patterns in *Rochalimaea quintana*, the agent of trench fever. Antimicrob Agents Chemother 1984;25:690–693.
234 Maurin M, Gasquet S, Ducco C, Raoult D: MICs of 28 antibiotic compounds for 14 *Bartonella* (formerly *Rochalimaea*) isolates. Antimicrob Agents Chemother 1995;39:2387–2391.
235 Maurin M, Raoult D: Antimicrobial susceptibility of *Rochalimaea quintana, Rochalimaea vinsonii* and the newly recognized *Rochalimaea henselae*. J Antimicrob Chemother 1993;32:587–594.
236 Wolfson C, Branley J, Gottlieb T: The E test for antimicrobial susceptibility testing of *Bartonella henselae*. J Antimicrob Chemother 1996;38:963–968.
237 Musso D, Drancourt M, Raoult D: Lack of bactericidal effect of antibiotics except aminoglycosides on *Bartonella* (*Rochalimaea*) *henselae*. J Antimicrob Chemother 1995;36:101–108.
238 Ives TJ, Manzewitsch P, Regnery RL, Butts JD, Kebede M: In vitro susceptibilities of *Bartonella henselae, B. quintana, B. elizabethae, Rickettsia rickettsii, R. conorii, R. akari*, and *R. prowazekii* to macrolide antibiotics as determined by immunofluorescent-antibody analysis of infected vero cell monolayers. Antimicrob Agents Chemother 1997;41:578–582.
239 Maurin M, Lepocher H, Mallet D, Raoult D: Antibiotics susceptibility of *Afipia felis* in axenic medium and in cells. Antimicrob Agents Chemother 1993;37:1410–1413.

240 Cockerell CJ, Bergstresser PR, Myrie-Williams C, Tierno PM: Bacillary epithelioid angiomatosis occurring in an immunocompetent individual. Arch Dermatol 1990;126:787–790.
241 Spach DH, Callis KP, Paauw DS, Houze YB, Schoenknecht FD, Welch DF, Rosen H, Brenner DJ: Endocarditis caused by *Rochalimaea quintana* in a patient infected with human immunodeficiency virus. J Clin Microbiol 1993;31:692–694.
242 Daly JS, Worthington MG, Brenner DJ, Moss WC, Hollis DG, Weyant RS, Steigerwalt AG, Weaver RE, Daneshvar MI, O'Connor SP: *Rochalimaea elizabethae* sp nov isolated from a patient with endocarditis. J Clin Microbiol 1993;31:872–881.
243 Lewis DE, Wallace MR: Treatment of adult systemic cat scratch disease with gentamicin sulfate. West J Med 1991;154:330–331.
244 Rappaport DC, Cumming WA, Ros PR: Treatment of adult systemic cat scratch disease with gentamicin sulfate. West J Med 1991;154:330–331.
245 Collipp PJ: Cat-scratch disease: Therapy with trimethoprim-sulfamethoxazole. Am J Dis Child 1992;146:397–399.
246 Holley HPJ: Successful treatment of cat scratch disease with ciprofloxacin. JAMA 1991;265:1563–1565.
247 Brouqui P, Raoult D: *Bartonella quintana* invades and multiplies within endothelial cells in vitro and in vivo and forms intracellular blebs. Res Microbiol 1996;147:719–731.

Pierre-Edouard Fournier, MD, Unité des Rickettsies, CNRS UPRESA 6020,
Faculté de Médecine, Université de la Méditerranée, 27, boulevard Jean-Moulin,
F–13385 Marseille Cedex 05 (France)
Tel. +33 04 91 38 55 17, Fax +33 04 91 83 03 90, E-Mail Didier.Raoult@medecine.univ-mrs.fr

Schmidt A (ed): *Bartonella* and *Afipia* Species Emphasizing *Bartonella henselae*.
Contrib Microbiol. Basel, Karger, 1998, vol 1, pp 63–76

# Human Diseases – Apart from Cat-Scratch Disease, Bacillary Angiomatosis, and Peliosis – and Carriership Related with *Bartonella* and *Afipia* Species

*Ingo B. Autenrieth, Michael Haimerl*

Max von Pettenkofer-Institut für Hygiene und Medizinische Mikrobiologie,
Ludwig Maximilians-Universität München, Deutschland

## Introduction

At present, eleven *Bartonella* species are known, four of which are pathogenic for humans: *B. bacilliformis, B. quintana, B. henselae* and *B. elizabethae.* While *B. bacilliformis* is related with a typical disease, called Carrion's disease, occurring exclusively in South America, two other *Bartonella* species, *B. quintana* and *B. henselae*, occur probably worldwide, and are related with various clinical manifestations including cat-scratch disease (CSD), bacillary angiomatosis (BA), peliosis, and others. *B. quintana* is well known from World War I as being the etiological agent of trench fever. *B. henselae* and *B. elizabethae* are new pathogens that were discovered only a few years ago. While *B. henselae* is related with various well-known diseases and has been detected frequently, *B. elizabethae* has been found in only one single case with endocarditis.

CSD might also be caused by a further bacterial species, subsumed in the genus *Afipia*: *A. felis, A. clevelandensis* and *A. broomeae* as well as three further *Afipia* species may possibly cause diseases in humans.

During the past few years, an increasing body of evidence revealed that *Bartonella* species, and possibly, but less clear, also *Afipia* species, may cause a broad spectrum of clinical manifestations other than the classical above-mentioned diseases. Thus, bacteremia, endocarditis, chronic lymphadenopathy, as well as systemic manifestations in various organs including liver, lungs, CNS, eyes and bones may be associated with *Bartonella* species. However, the etiology of such cases might often not be diagnosed due to the difficulties with laboratory methods required for detection of these bacterial agents or due to the fact that clinicians are not aware about the significance of *Bartonella* and *Afipia* species in differential diagnosis of infectious diseases. Thus, these bacterial species are often not considered as putative infectious agents in patients with the above-mentioned syndromes. In this chapter, human diseases, apart from CSD, BA and peliosis that are associated with *Bartonella* or *Afipia* species as well as the putative carriership with *Bartonella* and *Afipia* species will be discussed (table 1).

## Verruga peruana and Oroya Fever

*B. bacilliformis* was first described by Alberto Barton in 1909 in Peru. He identified *B. bacilliformis* as the etiological agent of a syndrome called Carrion's disease. Daniel Carrion was a medical student who wanted to elucidate the etiology of a since long time well-known clinical manifestation called verruga peruana endemic in the Andes mountain region of South America. This disease is manifested by multiple nodular vascular eruptions of the skin and mucosal surfaces accompanied by rheumatic pain and fever. Unfortunately, he was not aware that this disease is usually preceded by another entity called Oroya fever which is manifested as fever and severe anemia and which was associated with high mortality. In fact, today it is well established that *B. bacilliformis* causes a diphasic illness, namely febrile hemolytic anemia – acute Oroya fever – which may be followed by cranberry-like tumors of the cutis, chronic verruga peruana. Daniel Carrion's self-experimentation in which he inoculated himself with blood from a patient's verruca ended with a tragedy as he subsequently died from acute Oroya fever [Schultz, 1968]. About the actual relationship between both entities, however, he was only aware during the last few days of his short life.

Oroya fever is an acute systemic disease presenting with high fever, septicemia and hemolytic anemia. After an incubation time of 2–6 (even up to 14) weeks, the patients may usually suffer from high fever, chill-like symptoms and headaches. Rapid disease progression accompanied by rheumatic pain including myalgia and arthralgia, lymphadenopathy and an altered mental status, usually occurs. Moreover, complications such as meningoencephalitis, stroke and cardiovascular symptoms including angina and dyspnea may be associated with the disease. Most of the symptoms are probably related to invasion into and growth of *B. bacilliformis* within the erythrocytes, resulting finally into rapidly developing hemolysis, anemia, as well as microvascular thrombosis. In fact, *B. bacilliformis* has been clearly demonstrated to invade

*Table 1.* Human diseases other than CSD, BA, peliosis, and carriership related with *Bartonella* and *Afipia* species

| Species | Occurrence | Reservoir | Trans-mission | Carriership in humans | Diseases other than CSD, BA, peliosis or source of isolate |
|---|---|---|---|---|---|
| *B. bacilliformis* | Peru, Ecuador, Columbia | Humans | Sandfly, ticks? | Yes (in blood) | Carrion's disease (diphasic: acute Oroya fever, chronic verruga peruana) |
| *B. quintana* | Worldwide | Humans (e.g., alcoholics, homeless, HIV-patients), others likely | Body louse | In blood? | Trench fever, bacteremia, endocarditis, chronic lymphadenopathy, systemic manifestations in internal organs, bones, CNS diseases |
| *B. henselae* | Worldwide | Cats | Cat scratches or bites, cat flea | Unknown | Bacteremia, endocarditis, chronic lymphadenopathy, systemic manifestations in internal organs, lung, bones, CNS diseases |
| *B. elizabethae* | Unknown (1 case only) | Unknown | Unknown | Unknown | Endocarditis |
| *A. felis* | Unknown (US only?) | Unknown | Cat scratches? | Unknown | Unknown |
| *A. clevelandensis* | Unknown | Unknown | Unknown | Unknown | Tibia |
| *A. broomeae* | Unknown | Unknown | Unknown | Unknown | bone marrow, bone abscess, pleural fluid |
| *Afipia* genospecies 1–3 | Unknown | Unknown | Unknown | Unknown | Bronchial washing, water |

into erythrocytes, and the required genetic loci have been identified and cloned [Minnick et al., 1996]. Thus, *B. bacilliformis* can be considered a hemotropic bacterium [Dooley, 1980]. Death usually occurs only in this acute phase from acute hemolysis or from septicemia with, e.g., *Salmonella* species [Cuadra, 1956]. Oroya fever is fatal in up to 90% of cases without appropriate therapy [Gray et al., 1990]. After surviving Oroya fever, the patients are often compromised and may be susceptible to opportunistic infections.

Verruga peruana is a chronic, persistent disease primarily involving the skin. Within a few months after infection, skin lesions presenting as painless nodules, teleangiectatic granulomatous purple lesions resembling cranberry-like tumors primarily in the face, neck and extremities appear. Moreover, lesions of the mucosal surfaces and internal organs may occur. The histopathological hallmark of these nodule-like lesions is vascular with an endothelial cell proliferation. The factor produced by *B. bacilliformis* that accounts for endothelial cell proliferation has been partially characterized [Conley et al., 1994]. Bacteria may also be histologically evident in these lesions. After months or years, the lesions may become fibrotic, and usually disappear spontaneously. Recently, verruga peruana has also been described as a 'traveller disease' [Matteeli et al., 1994].

The fact that *B. bacilliformis* infections are transmitted by arthropod vectors such as sand flies (*Lutzomyia verrucarum* or *Phlebotomus* species) has been known for more than 200 years and was already mentioned by Cosme Bueno in 1764 [Herrer and Christensen, 1975]. However, other fly species and possibly ticks (*Dermacentor* species) might also be involved in transmission of *B. bacilliformis*.

Carriership with *B. bacilliformis* may occur in up to 8–15% of patients surviving acute Oroya fever. These patients may serve as a reservoir of *B. bacilliformis*. In fact, in these individuals, chronic asymptomatic bacteremia occurs, and latent infection may persist for long periods of time. However, the reservoir of *B. bacilliformis* infections apart from humans has not yet been completely elucidated. Nevertheless, a reservoir outside humans, e.g., possibly in small rodents, seems likely as Carrion's disease also occurs in regions with a very low human population density. Moreover, *B. bacilliformis* has been experimentally transmitted to *Macaca mulatta* via sand flies [Herrer and Christensen, 1975].

The prevalence of *Bartonella*-specific antibodies in sera of individuals from Peru is high. About 21.7–64% of sera from endemic areas were found to react with *B. bacilliformis* antigen [Knobloch et al., 1985; Gray et al., 1990]. However, possible cross-reactive antibodies directed against lipopolysaccharide of Chlamydiae as well as antibodies against conserved immunodominant proteins of *B. bacilliformis* such as a 65-kDa heat-shock protein [Knobloch et al., 1985; Knobloch and Schreiber, 1990] may occur and might account for nonvalid results of serological studies.

## Trench Fever

Trench fever (also known as 5-day fever, quintan fever, Wolhynia fever) is a self-limited disease caused by *B. quintana* that is well known from World

War I when about 1 million soldiers suffered from this disease. The term 'quintana' refers to the 5-day (4–8 days) interval between fever attacks that usually last for about 5 days.

After an incubation period of 2–3 (maximally 1–4) weeks, various mild or severe symptoms including fever, headache – mainly in the front region – and pain in the legs – typically tibia region – and back, myalgia as well as maculopapular erythematous rash may occur [McNee et al., 1916]. Symptoms may range from mild or asymptomatic to severe, and usually recur although less severe after 5 days of fever-free intervals.

Signs of a general infection including weakness, splenomegaly and joint pains, the latter of which might reflect reactive arthritis, may occur. Moreover, vomiting and diarrhea may be associated with trench fever. Laboratory findings usually reveal increased counts for white blood cells and other rather nonspecific changes.

After 4–6 weeks, symptoms disappear in most patients. Thus, trench fever is usually not fatal but may be associated with significant morbidity. However, few cases with chronic persistent infections including headache, pains and altered mental status may occur. Nowadays, classical trench fever does practically not occur or is a very rare condition, and *B. quintana* infections are rather associated with classical manifestations such as BA or with diseases such as bacteremia, endocarditis or chronic lymphadenopathy as outlined below. Whether the altered clinical appearance of *B. quintana* infections is due to changes in host factors, epidemiology or virulence is not yet known [Relman, 1995].

### Bacteremia and Endocarditis

Apart from classical trench fever, modern *B. quintana* infection may present as bacteremia. *Bartonella*-associated bacteremia has been reported in immunocompromised individuals such as HIV-infected patients and in a patient with chronic leukemia after bone marrow transplantation. In fact, homeless, alcoholics or immunocompromised patients such as HIV-infected individuals may be more often infected than individuals without obvious risk factors [Regnery et al., 1992a, b; Jackson et al., 1996; Spach et al., 1993, 1995a, b]. Thus, an outbreak of 10 cases of *B. quintana* bacteremia has been reported in homeless, alcoholic persons in Seattle [Jackson et al., 1996]. However, *B. henselae* bacteremia has also been reported in healthy men and a healthy young child [Lucey et al., 1992; Welch et al., 1993]. In the latter case, *B. henselae* was isolated from blood, and after 4 days of antibiotic therapy, symptoms rapidly disappeared.

The symptoms are usually those of 'nonspecific' chronic bacteremia including fever, fatigue, weight loss, anorexia, diarrhea and hepato-splenomegaly. Laboratory findings include thrombocytopenia, lymphocytopenia and granulocytosis, also hepatic enzymes might be elevated [Slater et al., 1990]. Bacteremic episodes of 10 days to 8 weeks, or even up to 1 year, may occur.

Endocarditis may be caused by *B. quintana*, *B. henselae* and *B. elizabethae* [Daly et al., 1993; Drancourt et al., 1995, 1996a, b; Spach et al., 1995a, b; Holmes et al., 1995; Jalava et al., 1995]. However, *B. elizabethae* was identified in a single case. Usually compromised patients with immunodeficiencies (e.g., HIV-infected individuals), homeless, alcoholics and heavy smokers are affected by *Bartonella*-related endocarditis. However, immunocompetent individuals might also be involved.

Both poor hygienic conditions and contact with cats appear to be the most important epidemiological factors in these patients. Clinical signs and symptoms of these patients resemble those usually observed in bacteremic patients including fever (38–39 °C), fatigue, weight loss, weakness and sweats. Moreover, splenomegaly, hepatomegaly, systolic heart murmurs, myocarditis, anemia, thromocytopenia and purpura, but also increased leukocyte counts and erythrocyte sedimentation rate etc. as well as glomerulonephritis including proteinuria and hematuria have been observed [Daly et al., 1993; Drancourt et al., 1995a, b; Spach et al., 1995a, b; Holmes et al., 1995; Jalava et al., 1995]. Thus, there are no *Bartonella*-specific symptoms in *Bartonella*-associated endocarditis. In most cases the infected valves had to be replaced by surgery.

In patients with *Bartonella*-associated endocarditis, *B. quintana* and *B. henselae* were isolated from blood cultures by both conventional agar cultures and cell culture techniques by using endothelial cell lines. Viable bacteria could not be isolated from valves so far. However, using PCR and immunohistochemistry techniques, *Bartonella* could be detected in affected valves. Interestingly, in some of these patients, *Bartonella* could be detected in lymph node tissue by PCR suggesting that endocarditis might have developed subsequently to asymptomatic CSD or subclinical chronic lymphadenopathy.

In *Bartonella*-associated endocarditis, high anti-*Bartonella* antibody titers in serum can usually be detected [Daly et al., 1993; Drancourt et al., 1995; Spach et al., 1995a, b; Holmes et al., 1995; Jalava et al., 1995]. Thus, in culture-negative endocarditis, serological tests should be appropriate for diagnosis of *Bartonella* infection. A recent report suggested that in about 3% of all cases of endocarditis, *Bartonella* species were diagnosed in patients tested in reference laboratories in three different countries [Maurin et al., 1997].

At present it is not clear whether the duration of bacteremia, preexisting defective valves or other factors such as strain differences are the most important risk factors for *Bartonella*-associated endocarditis. Nevertheless, while *B. quin-*

*tana* typically causes endocarditis in immunocompromised individuals living under poor hygienic conditions (e.g., homeless), *B. henselae* endocarditis usually occurs in individuals with preformed valvulopathy or occurs spontaneously.

## Chronic Lymphadenopathy

Chronic lymphadenopathy has been attributed to *B. quintana* infections in few cases although viable bacteria have not been isolated from the lymph nodes but from blood or bone marrow in these patients [Raoult et al., 1994a, b; Drancourt et al., 1996a, b]. However, in single cases, *Bartonella* DNA was detected in lymphoid tissues [Raoult et al., 1994a, b; Drancourt et al., 1996a, b]. In some of these cases, only few or no symptoms were reported. At present, it is unclear whether cases with chronic lymphadenopathy reflect a disease that resembles rather chronic CSD in possibly immunocompromised patients as a result of subclinical primary manifestations of CSD or whether chronic lymphadenopathy is a different entity from classical *Bartonella* infections such as CSD. Some of these patients had indeed contact with cats or were immunocompromised [Drancourt et al., 1996a, b].

Similar to CSD, usually cervical lymph nodes are involved in chronic lymphadenopathy. In some cases even mediastinal lymph nodes have been found to be affected and increased in size as revealed by computer tomography [Raoult et al., 1994a, b; Drancourt et al., 1996a, b]. Leukocyte counts, apart from decreased numbers in lymphocytes, were within normal limits. Histological investigation of biopsy specimens revealed typical granulomatous reactions resembling those described in CSD [Drancourt et al., 1996a, b]. After extirpation of lymph nodes, relapses may occur [Margileth et al., 1987].

## Rare Clinical Manifestations

Involvement of various organs such as liver, lungs, eyes and bones in disseminated *Bartonella* infections, particularly also in CSD, has been described [Koehler et al., 1988, 1992; Waldvogel et al., 1994; Le et al., 1994; Caniza et al., 1995; Sölder et al., 1995]. The lesions in bones are usually osteolytic and are located in the bones of the extremities including femur, tibia, fibula and radius. *B. quintana* has been isolated from bone tissue [Koehler et al., 1992]. Most cases can in fact be considered as systemic complications of CSD rather than a different entity associated with infection by *Bartonella* species.

A variety of neurologic syndromes have been associated with *Bartonella* infections. Thus, CNS diseases including chronic headache, encephalitis, myelitis, cerebral arteritis, optical neuritis and retinitis have been attributed to *Bartonella* infections. In HIV patients with neurologic diseases the prevalence for *Bartonella*-specific antibodies was increased from 4 to 5.5% in controls to 32% [Schwartzman et al., 1994]. Some of these patients showed *Bartonella*-specific IgM antibody production or *Bartonella*-specific DNA in cerebrospinal fluid. CNS manifestations by *Bartonella* might be accompanied by changes of the mental status including hallucinations, disorientation as well as progressive dementia [Schwartzman et al., 1994]. In some cases, neurological symptoms such as hyperreflexion, ataxia and altered mental status appeared 1–6 weeks after manifestation of lymphadenopathy [Schwartzman et al., 1994]. Furthermore, a case of a young boy with acute encephalopathy but without evident immunosuppression including HIV infection has been reported [Kusumanto et al., 1997].

Encephalopathy with dementia has also been reported in HIV-infected individuals. A case-control study performed in Los Angeles with HIV-infected patients revealed that at least 4% of cases of HIV-associated dementia and neuropsychological decline were due to *B. henselae* infections, and might therefore potentially be treatable [Schwartzman et al., 1995]. Moreover, neuroretinitis, pleurisy and arthritis have been associated with bartonellosis (CSD) [Margileth et al., 1987].

Taken together, the pattern of organ involvement in *Bartonella* infections including lymph nodes, bones, including bone marrow, CNS and lungs might reflect the organ tropism of *Bartonella* species, but is not completely understood. However, organs with high blood support are usually involved, and thus suggest that acute or chronic bacteremia might account for this pattern, which may be related to the ecological niche of these agents.

## Carriership, Reservoir, and Transmission of *Bartonella* Species

Until today, the epidemiology of *B. henselae*, *B. quintana* and *B. elizabethae* infections is poorly understood. Moreover, the reservoir of these agents has not yet been fully established. Furthermore, it is not clear whether a *Bartonella* carriership in humans exists or not. If at all, carriership in humans with *B. quintana*, *B. henselae* or *B. elizabethae* is probably a very rare condition. First, *Bartonella* species do probably not colonize surfaces such as skin or the bowel. Thus, *Bartonella* species are not part of the normal or transient flora in humans. Second, their ecological niche in humans, namely endothelial cells, blood, erythrocytes and lymphoid tissue, is usually related with the development of clinical manifestations and the development of immune responses leading either to resolution of the pathogen from the sites of infection or to clinical manifestations. However, similar to *B. bacilliformis* infections it might nevertheless well occur that in particular *B. quintana* bacteremia in humans persists for some time without initial symptoms or after clinical symptoms have disappeared. Moreover, *B. henselae* bacteremia occurs in up to 70% of healthy pet cats [Koehler et al., 1994; Chomel et al., 1995; Sander et al., 1997]. Therefore, particularly in immunocompromised patients, a balance between the host defense mechanisms and the virulence of the pathogen may result in chronic persistent infections which, if symptoms are not present, might be considered as carriership. The mechanisms by which *Bartonella* species may evade host immune responses are not yet known.

A reservoir of *B. quintana* apart from humans has not yet been identified. *B. quintana* infections are transmitted by the human body louse, *Pediculus humanis*, especially in trench fever. So far, humans, such as homeless, alcoholics and immunocompromised patients, appear to be the only typical reservoir currently known. However, in many cases no lice were found in patients with *B. quintana* infections. As poor hygienic conditions are nevertheless often reported in these cases, a reservoir outside humans, possibly in rodents, might well exist.

In contrast, it is well established that both cats (via scratches and/or bites) and arthropode vectors (cat fleas, especially *Ctenocephalides felis*) are probably involved in transmission of *B. henselae* from its natural reservoir, the cat [Koehler et al., 1994]. Seroprevalence of anti-*B. henselae* antibodies in cats varies from 3.7 to 54.6% [Jameson et al., 1995; Chomel et al., 1995; Autenrieth et al., 1998]. Up to 41% of cats were found to be bacteremic with *B. henselae* [Sander et al., 1997; Koehler et al., 1994; Heller et al., 1997]. Moreover, *B. henselae* has been detected in cat fleas [Koehler et al., 1994]. However, apart from fleas, also other vectors such as ticks might be involved in transmission. Both CSD and the presence of anti-*Bartonella* serum antibodies in humans are associated with contact to cats [Zangwill et al., 1993]. In contrast, reservoir, distribution, as well as the mode of transmission of *B. elizabethae*, are unclear as only one single case has been reported so far.

The seroprevalence of *B. quintana* in humans of different countries is about 2–20% [Regnery et al., 1992a, b; Jackson et al., 1996; Zbinden et al., 1995]. One of the first studies showed that 88% of patients with CSD have increased levels of anti-*B. henselae* serum antibodies but only 3% of healthy controls [Regnery et al., 1992a, b]. Others found that 0% of blood donors had *B. henselae*-specific serum antibodies but usually patients with CSD [Raoult et al., 1994a, b]. Recently, the presence of *Bartonella*-specific serum antibody levels of > 1:100 was reported in 0.58% of 12,000 patients with suspected *Bartonella* infections [Maurin et al., 1997]. The prevalence of anti-*B. henselae* antibodies in healthy blood donors ranges also from 2 to 20% [Jackson et al., 1996; Zbinden et al., 1995]. However, as some patients with typical bartonellosis such as CSD have sometimes negative antibody titers whereas patients without evident bartonellosis may have high antibody titers [Amrein et al., 1996; Drancourt et al., 1996a, b], the value of serological investigations as a single tool for diagnosis of *Bartonella* infections as well as for studies to assess the prevalence of a putative carriership is questionable. Whether this is due to inappropriate antigens used in serological assays or due to strain variants and different serotypes, remains to be elucidated. Interestingly, recent work has demonstrated that in CSD patients with negative conventional *Bartonella* serology, anti-*Bartonella* antibodies could nevertheless well be detected when a new isolate of *B. henselae*, which may represent a new serotype, was used as an antigen in the serological assays [Drancourt et al., 1996a, b]. Likewise, the prevalence of serum antibodies against *B. elizabethae* is unclear because most serological tests, such as immunofluorescence assays, cannot distinguish between the different *Bartonella* species. The single patient reported so far with a *B. elizabethae* infection had no contact with cats nor was he immunocompromised [Daly et al., 1993]. However, he suffered from intestinal strongyloidiasis and exhibited a poor dentition and might have been predisposed to endocarditis.

While *B. quintana* and *B. henselae* occur worldwide, the distribution of *B. elizabethae* (1 case only!) is unknown. In contrast, as mentioned above, epidemiology of *B. bacilliformis* is well established and appears to be restricted to South America.

### *A. felis, A. clevelandensis, A. broomeae* and *A.* Genospecies 1–3

*A. felis* was first isolated from a patient with CSD in 1988 [English et al., 1988]. The name *Afipia* is an acronym derived from the Armed Forces Institute of Pathology (AFIP). *A. felis* has been experimentally shown to attach to, to invade into and to grow intracellularly within phagosomes of primary human monocytes and HeLa cells [Birkness et al., 1992]. The natural reservoir, geographic distribution as well as the mode of transmission of *Afipia* species are unclear as only few isolates from the USA and one from New Zealand have been documented so far.

All but one, an isolate from water, of these isolates have been found in human materials including lymph nodes, bone marrow, tissue and synovium, sputum, pleural fluid and bronchial washing [Brenner et al., 1991]. Classical CSD has been related with *A. felis* infection as this pathogen had been isolated from lymph node specimens. *A. clevelandensis* has been isolated from a tibia tissue specimen from a 69-year-old man, and *A. broomeae* was found in sputum, bone marrow and synovium (wrist abscess) [Brenner et al., 1991]. *Afipia* genospecies 1 and 2 have been detected in bronchoalveolar and pleural fluid while *Afipia* genospecies 3 has been isolated from water in Indiana [Brenner et al., 1991]. All three genospecies are believed to be possibly pathogenic for humans.

Although the above-mentioned data might suggest that *Afipia* species may account for diseases other than classical CSD, such as infections of the lungs and bone tissues, the significance of *Afipia* in human medicine is still obscure and remains to be further elucidated [Bergmanns et al., 1995; Regnery et al., 1992a, b; Patnaik and Peter, 1995]. Moreover, serological studies with sera from patients with classical CSD, other diseases, and healthy control patients revealed the prevalence of serum IgG antibodies against *Bartonella* species but not against *Afipia* species [Patnaik and Peter, 1995; Amrein et al., 1996; Regnery et al., 1992a, b; Raoult et al., 1994a, b] suggesting that occurrence of *Afipia* species is very limited. On the one hand, it cannot be excluded that antibody responses might be suppressed in *Afipia* infection or that the serological tests used in these studies were not appropriate to detect anti-*Afipia* antibody responses. On the other hand, detection of bacterial *Bartonella* DNA by PCR and detection of *Bartonella*-specific serum antibodies correlates quite well in patients with CSD [Bergmans et al., 1995].

Only one study reported a high seroprevalence of anti-*Afipia* antibodies in human sera [Müller, 1993]. Thus, 5–7% of 430 sera were found to be reactive with *A. felis* antigen, 3% with *A. broomeae*, and 11% with *A. clevelandensis* as determined by microagglutination method that detected mainly IgM antibodies. However, others could not confirm these findings [Patnaik and Peter, 1995; Raoult et al., 1994a, b; Regnery et al., 1992a, b].

Prevalence of antibodies to *B. henselae* in cats varies tremendously (5–81%) but might be considerably high depending on geographic location and climate probably due to the occurrence of appropriate vectors [Allerberger et al., 1995; Jameson et al., 1995; Heller et al., 1997; Autenrieth et al., 1998]. In a German study, no antibodies against *Afipia* were found in pet cat sera [Autenrieth et al., 1998].

Taken together, both clinical and epidemiological data argue against a significant role of *Afipia* in human diseases although more sophisticated studies including specific and sensitive serological tests need to be performed and might reveal more insight into this question.

## References

Allerberger VF, Schonbauer M, Regnery RL, Dierich MP: Prävalenz von *Rochalimaea henselae* Antikörpern bei Katzen in Österreich. Wien Tierärztl Monatsschr 1995;82:40–43.

Amrein MP, Briel DD, Jaulhac B, Meyer P, Monteil H, Piemont Y: Diagnostic value of the indirect immunofluorescence assay in cat-scratch disease with *Bartonella henselae* and *Afipia felis* antigens. Clin Diag Lab Immunol 1996;3:200–204.

Autenrieth IB, Haimerl M, Tenter AM, Hilger J, Simon K, Rommel M, Mahle M: Prevalence of serum antibodies against *Bartonella* spp. and *Afipia felis* among pet cats in Germany. Submitted for publication.

Bergmanns AM, Groothedde JW, Schellekens JFP, von Embden JDA, Ossewaarde JM, Schouls LM: Etiology of cat-scratch disease: Comparison of polymerase chain reaction detection of *Bartonella* (formerly *Rochalimaea*) and *Afipia felis* DNA with serology and skin test. J Infect Dis 1995;171: 916–923.

Birkness KA, George VG, White EH, Stephens DS, Quinn FD: Intracellular growth of *Afipia felis*, a putative etiologic agent of cat-scratch disease. Infect Immun 1992;60:2281–2287.

Brenner DJ, Hollis DG, Moss CW, English CK, Hall GS, Vincent J, Radosevic J, Birkness KA, Bibb WF, Quinn FD, Swaminathan B, Weaver R, Reeves M, O'Connor S, Hayes P, Tenover F, Steigerwalt A, Perkins B, Daneshvar M, Hill B, Washington J, Woods T, Hunter S, Hadfield T, Ajillo G, Kaufmann A, Wear D, Wenger J: Proposal of *Afipia* gen. nov., with *Afipia felis* sp. nov. (formerly the cat-scratch disease bacillus), *Afipia clevelandensis* sp. nov. (formerly the Cleveland Clinic Foundation strain), *Afipia broomeae* sp. nov., and three unnamed genospecies. J Clin Microbiol 1991;29: 2450–2460.

Caniza MA, Granger DL, Wilson KH, Washington MK, Kordick DL, Frush DP, Blitchington RB: *Bartonella henselae*: Etiology of pulmonary nodules in a patient with depressed cell-mediated immunity. Clin Infect Dis 1995;20:1505–1511.

Chomel BB, Abbott RC, Kasten RW, Floydhawkins KA, Kass PH, Glaser CA, Pedersen NC, Koehler JE: *Bartonella henselae* prevalence in domestic cats in California: Risk factors and association between bacteremia and antibody titers. J Clin Microbiol 1995;33:2445–2450.

Conley T, Slater L, Hamilton K: *Rochalimaea* species stimulate human endothelial cell proliferation and migration in vitro. J Lab Clin Med 1994;124:521–528.

Cuadra M: Salmonellosis complication in human bartonellosis. Tex Biol Med 1956;14:97–113.

Daly JS, Worthington MG, Brenner DJ, Moss CW, Hollis DG, Weyant RS, Steigerwalt AG, Weaver RE, Daneshvar MI, O'Connor SP: *Rochalimaea elizabethae* sp. nov. isolated from a patient with endocarditis. J Clin Microbiol 1993;31:872–881.

Dooley JR: Haemotropic bacteria in man. Lancet 1980;ii:1237–1239.

Drancourt M, Birtles R, Chaumentin G, Vandenesch F, Etienne J, Raoult D: New serotype of *Bartonella henselae* in endocarditis and cat-scratch disease. Lancet 1996a;347:441–443.

Drancourt M, Mainardi JL, Brouqui P, Vandenesch F, Carta A, Lehnert F, Etienne J, Goldstein F, Acar J, Raoult D: *Bartonella (Rochalimaea) quintana* endocarditis in three homeless men. N Engl J Med 1995;332:419–423.

Drancourt M, Moal V, Brunet P, Dussol B, Berland Y, Raoult D: *Bartonella (Rochalimaea) quintana* infection in a seronegative hemodialyzed patient. J Clin Microbiol 1996b;34:1158–1160.

English CK, Douglas JW, Margileth AM, Lissner CR, Walsh GP: Cat-scratch disease. Isolation and culture of the bacterial agent. JAMA 1988;259:1347–1352.

Gray GC, Johnson A, Thornton SA, Smith WA, Knobloch J, Kelley PW, Escudero LO, Huayda MA, Wignall FS: An epidemic of Oroya fever in the Peruvian Andes. Am J Trop Med 1990;42:215–221.

Heller R, Artois M, Xemar V, DeBriel D, Gehin H, Jaulhac B, Monteil H, Piemont Y: Prevalence of *Bartonella henselae* and *Bartonella clarridgeiae* in stray cats. J Clin Microbiol 1997;35:1327–1331.

Herrer A, Christensen HA: Implication of *Phlebotomus* sand flies as vectors of Bartonellosis and Leishmaniasis as early as 1764. Science 1975;190:154–155.

Holmes AH, Greenough TC, Balady GJ, Regnery RL, Anderson BE, O'Keana JC, Fonger JD, McCrone LE: *Bartonella henselae* endocarditis in an immunocompetent adult. Clin Infect Dis 1995;21:1004–1007.

Jackson LA, Spach DH, Kippen DA, Sugg NK, Regnery RL, Sayers MH, Stamm WE: Seroprevalence to *Bartonella quintana* among patients at a community clinic in downtown Seattle. J Infect Dis 1996;173:1023–1026.

Jalava J, Kotilainen P, Nikkari S, Skurnik M, Vänttinen E, Lehtonen OP, Eerola E, Toivanen P: Use of polymerase chain reaction and DNA sequencing for detection of *Bartonella quintana* in the aortic valve of a patient with culture-negative infective endocarditis. Clin Infect Dis 1995;21:891–896.

Jameson P, Green C, Regnery R, Dryden M, Marks A, Brown J, Cooper J, Glaus B, Greene R: Prevalence of *Bartonella henselae* antibodies in pet cats throughout regions of North America. J Infect Dis 1995;172:1145–1149.

Knobloch J, Bialek R, Muller G, Asmus P: Common surface epitope of *Bartonella bacilliformis* and *Chlamydia psittaci*. Am J Trop Med Hyg 1988;39:427–433.

Knobloch J, Schreiber M: Bb65, a major immunoreactive protein of *Bartonella bacilliformis*. Am J Trop Med Hyg 1990;43:373–379.

Knobloch J, Solano L, Alvarez O, Delgado E: Antibodies to *Bartonella bacilliformis* as determined by fluorescence antibody test, indirect haemagglutination and ELISA. Trop Med Parasitol 1985;36:183–185.

Koehler JE, Glaser CA, Tappero JW: *Rochalimaea henselae* infection: A new zoonosis with the domestic cat as reservoir. JAMA 1994;271:531–535.

Koehler JE, LeBoit PE, Egbert BM, Berger TG: Cutaneous vascular lesions and disseminated cat-scratch disease in patients with the acquired immunodeficiency syndrome (AIDS) and AIDS-related complex. Ann Intern Med 1988;109:449–455.

Koehler JE, Quinn FD, Berger TG, LeBoit PE, Tappero JW: Isolation of *Rochalimaea* species from cutaneous and osseous lesions of bacillary angiomatosis. N Engl J Med 1992;327:1625–1631.

Kusumanto YH, Veenhoven RH, Bokma JA, Schellekens JF: Two patients with atypical manifestations of cat-scratch disease. Ned Tijdschr Geneeskd 1997;22:141–148.

Le HH, Palay DA, Anderson B, Steinberg JP: Conjunctival swab to diagnose ocular cat-scratch disease. Am J Ophthalmol 1994;118:249–250.

Lucey D, Dolan MJ, Moss CW, Hollis DG, Wegner S, Morgan G, Almeida R, Leong D, Greisen K, Welch D, Slater LN: Relapsing illness due to *Rochalimaea henselae* in normal hosts: Implication for therapy and new epidemiologic associations. Clin Infect Dis 1992;14:683–688.

Margileth AM, Wear DJ, English CK: Systemic cat-scratch disease: Report of 23 patients with prolonged or recurrent severe bacterial infection. J Infect Dis 1987;155:390–402.

Matteelli A, Castelli F, Spinetti A, Bonetti F, Graifenberghi S, Carosi G: Verruga peruana in an Italian traveler from Peru. Am J Trop Med Hyg 1994;50:143–144.

Maurin M, Birtles R, Raoult D: Current knowledge of *Bartonella* species. Eur J Clin Microbiol Infect Dis 1997;16:487–506.

McNee JW, Renshaw A, Brunt EH: Trench fever: A relapsing disease occurring with the British forces in France. Br Med J 1916;12:225–234.

Minnick MF, Mitchell SJ, McAllister SJ: Cell entry and the pathogenesis of *Bartonella* infections. Trends Microbiol 1996;4:343–347.

Müller HE: Detection of antibodies to *Afipia* species by the microagglutination test. Eur J Clin Microbiol Infect Dis 1993;12:951–954.

Patnaik M, Peter JB: Cat-scratch disease, *Bartonella henselae*, and the usefulness of a routine serological testing for *Afipia felis*. Clin Infect Dis 1995;21:1064.

Raoult D, Drancourt M, Carta A, Gastaut JA: *Bartonella (Rochalimaea) quintana* isolation in patients with chronic adenopathy, lymphopenia, and a cat. Lancet 1994a;343:977.

Raoult D, Dupont HT, Enea-Mutillod: Positive predictive value of *Rochalimaea henselae* antibodies in the diagnosis of cat-scratch disease. Clin Infect Dis 1994b;19:355.

Regnery RL, Anderson BE, Clarridge JE III, Rodriguez-Barradas MC, Jones DC, Carr JH: Characterization of a novel *Rochalimaea* species, *R. henselae* sp. nov., isolated from blood of a febrile, human immunodeficiency virus-positive patient. J Clin Microbiol 1992a;30:265–274.

Regnery RL, Olson JG, Perkins BA, Bibb W: Serological response to *Rochalimaea henselae* antigen in suspected cat-scratch disease. Lancet 1992b;339:1443–1445.

Relman DA: Has trench fever returned? N Engl J Med 1995;332:463–464.

Sander A, Bühler C, Pelz K, Cramm E, Bredt W: Detection and identification of two *Bartonella henselae* variants in domestic cats in Germany. J Clin Microbiol 1997;35:584–587.

Schultz MG: Daniel Carrion's experiment. N Engl J Med 1968;278:1323–1326.

Schwartzman WA, Patnaik M, Angulo FJ, Visscher BR, Miller EN, Peter JB: *Bartonella (Rochalimaea)* antibodies, dementia, and cat ownership among men infected with human immunodeficiency virus. Clin Infect Dis 1995;21:954–959.

Schwartzman WA, Patnaik M, Barka NE, Peter JB: *Rochalimaea* antibodies in HIV-associated neurologic disease. Neurology 1994;44:1312–1316.

Slater LN, Welch DF, Hensel D, Coody DW: A newly recognized fastidious gram-negative pathogen as a cause of fever and bacteremia. N Engl J Med 1990;323:1587–1593.

Sölder B, Allerberger F, Covi B, Maurer K, Scheminzky C, Kreczy A, Schön G, Dierich MP: Cat-scratch disease with *Bartonella henselae.* Infect Immun 1995;23:228–231.
Spach DH, Callis KP, Paauw SD, Houze YB, Schoenknecht FD, Welch DF, Rosen H, Brenner DJ: Endocarditis caused by *Rochalimaea quintana* in a patient with human immunodeficiency virus. J Clin Microbiol 1993;31:692–694.
Spach DH, Kanter AS, Daniels NA, Nowowieski DJ, Larson AM, Schmidt RA, Swaminathan B, Brenner DJ: *Bartonella (Rochalimaea)* species as a cause of apparent 'culture-negative' endocarditis. Clin Infect Dis 1995a;20:1044–1047.
Spach DH, Kanter AS, Dougherty MJ, Larson AM, Coyle MB, Brenner DJ, Swaminathan B, Matar GM, Welch DF, Root RK, Stamm WE: *Bartonella (Rochalimaea) quintana* in inner-city patients with chronic alcoholism. N Engl J Med 1995b;332:424–428.
Waldvogel K, Regnery RL, Andersen BE, Caduff R, Caduff J, Nadal D: Disseminated cat-scratch disease: Detection of *Rochalimaea henselae* in affected tissue. Eur J Pediatr 1994;153:23–27.
Welch DF, Hensel DM, Pickett DA, San Joaquin VH, Robinson A, Slater LN: Bacteremia due to *Rochalimaea henselae* in a child: Practical identification of isolates in the clinical laboratory. J Clin Lab 1993;31:2381–2386.
Zangwill KM, Hamilton DH, Perkins BA, Regnery RL, Plikaytis BD, Hadler JL, Cartter ML, Wenger JD: Cat-scratch disease in Connecticut. Epidemiology, risk factors, and evaluation of a new diagnostic test. N Engl J Med 1993;329:8–13.
Zbinden R, Höchli M, Nadal D: Intracellular location of *Bartonella henselae* cocultivated with Vero cells and used for an indirect fluorescent-antibody test. Clin Diag Lab Immunol 1995;2:693–695.

Prof. Dr. med. Ingo B. Autenrieth, Max von Pettenkofer-Institut für Hygiene und Medizinische Mikrobiologie, Ludwig Maximilians-Universität München, Pettenkofer Strasse 9a, D–80336 München, Germany
Tel. +49 89 5160 5200, Fax +49 89 5380584, E-mail autenrieth@m3140.mpk.med.uni-muenchen.de

Schmidt A (ed): *Bartonella* and *Afipia* Species Emphasizing *Bartonella henselae*.
Contrib Microbiol. Basel, Karger, 1998, vol 1, pp 77–86

# *Bartonella henselae* Infections in HIV and AIDS

*Michael T. Wong*

Medical College of Virginia Hospitals/Virginia Commonwealth University,
Richmond, Va., USA

## Introduction

In the era of the human immunodeficiency virus-type 1 (HIV) and the acquired immunodeficiency syndrome (AIDS), new and exotic organisms are being recognized as causes for various opportunistic infections. In this decade, one such organism, *Bartonella henselae*, has been identified as the causative agent of cat scratch disease (CSD), bacillary angiomatosis (BA), peliosis hepatis, aspetic meningitis, relapsing bacteremia, and Leber's stellate neuroretinitis. Other *Bartonella* species, including *B. quintana*, and *B. elizabethiae*, also cause human disease in North America (trench fever and BA, and subacute bacterial endocarditis, respectively) while *B. bacilliformis* has been well recognized as causing manifestations consistent with *B. henselae* (Arroyo fever, verruca peruna) in South America. While specific manifestations are more common in immunosuppressed persons, the spectrum is not confined to either immunocompetent or immunosuppressed populations. Indeed, BA has been described in an otherwise healthy individual, and we have reported classic CSD with noncaseating granulomata in patients with advanced infection with the HIV and absolute CD4+ T-lymphocyte counts of $<10$ cells/mm$^3$.

*The Organism and Diagnosis* [1–4]. *B. henselae* is a small, pleomorphic, weakly Gram-negative staining organism (fig. 1). It is highly inert as demonstrated by catalase, oxidase and indole benchside biochemical testing. The organism is very slow growing and requires hemin; reported clinical specimens have required incubation for up to 45 days to demonstrate growth. Growth has been demonstrated on chocolate, CDC-anaerobic blood, brain-heart infusion, and buffered-charcoal yeast agars, most automated blood-culture systems

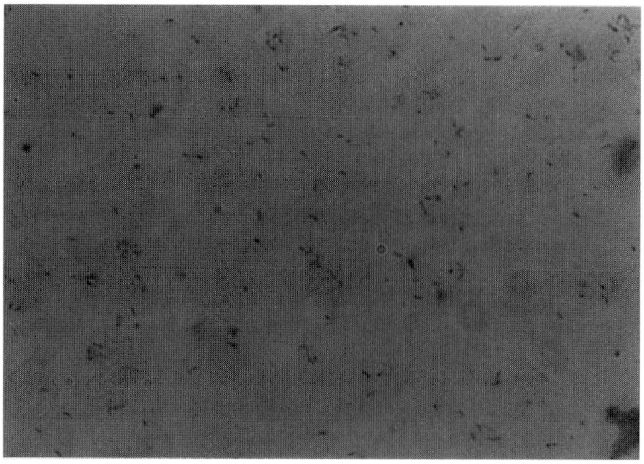

*Fig. 1. B. henselae* is a weakly Gram-negative staining organism as seen from this direct smear from a blood culture in a Bac-T-Alert® bottle, and demonstrates the coccobacillary nature of the organism. A carbol-fuchsin counterstain was used in place of the Gram's safarin to better highlight the organism.

(Bac-T-Alert® and Bac-Tec®) and liquid media (including HTM Broth®, BBL-Becton Dickinson), a variety of noncommercially available liquid media, and cell-monolayer cultures. The colonies may be pleomorphic on solid agars appearing either white to buff colored and dry, to creamy and somewhat mucoid. In liquid media, the colonies tend to coalesce near the surface of the media, and in highly hemin-enriched media, concentrate to a brownish color. Because of the slow growth patterns, the automated systems will not detect metabolic changes. Therefore, if suspicious, the bottles need to be held and blindly Gram-stained for evidence of the organism. It is now recommended that tissue and blood be obtained for culture in suspected cases. The blood should be processed by the lysis centrifugation method to improve yield. Presumptive identification may be made by colony morphology, Gram-staining characteristics, and biochemical inertness. Identification may be confirmed by measuring cellular fatty acid concentrations by gas-liquid chromatography demonstrating the characteristic C18:1, C18:0 and C16:0 fatty acid profile. Alternatively, polymerase chain reaction (PCR) amplification of the citrate synthase gene or 16S ribosomal subunit with restriction fragment length polymorphisms may also be employed.

Until recently, diagnosis of CSD or other manifestation was limited to clinical presentation and/or histopathologic findings. Classically, the organisms are demonstrated with the Warthin-Starry silver stain of biopsied materials (fig. 2). However, this is a technically very difficult stain to perform. In some

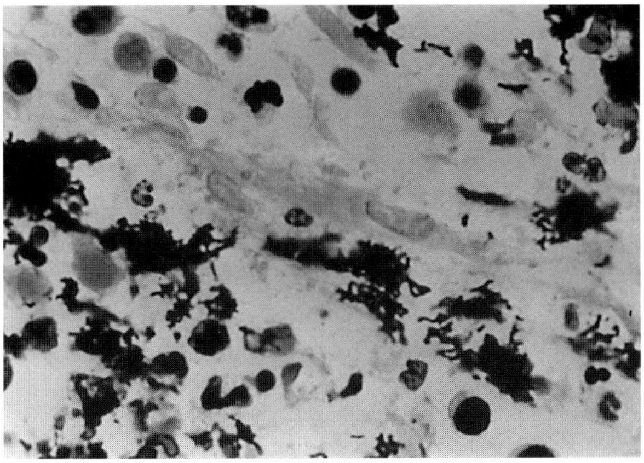

*Fig. 2.* Warthin-Starry silver stain. This patient presented with large isolated lymphadenopathy. Although the patient was HIV-positive, no cutaneous lesions were found. Excisional biopsy and histopathologic examination of the lymph node revealed changes consistent with BA. This Warthin-Starry silver stain highlights the nests of organisms, and diagnosis was confirmed both microbiologically and serologically.

cases, intradermal injection of purified CSD antigen was performed to elicit a delayed-type hypersensitivity response that was felt to be diagnostic. This material was heat-inactivated material obtained from the suppurative lymph nodes of persons with clinical CSD. While it was assumed that the antigens were those of *Afipia felis*, restriction fragment analysis of PCR products of the material revealed genetic material consistent with *B. henselae* and not with *A. felis*. Many of the associated manifestations were not recognized as part of the spectrum of *B. henselae* infection until improved culture methods and serologic diagnostic methods were developed. Because microbiologic evidence of infection is not very sensitive and may take many weeks before identification is made, serologic evidence of *Bartonella* antigens in clinically compatible disease is felt to be diagnostic. A noncommercially available immunofluorescent assay (IFA) for antibodies to *B. henselae* and *B. quintana* is performed by the Centers for Disease Control and Prevention (CDC). The presence of IFA-detected antibodies may indicate recent infection and provide supporting evidence of infection in a clinical syndrome associated with the organism. The duration of antibody response is not known although IFA reactivity has been documented to last for over 1 year in several longitudinally followed cases. It appears that these antibodies may only be markers of infection. Other serologic tests involving enzyme immunoassay format are commercially available, but lack the documented sensitivity and specificity studies that support the IFA.

*Physiology, Epidemiology and Hosts. Bartonella* species have been shown to be intraerythrocytic and intraneutrophilic which may explain its relative ease at escaping the human immune response. Cats appear to be a natural reservoir for *B. henselae*, and horizontal transmission by arthropod vectors (fleas) has been demonstrated. Other domestic animals have been implicated epidemiologically, but have not been found to harbor the organism to date. However, most companion cats appear to be unaffected by the organism. This has been demonstrated repeatedly by the culturing of *B. henselae* from seemingly healthy cats and kittens. Since most reliable diagnostic testing is not commercially available, blood culture appears to have a sensitivity of less than 70%, and prolonged antimicrobial therapy is unproved in treating otherwise well-appearing cats, it is not recommended that companion animals be treated. Likewise, the emotional, psychological and therapeutic benefits of companion animals has been well-founded, particularly in persons with chronic diseases. Thus, it is not recommended that persons with immunocompromising conditions, such as HIV infection or malignancy, give up their cat.

*Treatment.* Treatment in acute infection is controversial in the immunocompetent host. In most cases, the infection is localized, self-limited and results in minimal sequelae. However, in ocular and CNS disease, and in disseminated infection, treatment is clearly warranted. This is suggested in any manifestation of *Bartonella* infection in those persons with HIV infection or AIDS, regardless of stage of HIV disease. Various anecdotal studies had suggested the use of β-lactam agents with or without aminoglycosides for therapy. More recent data indicate that β-lactam agents are ineffective. Macrolides (erythromycin, azithromycin and clarithromycin) tetracyclines (principally, doxycycline) and rifampin appear to have the most reliable MIC and clinical data for therapy. Rifampin has been used as adjuvant therapy in difficult cases. The fluoroquinolones may have a role, but in some studies, the minimum inhibitory concentrations (MIC) were near their breakpoints. Duration of therapy is prolonged – often for many weeks or months. This is particularly true in HIV coinfection. However, unlike other opportunistic infections, eradication may be achieved, and life-long prophylaxis is not necessary.

## Clinical Manifestations

*BA Peliosis Hepatis* [5–10]. BA is a descriptive term for an infectious disease of the skin and organs characterized by vascular lesions. It was first described in 1983 in a patient with AIDS who presented with multiple lesions, fever, night sweats and weight loss. Biopsy and histopathology revealed characteristic vascular lakes with interstitial organisms by Warthin-Starry silver stain-

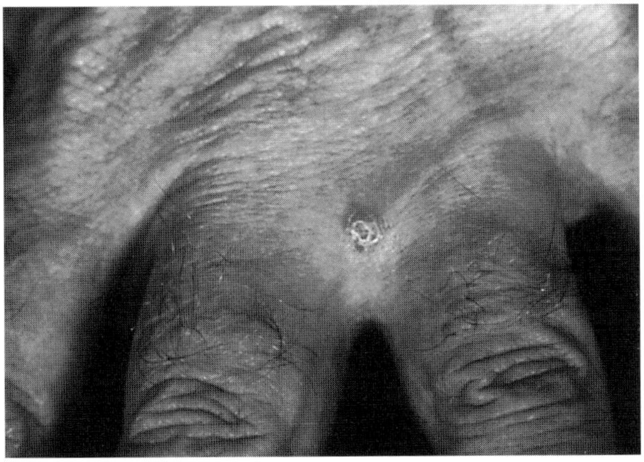

*Fig. 3.* BA: This is a typical cutaneous lesion of BA. Interestingly, it may also resemble the inoculation papule associated with CSD. Histopathologic findings of BA demonstrate lymphoproliferative epithelial changes with venous lakes.

ing, and the patient recovered with erythromycin therapy. Although BA may occur in non-HIV-infected persons, the degree of dissemination and severity of disease is clearly associated with the degree of immune dysfunction due to the HIV infection. Clinically, patients with BA also complain of fevers, sweats, malaise and fatigue, and symptoms referable to the organ system involved. Since this early report, the disease is more recognizable as an easily treatable process. However, untreated disease in this population is often fatal.

There are three major manifestations of BA. Most commonly it presents as a single or clustered reddish to brownish raised papular lesions on the skin and may be confused with Kaposi's sarcoma (fig. 3). Typically, they present as rare scattered lesions that may coalesce into larger papules. If left untreated, cutaneous dissemination may occur. Subcutaneous nodules are the second most common presentation. These tend to be larger, lack the vascular appearance grossly, and may be tender to palpation. Similar lesions have been described with disseminated fungal infections such as *Cryptococcus neoformans*, or occasionally pyogenic granulomata. These may ultimately break through the dermis and result in large, ulcerative tumors. In some cases, diffuse or isolated lymphadenopathy may occur without the associated rash. Finally, BA may present as a coalescent, cellulitic plaque. These are very tender and usually represent a cutaneous extension of deep osseous involvement. Plain roentgenographs of the bone will demonstrate lytic bone lesions and cysts. In all cases, histopathology demonstrates the typical BA findings with vascular epithelial proliferation, vascular lakes, and organisms on silver stain.

Systemic involvement may present as osteomyelitis with lytic bone lesions, parenchymal disease of the spleen, kidneys, and other visceral organs. Dissemination to mucosal surfaces including the conjunctiva, the lungs, and serosal surfaces as well as isolated CNS involvement have all been reported. Although disseminated disease is commonly associated with widespread cutaneous lesions, several case reports have demonstrated severe visceral involvement with the lack of any skin findings. Similarly, isolated or diffuse lymphadenopathy without skin lesions may occur. The differential diagnosis of such findings includes HIV-related malignancies, *Mycobacterium tuberculosis, M. avium-intracellulare* complex, suppurative adenitis associated with *Staphylococcus* or *Streptococcus* species, endemic mycoses, or HIV itself.

Perhaps one of the most profound visceral manifestations of BA is peliosis hepatis. This entity involves hepatomegaly that may be symptomatic, nausea and vomiting, and occasionally hypersplenism. Objective findings include modest elevations in serum transaminases, with substantial elevations in the alkaline phosphatase, and a new pancytopenia, which is largely due to sequestration, but may also reflect marrow involvement with *B. henselae*. Computerized tomograms of the abdomen will confirm organomegaly and associated adenopathy; occasionally, vascular lakes will coalesce and be visible with intravenous contrast enhancement.

Diagnosis of BA is made histologically with the characteristic vascular epithelioid hyperplasia, vascular lakes and occasionally an associated mixed inflammatory response. In some specimens, this may be confused with Kaposi's sarcoma or in the case of ulcerative lesions, pyogenic granulomata. However, unlike Kaposi's sarcoma, these are well-differentiated vascular elements. The histopathologic presentation in the liver and spleen is markedly different. Rather than vascular proliferation, large, blood-filled cystic spaces with myxoid stroma develop within the parenchyma. Interstitial bacteria may be visualized by Warthin-Starry silver staining. Serologic response with IFA for *Bartonella* antibodies may be extremely useful in this setting; a positive serology in this setting warrants antimicrobial therapy rather than antineoplastic agents. Ideally, microbiologic evidence with isolation of the organism will confirm the diagnosis.

Treatment for BA and peliosis hepatis involves the use of erythromycin or doxycycline. There is evidence that rifampin may be used in combination with these agents. All of these agents achieve reasonable intracellular levels. The duration of therapy may involve several months, but the results are often curative.

*Neuroretinitis* [11, 12]. Ocular manifestations of *B. henselae* infection include Parinaud's oculoglandular syndrome, BA of the conjunctiva, and Leber's stellate neuroretinitis. In the HIV-infected population, all three syndromes

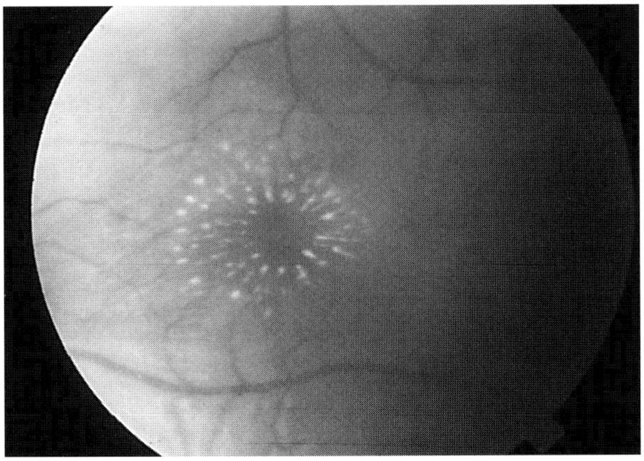

*Fig. 4.* Leber's stellate neuroretinitis. This photograph demonstrates the typical stellate hard exudates associated with *B. henselae* associated neuroretinitis. Early in this disease manifestation, significant retinal edema is present, probably the result of increased vascular permeability. As the edema resolves, lipids deposited in the choroid remain, producing the characteristic 'star' pattern. While visual acuity generally improves with resolution of edema, permanent impairment may occur.

may be observed. The role of *B. henselae* in Leber's stellate neuroretinitis (fig. 4) has only recently been confirmed. Patients usually complain of unilateral or sometimes bilateral diminished visual acuity. There may be a preceding febrile illness, and patients may have persistent constitutional symptoms of fever and malaise. Visual acuity may be diminished to light-dark discrimination. Direct retinoscopy demonstrates disc and retinal edema, and in more advanced disease, the presence of a macular star. As the edema and exudation spread to the macula, precipitation of plasma lipids produce the resultant macular star.

The mechanism by which this occurs in unclear. These fundoscopic changes may be the result of direct vascular invasion of the organism, or due to vascular incompetency due to a lymphocytic vasculitis similar to what is seen in BA and *B. henselae* associated lymphadenitis. Transmission and scanning electron microscopy of various *B. henselae* isolates demonstrated significant morphologic differences. In those organisms capable of invading HEp-2 cells (an epithelial cell line), filamentous and bundle-forming pili were identified. These were not seen in the noninvasive organisms. Thus, it is hypothesized that similar virulence mechanisms may attribute not only to the development of angioinvasive or angioproliferative disease versus granulomatous changes seen in classical CSD, but may also be responsible for tropism to retinal tissues. Alternatively, the fundoscopic changes may simply reflect vascular competency due to locally invasive organisms.

In most cases, these changes resolve slowly but spontaneously. Varying degrees of permanent loss of vision may occur. Retrospective reports suggest that most patients regain most of their sight, while others may go on to permanent visual impairment. Therapy typically involved the use of steroids to limit the extension of edema and local inflammation. However, with the demonstration of concurrent *B. henselae* bacteremia in several of these patients, directed antimicrobial therapy with doxycycline and rifampin in addition to systemic steroids helped improve resolution time and limit loss of vision. As in other manifestations, the duration of therapy has been as long as 6 weeks.

*Aseptic Meningitis and Invasive Central Nervous System (CNS) Disease* [11]. CNS involvement by *B. henselae* includes aseptic meningitis and CNS BA. Although some effort has been made to establish a link between AIDS dementia complex and *B. henselae*, this has not been borne out by well-developed serologic surveys.

Aseptic meningitis appears to occur in association with persistent bacteremia. In a described study, several patients infected with HIV developed symptoms of fevers, headaches and malaise. The symptoms progressed to frank meningismus and change in mental status. Patient histories revealed exposures to cats; in 1 case, the patient buried a kitten that died shortly after birth. Physical examination was unrevealing, and cerebral spinal fluid profile demonstrated a mild leukocytosis with mild to moderate elevation in protein and a mild suppression of glucose. These findings may not be different from CSF profiles associated with HIV infection alone. Blood cultures by lysis centrifugation may demonstrate *B. henselae* and peripheral serologies were positive by IFA. In the non-HIV-infected population, most cases of clinical aseptic meningitis associated with CSD resolved spontaneously. However, several cases of severe sequelae have been reported including seizures and encephalopathy.

In BA-associated disease, contrast-enhanced computerized tomograms of the head may reveal enhancing mass lesions with edema. These may have associated mass effects with cognitive dysfunction or focal neurologic deficits. In some cases, the presentation may mimic CNS toxoplasmosis or lymphoma.

Treatment of invasive CNS disease and aseptic meningitis appears to affect the clinical course substantially. Early therapy results with the abatement of symptoms and fevers, sometimes within the first few hours of initiation of therapy. Consideration for CNS penetrating antimicrobial regimens should be given. Although doxycycline and rifampin have well-established CNS penetration, reports indicate response and cure of intracerebral BA with erythromycin as well.

*Cat Scratch Disease* [13–16]. This manifestation has been discussed in more detail elsewhere in this book. However, it was previously felt that classical CSD with the development of noncaseating granulomata and pallisading epithelial cells would not be observed in HIV-infected persons with CD4+ T-lymphocyte counts of $<50$ cells/mm$^3$. This clearly is not the case, as several cases of confirmed CSD have been reported in patients with CD4+ counts of $<10$ cells/mm$^3$. The mechanism by which this occurs is unclear. However, it may be due, in part, to the morphologic lack of invasive pili as described previously. Therefore, this must be entertained within the differential diagnosis of those HIV-infected persons who present with isolated adenopathy and a distal inoculation papule.

## Conclusion

*B. henselae* is now recognized to produce a number of different clinical manifestations in humans. The spectrum ranges from local adenitis with inoculation papule to angioinvasive and angioproliferative disease that may involve any organ system. Any manifestation may occur in immunocompetent or immunosuppressed persons, but the severity of disease and the degree of dissemination appears to be closely associated with the health of the host's immune system. In addition, it appears that *B. henselae* may be dimorphic in nature with the propensity for invasive disease dependent on the expression of specific virulence factors. In general, most infections with *B. henselae* are self-limited. This is not the case in HIV-infected persons. In this group, therapy must be initiated as the infection may ultimately prove fatal if left untreated. Unlike other opportunistic organisms, however, *B. henselae* is curable in HIV co-infection, and does not require life-long prophylaxis. Treatment involves the use of antimicrobial agents that achieve intracellular concentrations. Those that have been proven effective both clinically and by MIC include erythromycin, doxycycline, rifampin, and theoretically, azithromycin and clarithromycin. The data regarding quinolone therapy are mixed at this time and should not be considered primary agents.

## References


1 Schwartman WA, Nesbit CA, Baron EJ: Development and evaluation of a blood-free medium for determining growth curves and optimizing growth of *Rochalimaea henselae*. J Clin Microbiol 1993; 31:1882–1885.

2 Wong MT, Thornton DC, Kennedy RC, Dolan MJ: A chemically defined liquid medium that supports the primary isolation of *Rochalimaea (Bartonella) henselae* from blood and tissue specimens. J Clin Microbiol 1995;33:742–744.

3 Moss CW, Holzer B, Wallace PL, Hollis DG: Cellular fatty acid composition of an unidentified organism and bacterium associated with cat scratch disease. J Clin Microbiol 1990;28:1071–1074.

4 Batterman HJ, Loutit JS, Peek A, Tompkins LS: Phenotypic characteristics of *Rochalimaea henselae* and *Rochalimaea quintana*. Clin Infect Dis 1993;17:534(abstr 21).
5 Relman DA, Loutit JS, Schmidt TM, Falkow S, Tompkins L: The agent of bacillary angiomatosis: An approach to the identification of uncultured pathogens. N Engl J Med 1990;323:1573–1578.
6 Tappero JW, Mohle-Boentani J, Koehler JE, Swaminathan B, Berger TG, LeBoit PE, Smith LL, Wenger JD, Pinner RW, Kemper CA: The epidemiology of bacillary angiomatosis and bacillary peliosis. JAMA 1993;269:770–775.
7 Stoler MH, Bonfiglio TA, Steigbigel RT, Pereira M: An atypical subcutaneous infection associated with acquired immune deficiency syndrome. Am J Clin Pathol 1983;80:714–718.
8 Spach DH, Panther LA, Thorning DR, Dunn JE, Piorde JJ, Miller RA: Intracerebral bacillary angiomatosis in a patient infected with human immunodeficiency virus. Ann Intern Med 1991;116: 740–742.
9 Koehler JE, Quinn FD, Berger TG, LeBoit PE, Tappero JW: Isolation of *Rochalimaea* species from cutaneous and osseous lesions of bacillary angiomatosis. N Engl J Med 1992;327:1625–1631.
10 Tappero JW, Koehler JE, Berger TG, Cockerell CJ, Lee TH, Busch MP, Stites DP, Mohle-Boentani J, Reingold AL, LeBoit PE: Bacillary angiomatosis and bacillary splenitis in immunocompetent adults. Ann Intern Med 1993;118:363–365.
11 Wong MT, Dolan MJ, Lattuada CP Jr, Regnery RP, Garcia ML, Mokulis EC, LaBarre RA, Ascher DP, Delmar JA, Kelley JW, Melcher GP: Neuroretinitis, aseptic meningitis and lymphadenitis associated with *Bartonella henselae* infection in immunocompetent patients and patients infected with human immunodeficiency virus type 1. Clin Infect Dis 1995;21:352–360.
12 Golnick KC, Marotto ME, Fanous MM, Heitter D, King LP, Halpern JI, Holley PH Jr: Ophthalmic manifestations of *Rochalimaea* species. Am J Ophthalmol 1994;118:145–151.
13 Dolan MJ, Wong MT, Regnery RL, Jorgensen JH, Garcia M, Peters J, Drehner D: Syndrome of *Rochalimaea henselae* adenitis suggesting cat scratch disease. Ann Intern Med 1993;118:331–336.
14 Zangwill KM, Hamilton DH, Perkins BA, Regnery RL, Plikaytis BD, Hadler JL, Cartter ML, Wenger JD: Cat scratch disease in Connecticut: Epidemiology, risk factors and evaluation of a new diagnostic test. N Engl J Med 1993;329:8–13.
15 Regnery RL, Oldson JG, Perkins BA, Bibb W: Serologic responses to *Rochalimaea henselae* antigen in suspected cat scratch disease. Lancet 1992;339:1443–1445.
16 Anderson B, Kelly C, Threlkel R, Edwards K: Detection of *Rochalimaea henselae* in cat-scratch disease skin test antigens. J Infect Dis 1993;168:1034–1036.

Michael T. Wong, MD, Assistant Professor, Quality Health Care and Infectious Diseases,
Associate Hospital Epidemiologist, Medical College of Virginia Hospitals,
PO Box 980019, Richmond, VA 23219 (USA)
Tel. (804) 828 2121, Fax (804) 828 2125, E-Mail miwong@gems.vcu.edu

Schmidt A (ed): *Bartonella* and *Afipia* Species Emphasizing *Bartonella henselae*.
Contrib Microbiol. Basel, Karger, 1998, vol 1, pp 87–97

# Bacillary Angiomatosis and Bacillary Peliosis: Histopathological Features and Differential Diagnosis

*Francesca M. Ruggiero*

Penn State College of Medicine, The Milton S. Hershey Medical Center, Hershey, Pa., USA

Bacillary angiomatosis (BA), a benign vascular proliferation in skin and visceral organs, has been identified as a response to infection by the *Bartonella* species of bacteria. Since the report of a case by Stoler et al. in 1983 [13], this lesion has provoked intense interest, linking the studies of AIDS, zoonoses, epidemiology and clinical laboratory and molecular diagnostics.

The histopathological features of BA, also called bacillary epithelioid angiomatosis, epithelioid angiomatosis, and, in the liver or spleen, bacillary peliosis, are relatively constant from site to site. This discussion will review the features in the two most common locations, skin and liver, with the understanding that they are applicable to lesions in the spleen [1–8], lymph nodes [2, 4, 5, 9], mucus membranes [10], larynx [10], esophagus [11], and multiple other sites [12].

The first description of a case of BA, attributed to Stoler et al. [13], continues to represent the commonly occurring features of this entity. That report described an immune compromised patient who had multiple 2–6 cm painless nodules on his skin. Subsequent authors [1, 3–10, 12, 14–18, 19–21] described violaceous papules and nodules ranging from 2 mm to 2 cm in size. The color and circumscription reflect that this is a vascular proliferation which grows in a lobular configuration. Even larger lesions retain a distinct lobularity at the microscopic level suggesting that separate growths coalesce (fig. 1). The clinical variability between papules and nodules corresponds to the microscopic variability in location in the lesion in either the superficial dermis, deep dermis, subcutis or combination thereof [17, 18]. Ulceration of the surface epithelium is possible [18]. The lobules consist of proliferated capillaries in a

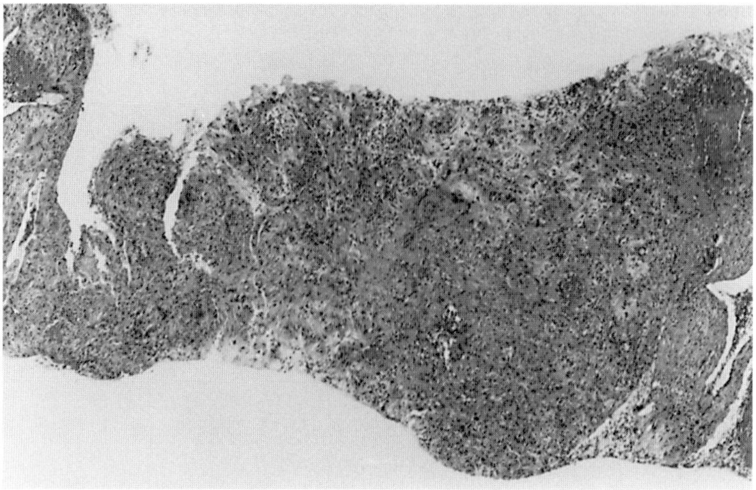

*Fig. 1.* BA in the deep soft tissue of the arm. The lobular configuration is retained even in a needle core biopsy. ×40.

fibromyxoid stroma. The capillaries are lined by plump 'epithelioid' endothelial cells. The surrounding stroma can be variably edematous containing mixed inflammatory cells, predominantly neutrophils, histiocytes, nuclear debris and amphophilic material (fig. 2).

The appearance of BA in the liver, also called bacillary peliosis hepatis, is similar to that in the skin [1, 2, 4–8, 12]. The hepatic architecture is disturbed by space-occupying lesions which are irregularly distributed in the hepatic parenchyma. Most are between 1 and 2 mm in diameter and are easily included in needle core biopsy specimens. As with the skin lesions, the liver lesions consist of a lobular proliferation of capillaries in a loose fibromyxoid stroma containing neutrophils, histiocytes, debris and amphophilic material (fig. 3). The liver lesions are separated from the remainder of the liver parenchyma by dilated and blood-filled sinusoids. Extravasated erythrocytes are also present within the lesions themselves. The latter features resemble those of classic peliosis hepatis, and that is the source of one of the original names for this lesion.

Several techniques have been used to provide evidence that BA is a tissue reaction to infection. Electron microscopy [2, 4, 6–8, 12, 13, 15, 17–19, 21] and the Warthin-Starry [1, 2, 4, 5, 7–9, 12, 13, 15–19, 21, 22] or modified Dieterle stains [23] have proven that the interstitial amphophilic clusters are groups of coccobacilli. The individual bacilli measure 0.2–0.5 μm in diameter and 0.5–2.5 μm in length and have trilaminar cell walls. They usually appear

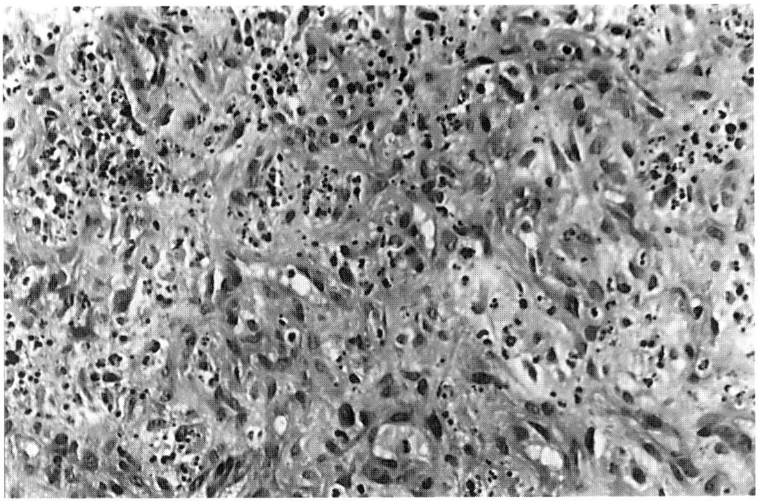

*Fig. 2.* Bacillary peliosis in the deep soft tissue of the arm. In this photograph, many capillaries are viewed longitudinally. They are surrounded by cuffs of neutrophils. The stroma is edematous and contains plump epithelioid cells. × 100.

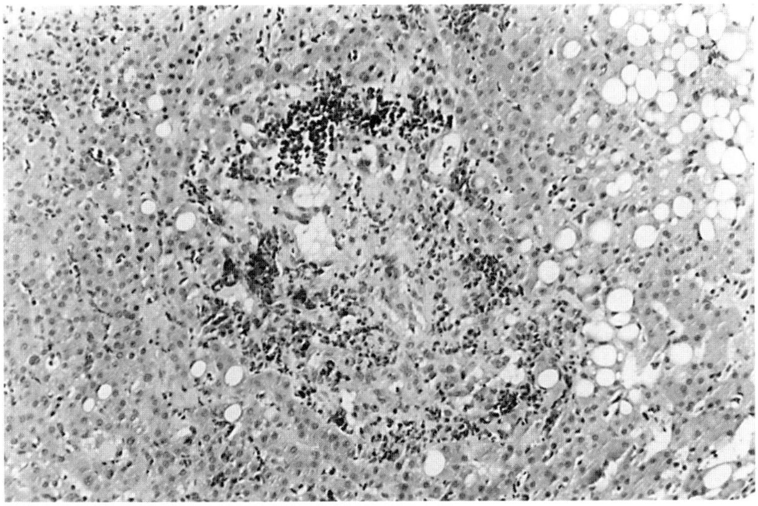

*Fig. 3.* Bacillary peliosis hepatis. This lesion demonstrates circumscription, peripheral dilated and congested sinusoids and central proliferated vessels in a loose stroma. This presents a more solid appearance than would be found in 'classic' peliosis hepatis. × 200.

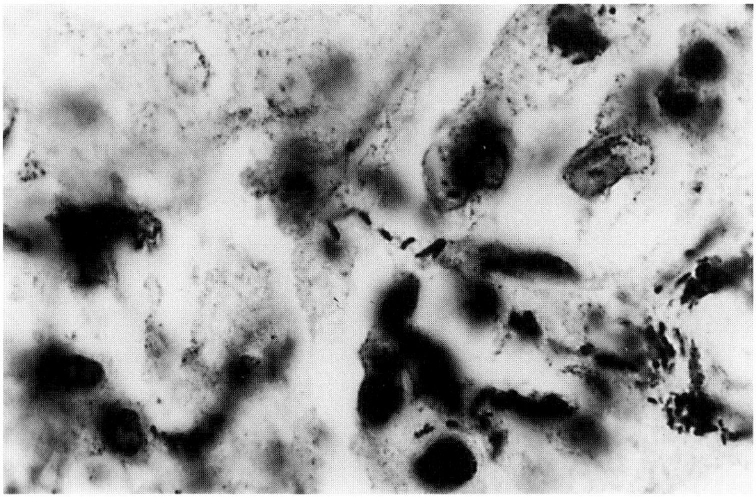

*Fig. 4.* Warthin-Starry-stained bacilli. Individual organisms are central and clusters are peripheral. × 1,000.

in clusters although they can be found singly or in small groups (fig. 4). Just as the HE appearance of these organisms may be mistaken for fibrin, the silver stain appearance may be mistaken for cellular debris. This is particularly problematic because they are most numerous in areas of necrosis. Examination of a less cellular, more edematous region provides a good opportunity to view the coccobacilli distinctly.

The Warthin-Starry stain is the most consistent cytochemical technique for demonstrating the organisms and this is necessarily performed on formalin-fixed tissue. B5 fixation, as might be used for lymph nodes, interferes with the Warthin-Starry staining. The Brown-Hopps variant of the tissue Gram stain has had variable success in decorating this Gram-negative organism [9, 15, 24]. Other versions of the tissue Gram stain, including the Brown-Brenn technique, have proven ineffective in demonstrating the bacilli. Stains for other organisms, including those for *Mycobacteria*, fungi, other bacteria or viral inclusions, have consistently been negative in these specimens.

Several authors have also used immunohistochemistry to identify the organism. Initially antibodies were raised to the 'cat scratch disease' bacillus, isolates from tissues of patients with a known diagnosis [15, 17]. Later, antibodies were raised to cultures of *Rochalimaea (Bartonella) henselae* [1, 2]. Further specific investigations included culturing the organism from fresh tissue, analysis of cell membrane protein by immunoblotting [2, 25] and finally DNA extraction, amplification and analysis [2, 3, 5, 21, 25–27]. These techniques

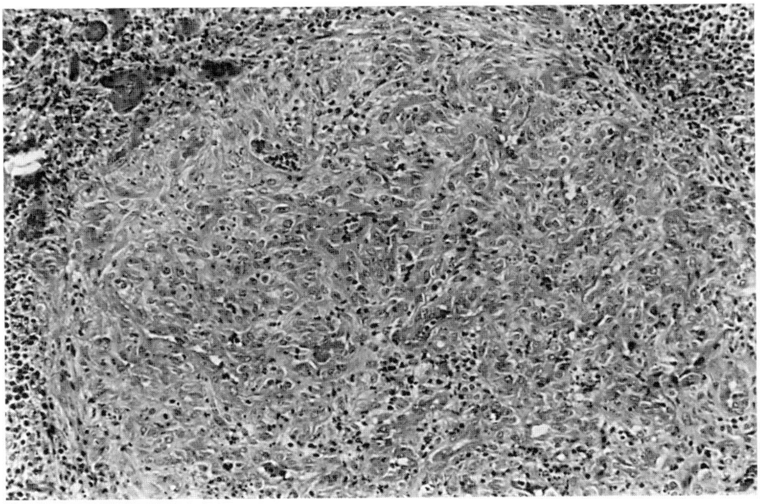

*Fig. 5.* Bacillary peliosis in a lymph node. The endothelial proliferation looks almost like solid sheets of cells. The lobular nature of the lesion is readily apparent. ×40.

have demonstrated that the organism which produces BA is of the *Bartonella* species and have linked BA with animal contact [3, 28, 29].

It is important to note that in any location there can be some variation in the appearance of BA. The endothelial cells, for example, may be so plump that they obscure the capillary lumena or impart a solid appearance to the proliferation [18, 22] (fig. 5). A reticulin stain may be useful to outline the vessels. LeBoit et al. [15, 18] and Axiotis et al. [22] also used immunohistochemistry to identify the endothelial cells and to prove continuity between the vascular lumena and the solid areas. The endothelial cells also may show nuclear enlargement, hyperchromasia and mitoses.

The composition of the stroma is also variable. Although the inflammatory infiltrate is most often described as containing neutrophils, some authors describe a lymphoplasmacytic infiltrate. Both LeBoit et al. [18] and Axiotis et al. [22], in demonstrating the nature of the endothelial cells, have also shown that some of the plump epithelioid cells are histiocytes. In addition, some cells decorate with both endothelial and histiocytic markers and others fail to mark with either [3, 10, 18, 22, 28, 29].

Finally, the lesions may resolve. This may occur spontaneously [16] or, more commonly, after antibiotic therapy [2, 5, 14, 15, 19, 25, 30] and has been supported by clinical observations and, in the case of parenchymal organs, imaging studies [17] or in autopsy examination [13]. The author believes that figure 6 represents an example of resolution in a liver biopsy. The patient,

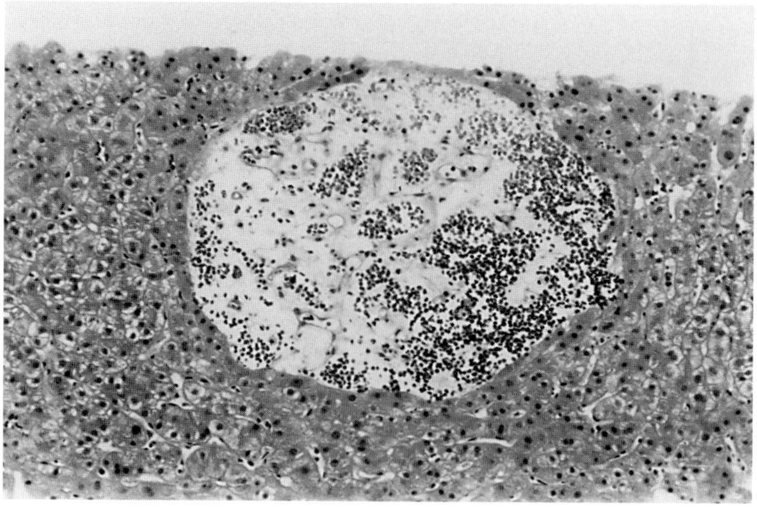

*Fig. 6.* Resolving bacillary peliosis hepatis. This was one of many hepatic lesions. The capillary lumena are small, the endothelial cells are flat and the interstitium has few inflammatory cells. Dilated, blood-filled spaces are still easily appreciated. × 200.

immune compromised because of organ transplantation, had a 2-week history of 'flu-like' symptoms and right upper quadrant pain. At the time of liver biopsy, he had received 2 weeks of plasmapheresis. As in ordinary BA, the liver parenchyma is disrupted by nodular shaped lesions. Examination of them shows that they are very neatly circumscribed. Small capillaries are present, but their endothelial cells are far less exuberant than in the typical lesion. The stroma is less cellular and has far fewer inflammatory cells and fewer extravasated erythrocytes. The picture is one of bland granulation tissue and conforms to a description of resolving bacillary peliosis offered by Steeper et al. [6]. A Warthin-Starry stain on the tissue did not show organisms but *B. henselae* DNA was present in blood samples and in DNA extracted from the tissue specimen. Following antibiotic therapy with erythromycin, the patient's clinical course improved and his blood did not contain *B. henselae* DNA.

The differential diagnosis of BA in the skin includes pyogenic granuloma, Kaposi's sarcoma, epithelioid variant of angiosarcoma and epithelioid hemangioma (table 1). Pyogenic granuloma [31] is a skin lesion with similar clinical features to BA: it occurs after injury or infection, presents as a bright red papule and is found on the extremities and the oral mucosa, and may also appear in groups or in a visceral form. It typically presents as a mass that protrudes above the skin, constricted by a collarette of thickened epidermis. The vascular tissue does grow in lobules separated by fibrous tissue. Central

*Table 1.* Histologic features of BA and its differential diagnosis [taken from 18]

| | Bacillary angiomatosis | Kaposi's sarcoma | Angiosarcoma | Lobular capillary hemangioma/ pyogenic granuloma | Epithelioid hemangioma |
|---|---|---|---|---|---|
| Circumscription | Good | Poor | Poor | Good | Good |
| Lobular capillary proliferation | Present | Absent | Absent | Present | Sometimes |
| Endothelial cell shape | Polygonal | Spindled | Spindled or polygonal | Usual flat, sometimes polygonal | Frequently polygonal |
| Protuberant endothelial cells | Present | Absent | Present | Variable | Present |
| Nuclear atypia | Present, nuclei vesicular, never hypochromatic | Sometimes, but usually in modular stage | Present, nuclei usually hyperchromatic | Usually absent | Slight |
| Smooth muscle around vessels | Absent | Absent | Absent | Absent | Present |
| Vascular spaces | Round | Slit-like, bizarre | Slit-like, sometimes bizarre | Round | Round |
| Hyaline globules | Absent | Present | Absent | Absent | Rare [P.E.L., pers. observation] |
| Neutrophils | Numerous, with debris | Absent unless ulcerated | Absent | Absent unless ulcerated | Absent |
| Eosinophils | Absent | Absent | Absent | Absent | Numerous in some |
| Granular material (bacteria) | Present in most cases on HE | Absent | Absent | Absent | Absent |
| Stromal edema | Present | Absent | Absent | Present | Absent, usually |
| Immunophenotype (FVIIIRAg/UEA) | +/+ | −/+ | +/+ | +/+ | −/+ |
| Enzyme histochemistry | $5'N^+$ $AlkP^+$ $ATPase^+$ | $5'N^+$ $AlkP^-$ $ATPase^-$ | | | |

ectatic vessels are a key feature. The endothelial cells are typically flat, there is less interstitial inflammation, and most important, there are no bacterial clumps.

The epithelioid hemangioma [32], also called angiolymphoid hyperplasia with eosinophilia or histiocytoid hemangioma, is commonly found in women between ages 20 and 40 years and presents as a small, red pruritic plaque around the ear which may ulcerate. Although the microscopic growth is of multiple dermal or subcuticular nodules composed of capillaries, a distinguishing feature is that they proliferate around a larger parent vessel. The endothelial cells are 'epithelioid' or plump. The inflammatory infiltrate, while mixed, characteristically contains numerous eosinophils.

The angiosarcoma of skin [33], including the epithelioid variant, may be distinguished from BA by its infiltrative pattern, the so-called 'dissection of collagen'. Similarly, the patch and plaque stages of Kaposi's sarcoma have an infiltrative pattern. The former is also characterized by angulated or jagged vessels. The nodular stage may present a diagnostic challenge. Features distinguishing Kaposi's sarcoma from BA include flatter endothelial cells, a honeycomb pattern of vascular channels, fibrous stroma, hemosiderin-laden macrophages, and intracellular and/or extracellular hyaline globules [31].

An unusual lesion considered in the discussion of BA is verruga peruana, the eruptive phase of Carrion's disease. Both entities are proliferative angiomatoses of the skin and mucus membranes which are produced by bacteria of the *Bartonella* species. Verruga peruana, caused by *B. bacilliformis*, is characterized by a lobular vascular proliferation in the papillary dermis, reticular dermis or subcutis which produce violaceous papules or nodules [34, 35]. The same features of plump endothelial cells, edematous stroma, and interstitial histiocyte-like cells are found. Electron microscopical examination also identifies a trilaminar bacterium of similar size to those seen in BA. The Warthin-Starry stain also outlines *B. bacilliformis*. Distinguishing histological features include a lymphoplasmacytic interstitial infiltrate, intracytoplasmic granular inclusions and phagocytized bacteria. Important to the diagnosis is geography. The *B. bacilliformis* is transmitted to humans by the *Lutzomyia* genus of flies which are endemic to the South American Andean valley of Peru, Columbia and Ecuador.

The differential diagnosis of BA or peliosis in the liver also includes (nonbacillary) peliosis hepatis. The classic definition of peliosis [36] is the presence of blood-filled spaces in the liver, spleen or lymph nodes. In the liver, these blood-filled spaces represent dilated sinusoids although some authors require additional evidence of reticulin fiber lysis. Classis peliosis hepatis has been associated with a variety of etiologies, including use of steroid hormones (anabolic, estrogenic or adrenocortical), infections with *Mycobacterium tuber-*

*culosis* or *M. leprae*, malnutrition and vasculitis. There are also reports of this lesion in patients with AIDS [37–39] and renal transplantation [40–42], the latter two of which would overlap with individuals most susceptible to BA. Distinguishing between these two lesions should include the observation of plump endothelial cells, a loose fibromyxoid stroma, interstitial neutrophils and particularly, proteinaceous clumps of Warthin-Starry decorated coccobaccili.

Finally, in lymph nodes, the differential diagnosis would include the abovementioned Kaposi's sarcoma, hemangioma, epithelioid hemangioma and vascular transformation of sinuses [43]. The latter is confined to the sinuses, and is characterized by proliferating and interanatomosing vascular channels which alternate with spindle cell fascicles. The endothelial cells are not as protuberant as in BA and bacterial colonies are absent.

In summary, BA is one manifestation of the diseases caused by the *Bartonella* genus of bacteria. Most cases of BA occur in immune compromised patients [2–10, 13, 15–17, 19–22, 24, 25, 27, 43, 44], although there have been reports in otherwise healthy individuals, and many are associated with animal contact [3, 7, 8]. The lesions of BA are most frequently found on the skin but visceral involvement may be extensive. Without antibiotic therapy, the consequences may range from discomfort to fatality [10]. Fortunately, most cases respond to antibiotic therapy with complete resolution of the lesions.


## Acknowledgements

The author gratefully acknowledges Drs. Nasimul Ahsan, Harold Yang and Michael Holman, and Dr. Deborah A. Belchis for contribution of cases.


## References


1 Reed JA, Brigati DJ, Flynn SD, McNuh NS, Min KW, Welch DF, Slater LN: Immunohistochemical identification of *Rochalimaea henselae* in bacillary (epithelioid) angiomatosis, parenchymal bacillary peliosis, and persistent fever with bacteremia. Am J Surg Pathol 1992;16:650–657.

2 Slater LN, Welch DF, Min K-W: *Rochalimaea henselae* causes bacillary angiomatosis and peliosis hepatis. Arch Intern Med 1992;152:602–606.

3 Tappero JW, Mohle-Boetani J, Koehler JE, Swaminathan B, Berger TG, LeBoit PE, Smith LL, Wegner JD, Pinner RW, Kemper CA, Reingold AL: The epidemiology of bacillary angiomatosis and bacillary peliosis. JAMA 1993;269:770–775.

4 Perkocha LA, Geaghan SM, Yen TSB, Nishimura LA, Chan SP, Carcia-Kennedy R, Honda G, Stoloff AC, Klein HZ, Goldman RL, Van Meter S, Ferrell LD, LeBoit PE: Clinical and pathological features of bacillary peliosis hepatis in association with human immunodeficiency virus infection. N Engl J Med 1990;323:1581–1586.

5 Relman DA, Loutit JS, Schmidt TML, Falcow S, Tompkins LS: The agent of bacillary angiomatosis. N Engl J Med 1990;323:1573–1580.

6 Steeper TA, Rosenstein H, Weiser J, Inampudi S, Snover D: Bacillary epithelioid angiomatosis involving the liver, spleen, and skin in an AIDS patient with concurrent Kaposi's sarcoma. Am J Clin Pathol 1992;97:713–718.

7 Kemper CA, Lombard CM, Deresinski SC, Tompkins LS: Visceral bacillary epithelioid angiomatosis: Possible manifestations of disseminated cat scratch disease in the immunocompromised host: A report of two cases. Am J Med 1990;89:216–222.

8 Chan JKC, Lewin KJ, Lombard CM, Teitelbaum S, Dorfman RF: Histopathology of bacillary angiomatosis of lymph node. Am J Surg Pathol 1991;15:430–437.

9 Angritt P, Tuur SM, Macher AM, Smith KJ, Park CS, Hobin FP, Myrie-Williams C: Epithelioid angiomatosis in HIV infection: Neoplasm or cat-scratch disease? Lancet 1988;i:996.

10 Cockerell CJ, Whitlow MA, Webster GF, Friedman-Kien AE: Epithelioid angiomatosis: A distinct vascular disorder in patients with the acquired immunodeficiency syndrome or AIDS-related complex. Lancet 1987;ii:654–656.

11 Chang AD, Drachenberg CI, James SP: Bacillary angiomatosis associated with extensive esophageal polyposis: A new mucocutaneous manifestation of acquired immunodeficiency disease (AIDS). Am J Gastroenterol 1996;91:2220–2223.

12 Adal K, Cockerell CJ, Petri WA Jr: Cat scratch disease, bacillary angiomatosis, and other infections due to *Rochalimaea*. N Engl J Med 1994;330:1509–1515.

13 Stoler MH, Bonfilio TA, Steigbigel RT, Pereira M: An atypical subcutaneous infection associated with acquired immune deficiency syndrome. Am J Clin Pathol 1983;80:714–718.

14 Groves MG, Harrington KS: *Rochalimaea henselae* infections: Newly recognized zoonoses transmitted by domestic cats. JAMA 1994;204:267–271.

15 LeBoit PE, Berger TG, Egbert B, Yen TSB, Stoler MH, Bonfiglio TA, Strauchen JA, English CK, Wear DG: Epithelioid haemangioma-like vascular proliferation in AIDS: Manifestation of cat scratch disease bacillus infection? Lancet 1988;i:960–963.

16 Knobler EH, Silvers DN, Fine KC, Lefkowitch JH, Grossman ME: Unique vascular skin lesions associated with human immunodeficiency virus. JAMA 1988;260:524–527.

17 Koehler JE, LeBoit PE, Egbert BM, Berger TG: Cutaneous vascular lesions and disseminated cat-scratch disease in patients with the acquired immunodeficiency syndrome (AIDS) and AIDS-related complex. Ann Intern Med 1988;109:449–455.

18 LeBoit PE, Berger TG, Egbert BM, Beckstead JH, Yen TSB, Stoler MA: Bacillary angiomatosis: The histopathology and differential diagnosis of a pseudoneoplastic infection in patients with human immunodeficiency virus disease. Am J Surg Pathol 1989;13:909–920.

19 Rudikoff D, Phelps RG, Gordon RE, Bottone EJ: Acquired immunodeficiency syndrome-related bacillary vascular proliferation (epithelioid angiomatosis): Rapid response to erythromycin therapy. Arch Dermatol 1989;125:706–707.

20 Mui BK, Mulligan ME, George WL: Response of HIV-associated disseminated cat scratch disease to treatment with doxycycline. Am J Med 1990;89:229–231.

21 Schlupen E-M, Schirren CG, Hoegl L, Schaller M, Volkenandt M: Molecular diagnosis of deep nodular bacillary angiomatosis and monitoring of therapeutic success. Br J Dermatol 1997;136:747–751.

22 Axiotis CA, Schwartz R, Jennings TA, Glaser N: AIDS-related angiomatosis. Am J Dermatopathol Pathol 1989;11:177–181.

23 Korbi S, Toccanier M-F, Leyvraz G, Stalder J, Kapanci Y: Use of silver staining (Dieterle's stain) in the diagnosis of cat scratch disease. Histopathology 1986;10:1015–1021.

24 Marasco WA, Lester S, Parsonnet J: Unusual presentation of cat scratch disease in a patient positive for antibody to the human immunodeficiency virus. Rev Infect Dis 1989;11:793–803.

25 Slater LN, Welch DF, Hensel D, Coody DW: A newly recognized fastidious gram-negative pathogen as a cause of fever and bacteremia. N Engl J Med 1990;323:1587–1593.

26 Dauga C, Miras I, Grimont PA: Identification of *Bartonella henselae* and *B. quintana* 16S rDNA sequences by branch-, genus- and species-specific amplification. J Med Microbiol 1996;45:192–199.

27 Bachelez H, Oksenhendler E, Lebbé C, Dauga C, Pinguier L, Mainguene C, Clauvell JD, Grimont PAD, Morel P, Lubertret L, Arlet G: Bacillary angiomatosis in HIV-infected patients: Report of three cases with different clinical courses and identification of *Rochalimaea quintana* as the etiologic agent. Br J Dermatol 1995;133:983–989.

28 English CK, Wear DJ, Margileth AM, Lissner CR, Walsh GP: Cat-scratch disease: Isolation and culture of the bacterial agent. JAMA 1988;259:1347–1352.
29 Koehler JE, Glaser CA, Tappero JW: *Rochalimaea henselae* infection: A new zoonosis with the domestic cat as reservoir. JAMA 1994;271:531–535.
30 Hall AV, Roberts CM, Maurice PD, McLean KA, Shousha S: Cat-scratch disease in patient with AIDS: Atypical skin manifestation. Lancet 1988;ii:453–454.
31 Calonje E, Wilson-Jones E: Vascular tumors: Tumors and tumor-like conditions of blood vessels and lymphatics; in Elder D, Elenitsas R, Jaworsky C, Johnson B Jr (eds.): Lever's Histopathology of the Skin, ed 7. Philadelphia, Lippincott-Raven, 1997, pp 889–932.
32 Enzinger FM, Weiss SW: Benign Tumors and Tumor-Like Lesions of Blood Vessels. Soft Tissue Tumors, ed 3. St Louis, Mosby, 1995, pp 579–626.
33 Enzinger FM, Weiss SW: Malignant Vascular Tumors. Soft Tissue Tumors, ed 3. St Louis, Mosby, 1995, pp 641–678.
34 Arias-Stella J, Lieberman PH, Erlandson RA, Arias-Stella J Jr: Histology, immunohistochemistry, and ultrastructure of the verruga in Carrion's disease. Am J Surg Pathol 1986;10:595–610.
35 Cárceres-Ríos H, Rodríguez-Tafur J, Bravo-Puccio F, Maguiña-Vargas C, Sanguineti-Diaz C, Carillo Ramos D, Patarca R: Verruga peruana: An infectious endemic angiomatosis. Crit Rev Oncogen 1995;6:47–56.
36 Wanless IR: Vascular disorders; in MacSween RNM, Anthony PP, Scheuer PJ, Burt AD, Portmann BC (eds.): Pathology of the Liver, ed 3. Edinburgh, Churchill Livingstone, 1994, pp 535–562.
37 Devars du Mayne J-F: Hepatic vascular lesions in AIDS. JAMA 1985;254:53–54.
38 Czapar CA, Weldon-Linne M, Moore DM, Rhone DP: Peliosis hepatis in the acquired immunodeficiency syndrome. Arch Pathol Lab Med 1986;110:611–613.
39 Scoazec J-Y, Marche C, Girard P-M, Houtman J, Durand-Schneider AM, Saimot AG, Benhamou JP, Feldman G: Peliosis hepatis and sinusoidal dilatations during infection by the human immunodeficiency virus (HIV). Am J Pathol 1988;131:38–47.
40 Degott C, Rueff B, Kreis H, Duboust A, Potet F, Benhamou JP: Peliosis hepatis in recipients of renal transplants. Gut 1978;19:748–753.
41 Izumi S, Nishiuchi M, Kameda Y, Nagano S, Fukunishi T, Kohro T, Shinji Y: Laparoscopic study of peliosis hepatis and nodular transformation of the liver before and after renal transplantation: Natural history and aetiology in follow-up cases. J Hepatol 1994;20:129–137.
42 Cavalcanti R, Pol S, Carnot F, Campos H, DeGoh C, Driss F, Legendre C, Kreis H: Impact and evolution of peliosis hepatis in renal transplant recipients. Transplantation 1994;58:315–316.
43 Juan R: Lymph Nodes. Ackerman's Surgical Pathology, ed 8. St Louis, Mosby, 1996, vol 2, pp 1743–1745.
44 Jerris RC, Regnery RL: Will the real agent of cat-scratch disease please stand up? Annu Rev Microbiol 1996;50:707–725.

Francesca M. Ruggiero, M.D., Assistant Professor of Pathology, Penn State College of Medicine, The Milton S. Hershey Medical Center, 500 University Drive, Hershey, PA 17033, USA

Schmidt A (ed): *Bartonella* and *Afipia* Species Emphasizing *Bartonella henselae*.
Contrib Microbiol. Basel, Karger, 1998, vol 1, pp 98–112

# Microbiological Diagnosis of *Bartonella* Species and *Afipia felis*

*Anna Sander*

Institut für Medizinische Mikrobiologie und Hygiene, Klinikum der Universität Freiburg, Deutschland

Until recently, the order *Rickettsiales* contained three families: *Rickettsiales, Bartonellaceae* and *Anaplasmataceae* [1]. In 1993, on the basis of molecular relatedness and phenotypic characteristics, the genus *Rochalimaea* (containing the species *R. quintana, R. vinsonii, R. henselae* and *R. elizabethae*) was removed from the order *Rickettsiales* and was united with the genus *Bartonella* (containing the only species *B. bacilliformis*) in the family *Bartonellaceae* [2]. Two years later, the genera *Bartonella* and *Grahamella* were unified [3]. However, the genus *Bartonella* includes presently 11 species, but only 5 of them are known to be pathogen to humans. *B. bacilliformis* is the causative agent of bartonellosis, *B. quintana* is the etiologic agent of trench fever and *B. henselae* the causative agent of cat scratch disease (CSD). Both species *B. henselae* and *B. quintana*, are known to cause bacillary angiomatosis (BA), bacillary peliosis hepatis, osteolytic lesions, relapsing fever with bacteremia, endocarditis and encephalitis [4, 5]. *B. elizabethae* was isolated from blood of a patient with endocarditis [6]. Recently, the first report of CSD associated with *B. clarridgeiae* has been published [7]. All other *Bartonella* species (*B. vinsonii, B. vinsonii* var. *berkhoffii, B. doshiae, B. grahamii, B. peromysci, B. talpae* and *B. taylorii*) have been isolated from various animals, but are not known to cause disease in humans [3].

The genus *Afipia* contains 6 species (*A. felis, A. clevelandensis, A. broomeae* and 3 unnamed species), from which only *A. felis*, formerly the 'cat scratch disease bacillus', was discussed to be pathogenic to humans [8].

The etiology of CSD was for a long time a subject of speculation. In 1988 [9] a Gram-negative bacillus, characterized as *A. felis*, was isolated from the lymph nodes of patients suffering from CSD and the etiologic agent of the disease seemed to be identified. However, many subsequent serological [10–12] and molecular detection-based studies [13, 14] confirmed *B. henselae* and not *A. felis* as the main agent of CSD.

## Collection and Transport of Specimens

Until now, only few clinical isolates have been obtained from patients suffering from CSD or other *Bartonella*-induced infections. Most *Bartonella* isolates are obtained from blood or tissue of HIV-infected patients. However, specimens should be taken from all patients suspected to be infected with *Bartonella* or *Afipia* species. Reasonable specimens are blood cultures and affected tissue such as lymph node, liver, spleen, skin, pus and bone marrow.

Successful isolation of *Bartonella* species depends on the origin and the number of specimens. Blood cultures from patients suffering from typical CSD often remain sterile, whereas isolation of *Bartonella* species from blood cultures of immunosuppressed patients, of patients with fever and patients with atypical CSD seems to be more efficient. In cases of typical CSD, lymph node biopsies or aspirates, pus of suppurated lymph nodes, or biopsies from other affected tissues should be obtained for culture.

In contrast to *A. felis, Bartonella* species are very fastidious organisms. Primary isolation of these bacteria is rather difficult and only successful if the interval from collection to culturing is as short as possible. The specimens should be transported to the laboratory immediately. If this is not possible, they could be frozen at $-70$ °C or stored at 4 °C.

## Isolation Procedures

*Bartonella* species are fastidious, slowly growing bacteria and routine bacterial culture protocols usually would not allow detection of these organisms. Successful isolation of *Bartonella* species depends on a number of key factors, including prolonged incubation time, the use of blood-enriched media, and cell lysis in blood cultures systems.

### *Microscopic Examination*

Microscopic examination of Gram-stained members of the genus *Bartonella* shows pleomorphic, thin and short ($0.6 \times 1.0$ μm), weakly stained Gram-negative rods. They are often slightly curved (fig. 1) and microscopically indistinguishable from *Afipia* species. Most of the members of *Bartonella* species are nonmotile. *B. henselae* and *B. quintana* can produce a twitching

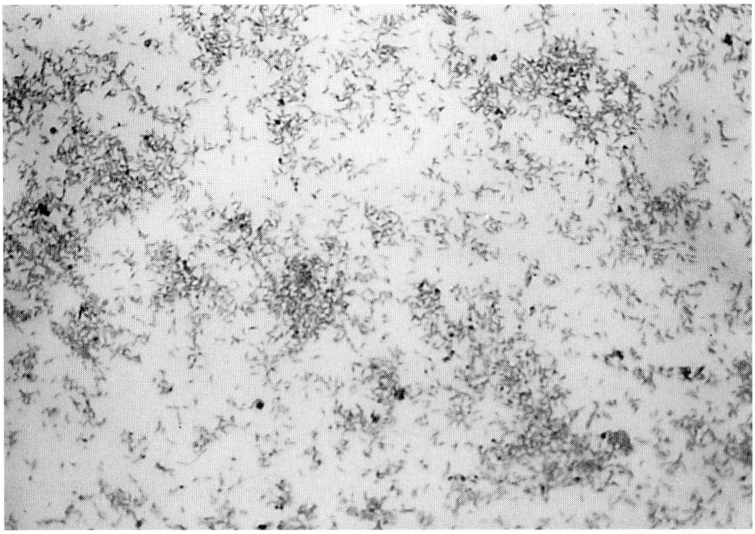

*Fig. 1.* Microscopic morphology of Gram-stained *B. henselae.*

motility, caused by fine fimbriae (pili) which could be seen on the electron microscope [15]. *B. bacilliformis* and *B. clarridgeiae* have been shown to have flagella in culture [16, 17]. All *Afipia* species are motile having a single polar, subpolar, or lateral flagellum [8].

*Culture*

Isolation of *Bartonella* species from human specimens is quite difficult, time-consuming, unreliable and requires some special laboratory procedures. *Bartonella* species are very fastidious organisms, and sterile cultures after a longer period of incubation do not exclude a suspected *Bartonella* infection. To obtain best growth conditions, tissues should be homogenized and CSF concentrated by centrifugation. For isolation of *Bartonella* species from blood specimens, Isolator™ blood-lysis tubes (Wampole, Cranbury, N.J., USA) and tubes containing EDTA are the most reliable systems. For *B. henselae* it was shown that if the specimens are plated immediately or within 24 h onto agar plates, the Isolator™ system is more sensitive than tubes containing EDTA. However, if the specimens are stored for a longer time (26 days) frozen at −65 °C the sensitivity of detection of *B. henselae* improved in both methods, and the isolation rate in the EDTA tubes was higher than that in the Isolator™ tubes [18]. Isolator™ tubes contain sodium polyanetholsulfonate, an anticoagulant that inhibits the antibacterial effects of blood, and saponin, which

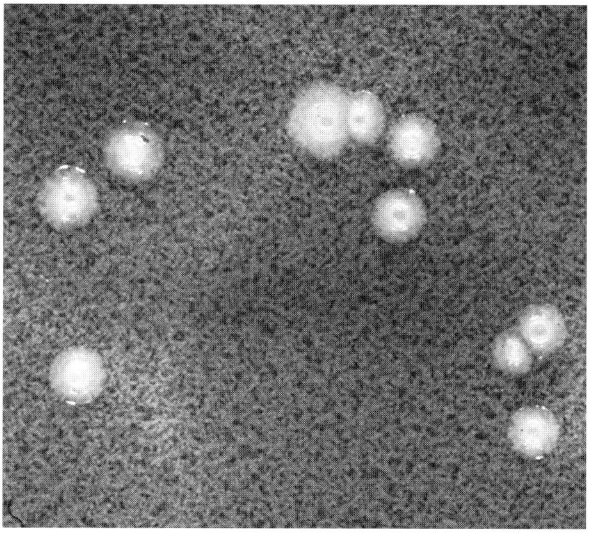

*Fig. 2.* Rough colonies of *B. henselae* cultured on chocolate agar plates for 14 days at 37 °C.

lyses erythrocytes and leukocytes. Blood cells collected in EDTA tubes remain unlysed. *B. henselae* and *B. bacilliformis* are shown to be intracellular and reside within erythrocytes [19, 20]. Therefore, blood cell lysis by saponin or by freezing improves *B. henselae* recovery [18]. Detection of *Bartonella* species in conventional automated blood culture systems is less reliable, as the organisms produce little or no $CO_2$ to indicate bacterial growth. However, *B. henselae* could be detected in 5 immunosuppressed patients using BacT/Alert™ (Organon) blood culture system. Positive growth algorithms were obtained and wet preparations demonstrated a pleomorphic bacillus with a twitching motility. By subculturing on solid media, more isolates could be obtained if the blood culture broth from the BacT/Alert™ bottle was injected and lysed into an Isolator™ tube [21]. Additionally, *B. quintana* was detected in 34 of 6,000 Bactec™ aerobic blood cultures by routine acridine orange staining [22].

Intracellular growth within the phagosomes of human monocytes and HeLa cells was also demonstrated for *A. felis*, formerly thought to be a putative etiologic agent of CSD [23]. Direct plating onto solid media or cocultivation in cell cultures are the two possible methods for culturing of *Bartonella* species.

*Culture on Solid Media.* Growth of *Bartonella* species is hemin-dependent [24] and best growth occurs on blood-enriched agar in a humid atmosphere containing 5–10% $CO_2$ at 35 °C. *B. henselae* and *B. quintana* grow well on standard chocolate agar, on commercial brain heart infusion agar (BHIA) contain-

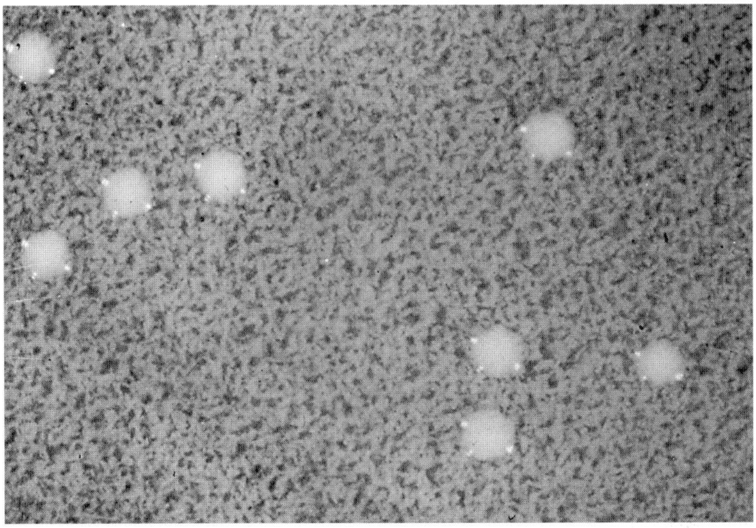

*Fig. 3.* Smooth colonies of *B. henselae* cultured on chocolate agar plates for 12 days at 37 °C. (From Sander [49], with permission).

ing 5% sheep blood, tryptic soy agar (TSA) supplemented with 5% sheep blood, heart infusion agar (HIA) containing 5% rabbit blood, and on Columbia blood agar [25, 26]. The type of blood and the age of medium seem to be important factors for cultures. Best growth occurs on fresh agar plates (as fresh as possible, in general less than 12 days old). Rabbit blood was discussed to be more effective than sheep blood [27]. However, primary isolation of *B. henselae* using sheep blood was successful in many cases [25–28]. Growth of *B. henselae* can be improved by cocultivation with certain strains of coagulase-negative staphylococci, *B. henselae* forming satellite colonies around these bacteria [26]. On blood agar, better growth was also seen near cocultivated *Staphylococcus aureus* colonies [28, 29]. Primary isolates of non-*bacilliformis* species of *Bartonella* grow very slowly. On solid media, first visible growth of the colonies occurs at the earliest after 5–15 days of incubation [25–27, 30] but primary isolation from human specimens may require up to 21–45 days [28, 31]. The risk of losing the isolates during these long incubation periods in humid atmosphere due to environmental contamination of the blood agar plates with moulds or rapid growing bacteria is considerable. Therefore, addition of an antimycotic such as amphotericin B to the culture medium and sealing the plates with Parafilm or Shrink Seal after the first 24 h of incubation may be beneficial [15, 32]. Primary colonies are whitish-cream colored, often highly adherent, deeply embedded into the agar, hard to break up and very small with an average size of 0.3–2.0 mm. First sub-

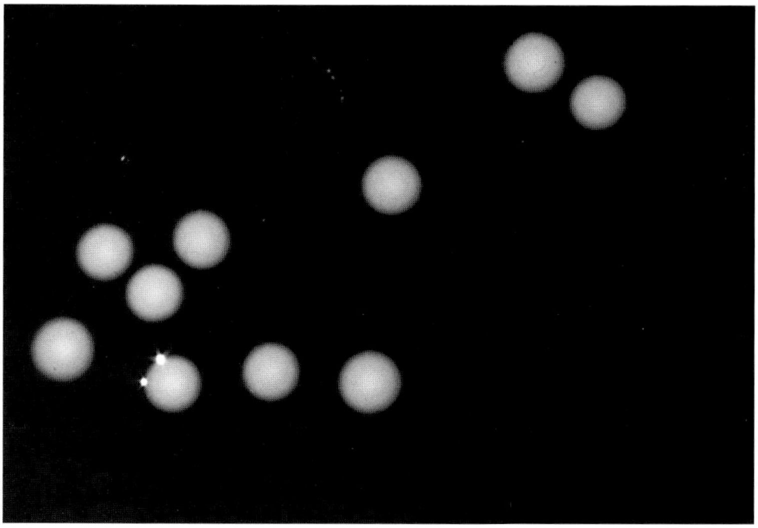

*Fig. 4.* *A. felis* colonies on BCYE agar for 7 days at 30 °C.

cultivation can be quite difficult, but after multiple passages of 4–5 subcultures, the time necessary for visible growth decreases to 3–5 days [25–27]. In primary cultures and in the first subcultures, *B. henselae* and *B. quintana* generally grow very heterogeneously, forming irregular, rough and/or circular, smooth colonies (fig. 2). However, after several passages, the colonies become smooth, shiny and less adherent (fig. 3). Primary isolation of *B. henselae* from blood and tissue specimens within 10–16 days was additionally reported by using a cell-free, extract-free, defined liquid medium [33].

*A. felis* grows best on buffered charcoal yeast extract (BCYE) plates, the standard for isolation of *Legionella* species. *Afipia* colonies of 1–3 mm in diameter occur after 72 h of incubation at 25–30 °C. They are smooth, glossy and white to cream-colored (fig. 4).

*Culture on Cell Culture Systems.* Cocultivation of *Bartonella* species in different cell cultures, including endothelial cells [34], Vero cells [35] and HeLa human cervical carcinoma cells [36] is reported. *B. quintana* was successfully isolated by these methods from blood and tissues of patients with BA, endocarditis or chronic lymphadenopathy [34, 35, 37]. Subcultivation of *Bartonella* species isolated in cell cultures onto agar plates is reported to be difficult [32] and cell culture systems are not used routinely in many microbiological laboratories. Therefore, most *Bartonella* isolates were obtained by direct cultivation on blood agar. Cocultivation in cell culture systems could be an additional method to enhance the recovery rate of *Bartonella* species.

*Table 1.* Biochemical characteristics of *Bartonella* species and *A. felis*

| | *B. henselae* | *B. quintana* | *B. clarridgeiae* | *B. elizabethae* | *B. bacilliformis* | *A. felis* |
|---|---|---|---|---|---|---|
| Gram reaction | – | – | – | – | – | – |
| Capnophilia | + | + | + | + | – | – |
| Catalase | – | – | – | – | + | – |
| Oxidase | – | – | – | – | – | + |
| Urea | – | – | – | – | – | + |
| Nitrate reduction | – | – | – | – | – | + |
| Growth at: | | | | | | |
| 25 °C | – | – | – | – | + | + |
| 30 °C | + | + | + | + | + | + |
| 35–37 °C | + | + | + | + | – | +[W] |
| 42 °C | – | – | – | – | – | – |
| Optimal growth temperature, °C | 35–37 | 35–37 | 35–37 | 35–37 | 25–30 | 25–30 |
| Flagella | – | – | + | – | + | + |
| Hemolysis | – | – | – | – | +[a] | – |
| Gelatin hydrolysis | – | – | – | – | – | – |
| Indole production | – | – | – | – | – | – |
| Citrate (Simmons) | – | – | – | – | – | – |
| Esculin hydrolysis | – | – | – | – | – | – |
| Voges-Proskauer (Rosco) | – | – | – | – | – | – |

[W] weak; [a] after a longer incubation time (7–10 days).

*Biochemical Characteristics*

Identification of *Bartonella* species in the routine microbiology laboratory is quite difficult, because they are phenotypically and genotypically very similar. *Bartonella* species should be suspected, when after prolonged incubation on blood-enriched media small mostly adherent colonies of Gram-negative pleomorphic bacilli were recovered. Biochemical tests are of little use in the differentiation of *Bartonella* species. The species are biochemically inert in almost all conventional tests, and commercially available identification kits do not contain *Bartonella* species in their diagnostic databases. Differentiation criteria on the genus and species level between *Bartonella* and *Afipia* species are shown in table 1. *Bartonella* and *Afipia* species do not produce acid from carbohydrates such as fructose, glucose, inositol, lactose, maltose, mannitol, mannose, melibiose, raffinose, rhamnose and sucrose in conventional biochemical tests. Test kits which are primarily designed for the identification of anaer-

*Table 2.* Comparison of commercial systems (biotype codes) for identification of *Bartonella* species

| System | Biotype code(s) | | | | | Ref. |
|---|---|---|---|---|---|---|
| | *B. henselae* | *B. quintana* | *B. vinsonii* | *B. elizabethae* | *B. bacilliformis* | |
| RapID ANA II System | 000671 | 000671 | 000661 | 00067/61 | 000641 | Clarridge [38] |
| | 000671 | nd | nd | nd | nd | Regnery [25] |
| | 000671 | 000671 | nd | 000671 | 000671 | Sander [26, and unpubl. data] |
| | 000671 | 000671 | nd | nd | nd | Schmidt [28] |
| | 000661 | 000641 | 000441 | nd | 000641 | Welch [27] |
| MicroScan Rapid | 10077640 | 10073640 | 10073200 | nd | 10077240 | Welch [27] |
| Anaerobe Panel | 10077640 | 10077640 | nd | nd | nd | Schmidt [28] |
| Rapid ID 32 A | 0000 0737 05 | 0000 0737 05 | nd | 0000 0737 05 | 0000 0126 00 | Sander [26, and unpubl. data] |
| An-IDENT System | 0004032 | 0004032 | 0004032 | nd | 0004032 | Welch [27] |

nd, not done.

obic organisms are useful for detection of enzyme activities (table 2). Enzymatic hydrolysis of proline-β-naphthylamide (PRO) and phenylalanine-β-naphthylamide (PAL) is often less pronounced than hydrolysis of leucyl-glycine-β-naphthylamide (LGY), glycine-β-naphthylamide (GLY), arginine-β-naphthylamide (ARG) and serine-β-naphthylamide (SER) in the RapID ANA II System, but they should be clearly scored as positive by comparing the color development with the IDS RapID ANA II color chart. Biochemical tests may be useful for identification to the genus level, but it does not allow a reliable differentiation between the *Bartonella* species.

*Whole-Cell Fatty Acid (CFA) Analysis*

CFA analysis is useful for identifying members of the genus *Bartonella*. Fatty acid methyl esters are prepared from cultures grown on BHIA containing 5–10% of rabbit or sheep blood [38] or on chocolate agar plates [25, 26], incubated at 35–37 °C for 4–6 days. CFA analysis was performed by separating fatty acid methyl ester derivatives on a gas chromatograph and identification by using a computer-assisted comparison of the retention time of the fatty acids with that of a standard calibration mixture (Microbial-Identification System, Neward, Del., USA). The major fatty acids observed for *B. henselae* (fig. 5) and *B. quintana* are *cis*-11-octadecanoic acid (C18:1ω7c), octadecanoic acid (C18:0), and hexadecanoic acid (C16:0) [6, 25, 26, 28, 30, 38, 39]. However,

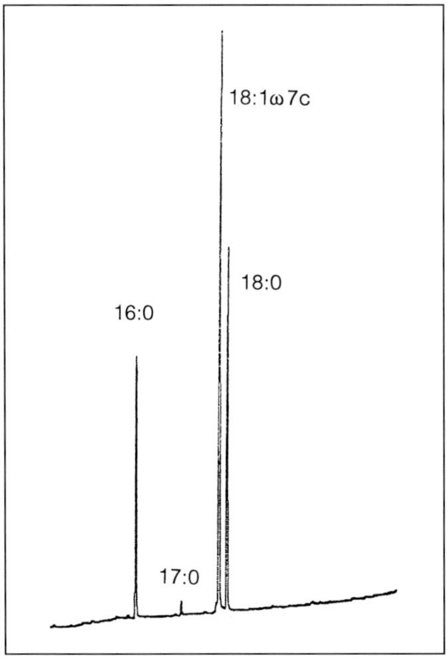


*Fig. 5.* Gas chromatogram of methylated fatty acids of *B. henselae* grown on chocolate agar for 6 days at 37 °C.

*Table 3.* Percent CFA methyl ester in *Bartonella* species and *A. felis*

| | 16:1ω7c | 16:0 | 17:0 | 17:0 Cyclo | Summed feature 7[a] | 18:0 | 19:0 Cyclo |
|---|---|---|---|---|---|---|---|
| *B. henselae*[b] | 0–1 | 16–23 | 0–3 | 0 | 48–59 | 19–36 | 0 |
| *B. quintana*[c] | 0–1 | 15–23 | 0–5 | 0 | 48–56 | 16–32 | 0 |
| *B. elizabethae*[c] | 1 | 24–25 | 14–19 | 0 | 38–41 | 11–12 | 0 |
| *B. bacilliformis*[c] | 17–21 | 22–28 | 0 | 0 | 40–52 | 2 | 0 |
| *A. felis*[d] | 12.92 | 3.67 | 0 | 3.33 | 64.40 | 10.74 | 4.13 |

[a] Summed feature 7 containing the CFAs 18:1 ω7c/ω9t/ω12t.
[b] CFA methyl ester of 12 *B. henselae* isolates [26] grown on chocolate agar (6 days at 37 °C).
[c] Adapted from Clarridge et al. [38].
[d] *A. felis* grown on BCYE agar (3 days at 30 °C) [Sander, unpubl. data].

there are only small differences between *B. henselae* and *B. quintana* species and the two species cannot be distinguished from each other by CFA analysis [6, 25, 26, 28, 30, 38]. *B. elizabethae* contains a greater amount of C17:0 and less 18:0 CFAs. *B. bacilliformis* is more distantly related having more C16:1ω7c and less C18:0 fatty acids than other *Bartonella* species (table 3). No

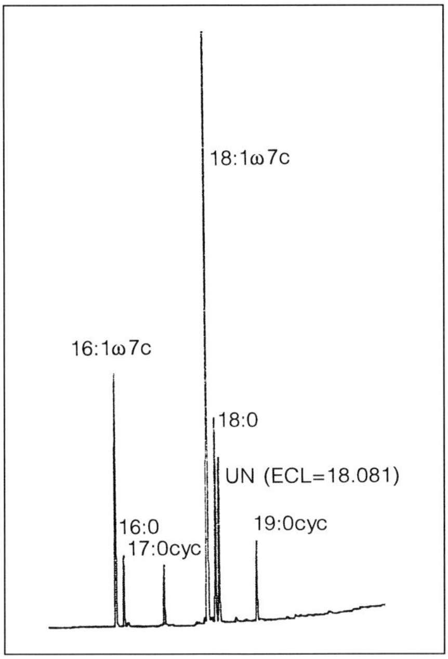


*Fig. 6.* Gas chromatogram of methylated fatty acids of *A. felis* grown on BCYE agar for 3 days at 30 °C. UN, unnamed fatty acid.

hydroxy or cyclopropane fatty acids were found in *Bartonella* species. The fatty acid patterns of *A. felis* is clearly different from all *Bartonella* species, containing large amounts of C18:1ω7c and two cyclopropane acids (fig. 6, table 3) [8, 39, 40, Sander, unpubl. data]. Separate preparations of bacterial cells on either heart infusion agar or buffered charcoal yeast extract agar were shown to give similar fatty acid results [40].

*Protein Profiles (SDS-Page Analysis)*

One-dimensional analytical sodium dodecyl sulfate-polyacrylamide gel electrophoresis (SDS-PAGE) shows unique protein profiles for each *Bartonella* species (fig. 7), which were different from those of *Afipia* species. Distinct protein profiles were demonstrated for *B. henselae, B. quintana* and *B. vinsonii* [26, 28, 31], and identical protein profiles were found between different *B. quintana* isolates [28, 31]. Recently, three major heat-shock proteins produced by *B. henselae* and *B. quintana* of 70, 60 and 10 kD were described [41]. A fourth major heat-shock protein (Mhsp4) was found to be larger in *B. quintana* (20 kD) than in *B. henselae* (17 kD). However, an immunoreactive 17-kD antigen described by Anderson et al. [42] seems to be the same protein as the *B. henselae* Mhsp4 [41].

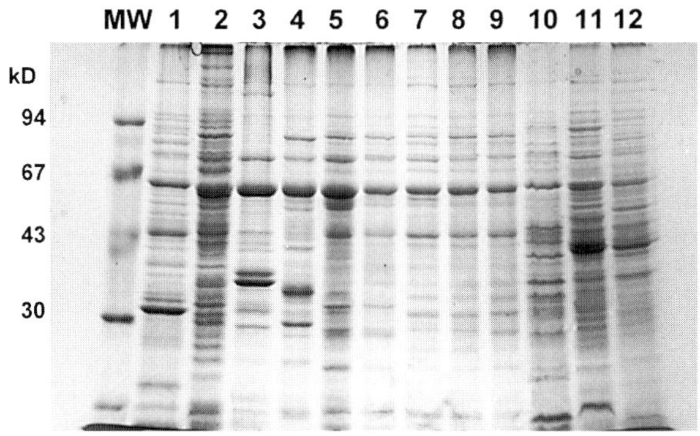


*Fig. 7.* Protein profiles of *Bartonella* and *Afipia* species: Lane MW, molecular mass standard; lane 1, *B. bacilliformis*; lane 2, *B. elizabethae*; lane 3, *B. clarridgeiae*; lane 4, *B. quintana*; lanes 5–9, *B. henselae*; lane 10, *A. felis*; lane 11, *A. broomeae*; lane 12, *A. clevelandensis.*

## DNA Fingerprinting

*DNA Macrorestriction Patterns (PFGE)*

Pulsed-field gel electrophoresis (PFGE) has been shown to be a suitable method for inter- and intraspecies identification of *Bartonella* species [31, 43, 44]. Digestion with the restriction enzymes *Sma*I and *Eag*I showed specific patterns for *B. henselae, B. quintana, B. elizabethae* and *B. vinsonii* and subtyping of 7 *B. quintana* isolates and 4 *B. henselae* isolates could be demonstrated [31, 44]. A total of 11 different patterns was found among 18 *B. henselae* isolates with PFGE by *Sma*I digestion of the DNA [44].

*Rep-PCR (ERIC- and REP-PCR)*

Repetitive-element PCR (rep-PCR) such as ERIC (enterobacterial repetitive intergenic consensus)-PCR and REP (repetitive extragenic palindromic)-PCR are useful techniques for identification of *Bartonella* organisms to the species level, showing different pattern for *B. henselae, B. quintana, B. elizabethae, B. vinsonii* and *B. bacilliformis* [26, 28, 45]. Discrimination between strains within the species was demonstrated for *B. henselae.* Five different fingerprint profiles were identified among 17 isolates of *B. henselae* by combining the results of both methods, whereas among 5 *B. quintana* isolates only a unique profile was found [45]. Subtyping of 18 *B. henselae* isolates by both techniques in another study revealed four different fingerprint profiles of these strains [46]. The ERIC-PCR banding patterns were less complex than those obtained by REP-PCR but allowed better discrimination between the isolates

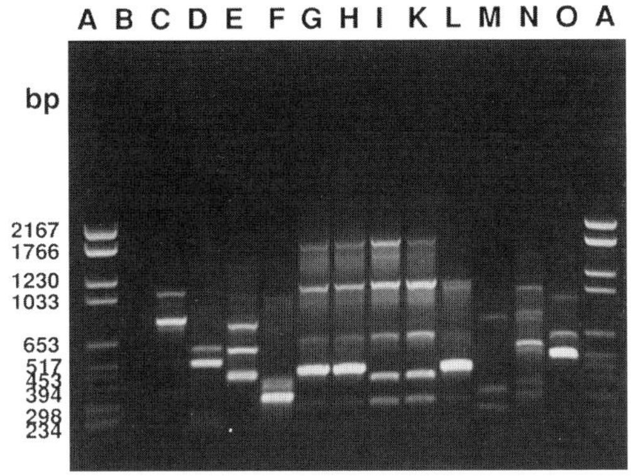


*Fig. 8.* RAPD-PCR (Primer M13) of *Bartonella* and *Afipia* species: Lanes A, DNA molecular size markers; lane B, negative control; lane C, *B. bacilliformis*; lane D, *B. elizabethae*; lane E, *B. clarridgeiae*; lane F, *B. quintana*; lanes G–L, *B. henselae* (3 different subtypes); lane M, *A. felis*; lane N, *A. broomeae*; lane O, *A. clevelandensis.*

in both studies. Different subtypes of *B. henselae* were obtained by ERIC-PCR from isolates obtained from 3 patients with BA and from the cats to which the patients were exposed [47]. REP-PCR could not discriminate in these cases and similar patterns were obtained for all *B. henselae* isolates.

*Random Amplified Polymorphic DNA (RAPD)*

Random amplified polymorphic DNA (RAPD) typing uses a short (usually 10- to 15-bp) arbitrarily chosen primer to amplify sequences of the genomic DNA under low-stringency conditions. By using this technique, different patterns were obtained from 18 *B. henselae* isolates [46], and differentiation between *Bartonella* and *Afipia* species is possible (fig. 8) [Sander, unpubl. data].

*Restriction Fragment Length Polymorphism Analysis (RFLP)*

Restriction endonuclease analysis of a PCR-based DNA fragment including the spacer region between the 16S and 23S rRNA genes and a portion of the gene coding for 23S rRNA were performed for differentiation between *Bartonella* species and subtyping of *B. henselae* [48]. Digestion of the amplicons with *Alu*I, *Hae*III, *Taq*I, *Hinf*I, and *Mse*I allowed species differentiation between *B. henselae, B. quintana, B. vinsonii* and *B. bacilliformis.* Of the 11 *B. henselae* isolates investigated, six different restriction patterns were found by digestion with *Alu*I and four patterns with *Hae*III, respectively. Combining the different PCR-RFLP types obtained with both restriction endonucleases, seven subtypes within *B. henselae* isolates were determined [48].

*Present Status of Subtyping*

Only limited data on subtyping of *Bartonella* species are available. Strains of *B. henselae* seem to be highly heterogeneous. The combined use of different molecular techniques is needed for optimal differentiation and for establishing the most promising methods for subtyping of *Bartonella* isolates. Such studies may be useful to determine the role of *B. henselae* and/or *B. quintana* in BA, CSD and other diseases, and the involvement of different vectors in the transmission of *Bartonella* species.

In conclusion, isolation of *Bartonella* species, although very difficult in many cases, is highly important, not only for the etiological diagnosis, but also for genetical investigations on the isolates. Analyses of the strain relatedness of clinical and nonclinical (e.g. vectors, cats, parasites) isolates will provide the basis for further studies on the epidemiology and the pathogenicity of these agents.

## References


1 Weiss E, Moulder JW: Order I. *Rickettsiales* Gieszczkiewicz (sic) 1939, $25^{AL}$; in Krieg NR, Holt JG (eds): Bergey's Manual of Systematic Bacteriology. Baltimore, Williams & Wilkins, 1984, vol 1, pp 687–688.

2 Brenner DJ, O'Connor SP, Winkler HH, Steigerwalt AG: Proposals to unify the genera *Bartonella* and *Rochalimaea*, with descriptions of *Bartonella quintana* comb. nov., *Bartonella vinsonii* comb. nov., *Bartonella henselae* comb. nov., and *Bartonella elizabethae* comb. nov., and to remove the family *Bartonellaceae* from the order *Rickettsiales*. Int J Syst Bacteriol 1993;43:777–786.

3 Birtles RJ, Harrison TG, Saunders NA, Molyneux DH: Proposals to unify the genera *Grahamella* and *Bartonella*, with descriptions of *Bartonella talpae* comb. nov., *Bartonella peromysci* comb. nov., and three new species, *Bartonella grahammii* sp. nov., *Bartonella taylorii* sp. nov., and *Bartonella doshiae* sp. nov. Int J Syst Bacteriol 1995;45:1–8.

4 Anderson BE, Neuman MA: *Bartonella* ssp. as emerging human pathogens. Clin Microbiol Rev 1997;10:203–219.

5 Sander A, Kaliebe T, Bredt W: *Bartonella* (*Rochalimaea*)-Infektionen: Katzenkratzkrankheit und bazilläre Angiomatose. Dtsch Med Wochenschr 1996;121:65–69.

6 Daly JS, Worthington MG, Brenner DJ, Moss CW, Hollis DG, Weyant RS, Steigerwalt AG, Weaver RE, Daneshvar MI, O'Connor SP: *Rochalimaea elizabethae* sp. nov. isolated from a patient with endocarditis. J Clin Microbiol 1993;31:872–881.

7 Kordick DL, Hilyard EJ, Hadfield TL, Wilson KH, Steigerwald AG, Brenner DJ, Breitschwerdt EB: *Bartonella clarridgeiae*, a newly recognized zoonotic pathogen causing inoculation papules, fever, and lymphadenopathy (cat scratch disease). J Clin Microbiol 1997;35:1813–1818.

8 Brenner DJ, Hollis DG, Moss CW, English CK, Hall GS, Vincent J, Radosevic J, Birkness KA, Bibb WF, Quinn FD, Swaminathan B, Weaver R, Reeves MW, O'Connor SP, Hayes PS, Tenover FC, Steigerwald AG, Perkins BA, Daneshvar MI, Hill BC, Washington JA, Woods TC, Hunter SB, Hadfield TL, Ajello GW, Kaufmann AF, Wear DJ, Wenger JD: Proposals of *Afipia* gen. nov., with *Afipia felis* sp. nov. (formerly the cat scratch disease bacillus), *Afipia clevelandensis* sp. nov. (formerly the Cleveland Clinic Foundation strain), *Afipia broomeae* sp. nov., and three unnamed genospecies. J Clin Microbiol 1991;29:2450–2460.

9 English CJ, Wear DJ, Margileth AM, Lissner CR, Walsh GP: Cat-scratch disease; isolation and culture of the bacterial agent. JAMA 1988;259:1347–1352.

10 Zangwill KM, Hamilton DH, Perkins BA, Regnery RL, Plikaytis BD, Hadler JL, Cartter ML, Wenger JD: Cat scratch disease in Connecticut. N Engl J Med 1993;329:8–13.

11 Szelc-Kelly CM, Goral S, Guillermo I: Serologic responses to *Bartonella* and *Afipia* antigens in patients with cat scratch disease. Pediatrics 1995;96:1137–1142.
12 Dalton MJ, Robinson LE, Cooper J, Regnery RL, Olson JG, Childs JE: Use of *Bartonella* antigens for serologic diagnosis of cat-scratch disease at a national referral center. Arch Intern Med 1995; 155:1670–1676.
13 Bergmans AMC, Groothedde JW, Schellekens JFP, von Embden JDA, Ossewaarde JM, Schouls LM: Etiology of cat scratch disease: Comparison of polymerase chain reaction detection of *Bartonella* (formerly *Rochalimaea*) and *Afipia felis* DNA with serology and skin test. J Infect Dis 1995;171: 916–923.
14 Goldenberger D, Zbinden R, Perschil I, Altwegg M: Nachweis von *Bartonella (Rochalimaea) henselae/B. quintana* mittels Polymerase-Kettenreaktion (PCR). Schweiz Med Wochenschr 1996; 126:207–213.
15 Welch DF, Slater LN: *Bartonella*; in Murray PR (ed): Manual of Clinical Microbiology, ed 6. Washington, ASM Press, 1995, pp 690–695.
16 Scherer DC, DeBuron-Connors I, Minnick MF: Characterization of *Bartonella bacilliformis* flagella and effect of antiflagellin antibodies on invasion of human erythrocytes. Infect Immun 1993;61: 4962–4971.
17 Lawson PA, Collins MD: Description of *Bartonella clarridgeiae* sp. nov. isolated from the cat of a patient with *Bartonella henselae* septicemia. Med Microbiol Lett 1996;5:64–73.
18 Brenner SA, Rooney JA, Manzewitsch P, Regnery RL: Isolation of *Bartonella (Rochalimaea) henselae*: Effects of methods of blood collecting and handling. J Clin Microbiol 1997;35:544–547.
19 Benson LA, Kar S, McLaughlin G, Ihler GM: Entry of *Bartonella bacilliformis* into erythrocytes. Infect Immun 1986;54:347–353.
20 Kordick DL, Wilson KH, Sexton DJ, Hadfield TL, Berkhoff HA, Breitschwerdt EB: Intraerythrocytic presence of *Bartonella henselae*. J Clin Microbiol 1995;33:1655–1656.
21 Tierno PM, Inglima K, Parisi MT: Detection of *Bartonella (Rochalimaea) henselae* bacteremia using BacT/Alert blood culture system. Am J Clin Pathol 1995;104:530–536.
22 Larson AM, Dougherty MJ, Nowowiejski DJ, Welch DF, Matar GM, Swaminathan B, Coyle MB: Detection of *Bartonella (Rochalimaea) quintana* by routine acridine orange staining of broth blood cultures. J Clin Microbiol 1994;6:1492–1496.
23 Birkness KA, George VG, White EH, Stephens DS, Quinn FD: Intracellular growth of *Afipia felis*, a putative etiologic agent of cat scratch disease. Infect Immun 1992;60:2281–2287.
24 Drancourt M, Raoult D: Proposed tests for the routine identification of *Rochalimaea* species. Eur J Clin Microbiol Infect Dis 1993;12:710–713.
25 Regnery RL, Anderson BE, Clarridge JE, Rodriguez-Barradas MC, Jones DC, Carr JH: Characterization of a novel *Rochalimaea* species, *R. henselae* sp. nov., isolated from blood of a febrile, human immunodeficient virus-positive patient. J Clin Microbiol 1992;30:265–274.
26 Sander A, Bühler C, Pelz K, von Cramm E, Bredt W: Detection and isolation of two *Bartonella henselae* variants in domestic cats in Germany. J Clin Microbiol 1997;35:584–587.
27 Welch DF, Hensel DM, Pickett DA, San Joaquin VH, Robinson A, Slater LN: Bacteremia due to *Rochalimaea henselae* in a child: Practical identification of isolates in the clinical laboratory. J Clin Microbiol 1993;31:1882–1885.
28 Schmidt HU, Kaliebe T, Poppinger J, Bühler C, Sander A: Isolation of *Bartonella quintana* from an HIV-positive patient with bacillary angiomatosis. Eur J Clin Microbiol Infect Dis 1996;15:736–741.
29 Slater LN, Welch DF, Hensel D, Coody DW: A newly recognized fastidious Gram-negative pathogen as a cause of fever and bacteremia. N Engl J Med 1990;323:1587–1593.
30 Welch DF, Pickett DA, Slater LN, Steigerwalt AG, Brenner DJ: *Rochalimaea henselae* sp. nov., a cause of septicemia, bacillary angiomatosis, and parenchymal bacillary peliosis. J Clin Microbiol 1992;30:275–280.
31 Maurin M, Roux V, Stein A, Ferrier F, Viraben R, Raoult D: Isolation and characterization by immunofluorescence, sodium dodecyl sulfate-polycrylamide gel electrophoresis, Western blot, restriction fragment length polymorphism-PCR, 16S rRNA gene sequencing, and pulsed-field gel electrophoresis of *Rochalimaea quintana* from a patient with bacillary angiomatosis. J Clin Microbiol 1994;32:1166–1171.

32 Maurin M, Birtles R, Raoult D: Current knowledge of *Bartonella* species. Eur J Clin Microbiol Infect Dis 1997;16:487–506.
33 Wong MT, Thornton DC, Kennedy RC, Dolan MJ: A chemically defined liquid medium that supports primary isolation of *Rochalimaea (Bartonella) henselae* from blood and tissue specimens. J Clin Microbiol 1995;33:742–744.
34 Koehler JE, Quinn FD, Berger TG, LeBoit PE, Tappero JW: Isolation of *Rochalimaea* species from cutaneous and osseous lesions of bacillary angiomatosis. N Engl J Med 1992;327:1625–1631.
35 Zbinden R, Höchli M, Nadal D: Intracellular location of *Bartonella henselae* cocultivated with Vero cells and used for an indirect fluorescent-antibody test. Clin Diagn Lab Immunol 1995;2: 693–695.
36 Drancourt M, Mainardi J, Brouqui P, Vandenesch F, Carta A, Lehnert F, Etienne J, Goldstein F, Acar J, Raoult D: *Bartonella (Rochalimaea) quintana* endocarditis in three homeless men. N Engl J Med 1995;332:419–423.
37 Raoult D, Drancourt M, Carta A, Gastaut JA: *Bartonella (Rochalimaea) quintana* isolation in a patient with chronic adenopathy, lymphopenia and a cat. Lancet 1994;343:977.
38 Clarridge JE, Raich TJ, Pirwani D, Simon B, Tsai L, Rodriguez-Barradas MC, Regnsery R, Zollo A, Jones DC, Rambo C: Strategy to detect and identify *Bartonella* species in a routine clinical laboratory yields *Bartonella henselae* from human immunodeficiency virus-positive patient and a unique *Bartonella* strain from his cat. J Clin Microbiol 1995;33:2107–2113.
39 Dolan MJ, Wong MT, Regnery RL, Jorgensen JH, Garcia M, Peters J, Drehner D: Syndrome of *Rochalimaea henselae* adenitis suggesting cat scratch disease. Ann Intern Med 1993;118:331–336.
40 Moss CW, Holzer G, Wallace PL, Hollis DG: Cellular fatty acid compositions of an unidentified organism and a bacterium associated with cat scratch disease. J Clin Microbiol 1990;28:1071–1074.
41 Haake DA, Summers TA, McCoy AM, Schwartzman W: Heat-shock response and groEL sequence of *Bartonella henselae* and *Bartonella quintana*. Microbiology 1997;143:2807–2815.
42 Anderson B, Lu E, Jones D, Regnery R: Characterization of a 17-kilodalton antigen of *Bartonella henselae* reactive with sera from patients with cat scratch disease. J Clin Microbiol 1995;33:2358–2365.
43 Roux V, Raoult D: Inter- and intraspecies identification of *Bartonella (Rochalimaea)* species. J Clin Microbiol 1995;33:1573–1579.
44 Sander A, Ruess M, Steinbrueckner B, Bredt W: DNA-Fingerprinting of *Bartonella henselae* by PFGE, ERIC-PCR, REP-PCR and AP-PCR. 13th Sesqui-Annual Meeting, American Society for Rickettsiology, Seven Springs Mountain Resort, Pa., 1997.
45 Rodriguez-Barradas MC, Hamill RJ, Houston ED, Georghiou PR, Clarridge JE, Regnery RL, Koehler JE: Genomic fingerprinting of *Bartonella* species by repetitive element PCR for distinguishing species and isolates. J Clin Microbiol 1995;33:1089–1093.
46 Sander A, Ruess M, Schuppler M, Bereswill S, Steinbrueckner B: Comparison of different DNA fingerprint techniques for molecular typing of *Bartonella henselae* isolates. Submitted 1998.
47 Koehler JE, Sanchez MA, Garrido CS, Whitfeld MJ, Chen FM, Berger TG, Rodriguez-Barradas MC, LeBoit PE, Tappero JW: Molecular epidemiology of *Bartonella* infections in patients with bacillary angiomatosis-peliosis. N Engl J Med 1997;337:1876–1883.
48 Matar GM, Swaminathan B, Hunter SB, Slater LN, Welch D: Polymerase chain reaction-based restriction fragment length polymorphism analysis of a fragment of the ribosomal operon from *Rochalimaea* species for subtyping. J Clin Microbiol 1993;31:1730–1734.
49 Sander A: Katzenkratzkrankheit IV-1.19. In: Hofmann (Hrsg) Infektiologie. ecomed Verlag, 24. Erg. Lfg. 2/1998.

Anna Sander, Institut für Medizinische Mikrobiologie und Hygiene,
Klinikum der Universität Freiburg, PO Box 820, D–79008 Freiburg (Germany)

Schmidt A (ed): *Bartonella* and *Afipia* Species Emphasizing *Bartonella henselae*.
Contrib Microbiol. Basel, Karger, 1998, vol 1, pp 113–129

# Diagnostics of Human Infections Caused by *Bartonella henselae*

*Philip M. Tierno, Jr.*

Microbiology Department, New York University Medical Center, Tisch Hospital, New York, N.Y., USA

## Introduction

Historically, organisms of the genus *Bartonella* (including former *Rochalimaea*) cause a number of different disorders, most of which are thought to be zoonoses. Diseases caused by these organisms range from the relatively innocuous trench fever to the potentially fatal bacillary angiomatosis. Although the classical *Bartonella* disease called Carrion's disease, also known as bartonellosis, and its vascular proliferative phase, verruga peruana, which has been recognized for more than a century, is a disease largely of academic interest, it is confined to only a small endemic area in South America. Interest in bartonellosis was rekindled in 1983 when a febrile illness manifest as subcutaneous nodules containing non-Gram-staining, argyrophilic bacteria was first reported by Stoler et al. [1]. They described an unusual subcutaneous vascular proliferative condition in an AIDS patient. Light microscopic examination of tissue stained with the Warthin-Starry method as well as examination of tissue using electron microscopy (EM) revealed clusters of bacilli within the vascular lesion. Treatment with oral erythromycin resulted in resolution of the process. This report was followed by those of a number of other patients with a similar condition in which bacteria have also been demonstrated [2–9]. All of these patients had documented HIV infections. Although similar vascular proliferations have been found in immunocompetent individuals [10, 11] and in one patient with an underlying malignancy [11], the first known reported case of this infectious condition occurring in a patient without HIV infection or without risk factors for its development was reported by Cockerell et al. [10]. Numerous additional cases were described primarily in a number of patients with HIV infection on whom red to purple papules and nodules of the skin had been mistakenly diagnosed as Kaposi's sarcoma and/or pyogenic granulomata [2]. Organisms similar to those described above were found when Warthin-Starry staining and EM were employed for diagnosis. Because of the vascular nature of the skin lesions, the condition was termed bacillary (epithelioid) angiomatosis (BA). Multiple attempts at culture of the causative organism were made, at that time, in an effort to isolate it, without success. As the then proposed organism of cat scratch disease (CSD), *Afipia felis*, had been cultured and characterized, and demonstrated morphologic features similar to the causative agent of BA, a number of articles appeared in the literature suggesting the two diseases were identical [3–5]. With greater awareness of this disorder, it was discovered that in addition to involvement of the skin and soft tissue lymph nodes, spleen, liver, bone, the central nervous system, and other organ systems were also commonly affected. Further demonstration of the causative agent of BA was successfully undertaken by Relman et al. [12] who used oligonucleotide primers complementary to 16S ribosomal RNA genes of eubacteria to amplify 16S ribosomal RNA genes of bacteria extracted from BA tissue samples. They determined that the organism was closely related to *B. quintana* (formerly *Rochalimaea quintana*) and was distinct from *A. felis*. The organism was eventually named *B. henselae* after Diane Hensel, a technician who was highly instrumental in the final identification of the organism [13]. Subsequently, Regnery et al. [14] developed a specific polymerase chain reaction (PCR) assay that detects DNA sequences of both *B. henselae* and *B. quintana* in lymph nodal tissue obtained from patients with CSD. These authors demonstrated that *B. henselae*, rather than either *B. quintana* or *A. felis*, was the major etiologic agent of CSD. In one study, *B. henselae* was found in blood samples of up to 61% of tested domestic cats, *Felis domesticus*, as well as in their fleas *Ctenocephalides felis* [15]. The authors suggest that because about 57 million pet cats reside in the USA, a vast risk for acquiring *B. henselae* infection exists.

*B. bacilliformis* and related organisms such as *B. quintana, B. henselae* and *B. elizabethae* are all members of the family *Rickettsiaceae*. Members of this family are usually transmitted by arthropod vectors, such as lice, fleas, flies, ticks and mites. *B. bacilliformis* is endemic only to certain areas of South America and is trasmitted by the bite of a local sandfly, *Phlebotomus* [16]. In vitro, *B. bacilliformis* induces endothelial proliferation, and causes angiogenesis in animals [17]. However, there is no current evidence that this species infects patients in the USA or Eurasia.

*B. quintana*, transmitted by the human louse *Pediculus humanus*, has been known to cause disease in humans since 1916, when epidemics of louse-borne trench fever were rampant among soldiers of World War I. During World

*Table 1.* Ectoparasites versus *Bartonella*

| | | |
|---|---|---|
| Sandfly | *Phlebotomis* | *B. bacilliformis* |
| Scabies | *Sarcoptes scabei* | *B. vinsonii, B. henselae* |
| Body lice | *Pediculus humanus corporis* | *B. quintana, B. henselae* |
| Head lice | *Pediculus humanus capitis* | *B. quintana* |
| Pubic lice | *Pediculus humanus pubis* | *B. quintana* |
| Ear mite | *Trombicula microti* | *B. vinsonii* |
| Pigeon mite | *Dermanyssus gallinae* | *B. henselae* |
| Rat mite | *Laelops nuttalli* | *B. henselae* |
| Cat fleas | *Ctenocephalides felis* | *B. henselae* |
| Dog fleas | *Ctenocephalides canis* | *B. henselae* |

War II, trench fever re-emerged and large-scale epidemics were once again reported [18].

*B. elizabethae* is most related to, and might be a variant of, *B. vinsonii* [15], which has been isolated from the spleen of the vole-mouse and then experimentally transmitted by the ear mite, *Trombicula microti*, to a hamster [19]. *B. elizabethae* has been reported to cause endocarditis in humans [20].

It is not difficult to propose that because of the ubiquitous nature of these bacteria, immunocompromised patients are very susceptible to diseases caused by *Bartonella* species that can be transmitted by either animal or arthropod, or both (table 1).

While *B. henselae* (and a variant species *clarridgeiae*), *B. quintana* and *B. elizabethae* have been reported to cause a variety of clinical infections (i.e. BA [10, 12, 16, 20], hepatic and splenic peliosis [21, 22], septicemia [20–25], endocarditis [26], as well as CSD [15], primary isolation of *Bartonella* species, other than *B. bacilliformis*, is a difficult task in the routine clinical laboratory and has only been accomplished by a handful of investigators, primarily because these bacteria are fastidious as well as slow growing with 2–7 weeks, if they grow at all. Isolator lysis concentration technique has been reported to be useful when septicemia is suspected [24]. *Bartonella* species have also been isolated from blood specimens by methods including direct plating of whole blood onto agar [24], as well as Septi-Chek biphasic system, and the automated Bactec 460 and Bactec NR 660 systems [25]. A relatively new, more rapid automated technique for the detection of bacteremia, BacT/Alert, has been commercially available for the past few years and has been reported to facilitate recovery of *B. henselae* [27]. Growth from tissue sources other than blood, spleen or lymph had not been successful.

There are presently 11 species in the genus *Bartonella* (table 2). In addition to the 6 aforementioned *Bartonella*, Birtles et al. [28] proposed a unification

*Table 2.* The species of *Bartonella*

| |
|---|
| *B. bacilliformis* |
| *B. quintana* |
| *B. henselae* |
| *B. clarridgeiae* |
| *B. elizabethae* |
| *B. vinsonii* |
| *B. doshiae* |
| *B. grahami* |
| *B. peromysci* |
| *B. taylorii* |
| *B. talpoe* |

*Table 3.* Diagnostic methods for human infections caused by *B. henselae*

| |
|---|
| Direct demonstration of *B. henselae* or its antigens: |
| (a) Histologic staining (e.g. HE, Warthin-Starry) |
| (b) Phase microscopy of wet preparations |
| (c) Acridine orange staining |
| (d) Electron microscopic examination |
| (e) Bacteriologic culture (e.g. blood, tissue, lymph) |
| (f) Fatty Acid Methyl Esters (FAME) analysis |
| (g) Immunofluorescence technique |
| (h) Immunoperoxidase technique |
| (i) PCR amplification of 16S ribosomal DNA |
| Serologic detection of *B. henselae* antibodies by immunoassays: |
| (a) Indirect immunofluorescence assay (IFA) |
| (b) Immunoperoxidase assay (IPA) |
| (c) Enzyme immunoassay (EIA) |

of the genera *Bartonella* and *Grahamella*. The two established *Grahamella* species, *G. peromysci* and *G. talpoe*, were renamed as *Bartonella* species. Additionally, Birtles et al. [28] described three new *Bartonella* species which were isolated from animals: *B. doshiae, B. grahamii* and *B. taylorii*.

In light of the difficulties involved with growing *Bartonella* in general and *B. henselae* specifically, a useful approach for the isolation and/or identification of this organism from patients is outlined below.

Two main types of laboratory procedures can be performed in order to diagnose human infections caused by *B. henselae* (table 3) namely: direct demonstration of *B. henselae* or its antigens and serologic detection of *B. henselae* antibodies by immunoassay.

## Direct Methods

*Histologic Stains*

Tissue from infections such as BA, hepatic or splenic peliosis, lymphadenitis, etc., should be biopsied and stained first with hematoxylin and eosin: Lobular proliferations of capillaries with large cuboidal endothelial cells lining individual vessels as well as interstitially are usually seen. A mixed inflammatory cell infiltrate consisting of lymphocytes, histiocytes and abundant neutrophils are seen especially in BA lesions. Note the difference between histology of CSD versus BA. In CSD the primary inoculation lesion are areas of frank necrosis surrounded by concentric layers of histocytes, lymphocytes and multinucleated giant cells. Lymph nodes are characterized by necrotizing granulomas ringed by lymphocytic infiltrates and multinucleated giant cells. In BA lesions there is a proliferative vascular lesions without granuloma.

Warthin-Starry staining performed on BA lesions usually demonstrate abundant masses of darkly staining pleomorphic bacteria between blood vessels. Bacilli can vary from thin, straight, curved and short. Some can be tapered at one end and small clumps or clusters can also usually be observed. Gram, Acid-fast and PAS stains usually fail to demonstrate the organism. A bacterium which is a non-Gram and non-Acid-fast staining, pleomorphic, argyrophilic bacillus isolated from a patient with a history and clinical symptomatology as described above and which does not grow using 'routine' bacteriologic methods is presumptively a *Bartonella* species. A wet preparation as described below should now be performed in order to detect 'rachety' or 'twitching' motility, characteristic of *Bartonella*, and thusly adding further support to the presumptive identification of *Bartonella* species.

Warthin-Starry staining of blood from blood culture bottles should be processed differently, as follows: 7.5 ml of homogenized blood culture broth from each 'positive' automated blood culture bottle should be injected into a separate Isolator tube (Wampole, Cranbury, N.Y., USA) and concentrated according to the manufacturer's instructions. A simple cell block procedure can then be performed using 0.5 ml of this lysed concentrated blood culture broth. After the cell block is solidified, sections can be made and stained by the Warthin-Starry technique as previously reported [27]. Darkly staining pleomorphic bacilli can be seen as shown in figure 1. Apparently lysing the RBCs free the intracellular bacilli.

*Phase Microscopy of Wet Preparations*

Tissue can be ground and added to about 1 ml of supplemented (250 μg/ml and 8% Fildes solution) brain heart infusion (BHI), trypticase soy broth

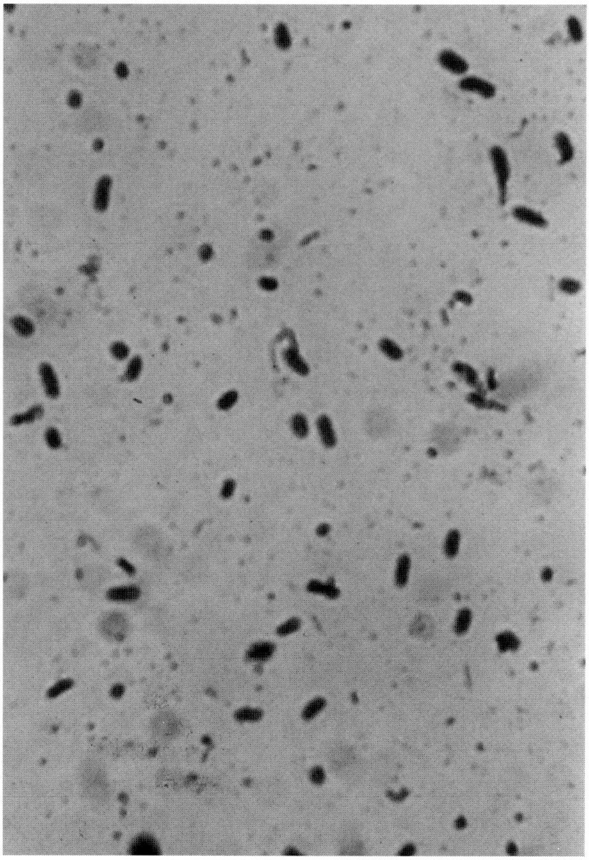

*Fig. 1.* Warthin-Starry technique revealing darkly staining pleomorphic bacilli of *B. henselae.*

(TSB) or aerobic blood culture medium, then incubated aerobically under 5% $CO_2$ tension at 36 °C for 48 h or longer. This will facilitate observation of the organism, after which one drop of broth should be placed on a glass slide followed by a coverslip.

One drop of suspected positive blood culture can be applied directly to a glass slide followed by a coverslip. An examination of smears can be made using either phase microscopy or routine light microscopy under oil immersion. A characteristic 'rachety' or 'twitching' clockwise, alternating to counterclockwise, motility of pleomorphic bacilli can then be observed [27]. With careful observation, on occasion, elongated bacilli can be seen exiting or entering RBCs as shown in figure 2.

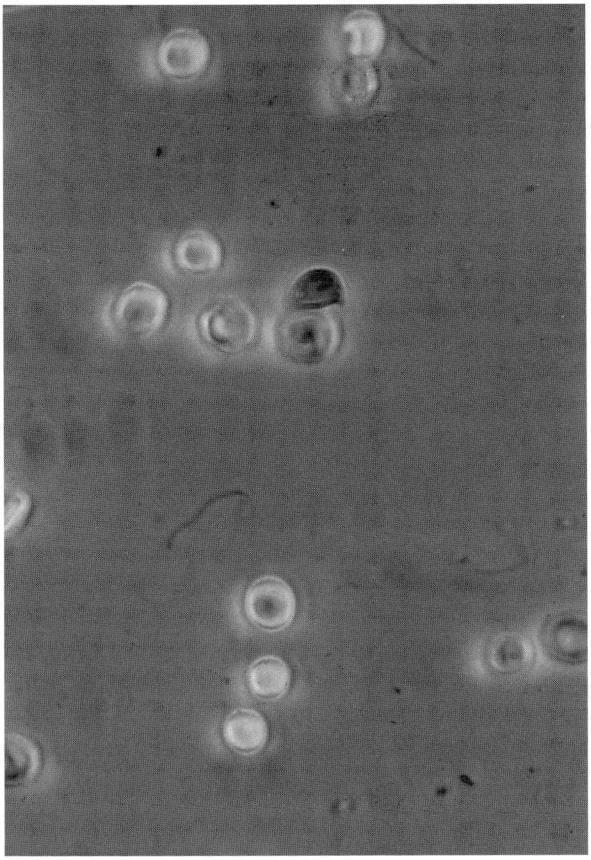

*Fig. 2.* Elongated bacilli of *B. henselae* seen exiting and entering erythrocytes.

*Acridine Orange Staining*

An alternative to Warthin-Starry staining is the acridine orange stain [27]. 7.5 ml of homogenized blood culture broth from each 'positive' bottle should be injected into an Isolator tube (Wampole) and concentrated according to the manufacturer's instructions. One drop of the lysed concentrate can be placed onto a glass slide, dried at room temperature, and fixed for 2 min with methanol. Acridine orange (0.01%) stain in buffer at pH 3.5–4.0 (BBL, Cockeyville, Md., USA) should be added to the air-dried slide and left for 2 min. Each slide should then be rinsed with water and air dried again.

Alternatively, one drop of ground tissue broth preparation, as described above, can be processed in a similar manner.

An examination of smears can be made by epifluorescence microscopy. Acridine orange-stained slides will reveal small orange-colored pleomorphic bacilli that can vary from thin, straight to ovoid and short bacilli. Some can be tapered at one pole, whereas others can be slightly curved. Occasional filamentation forms will be observed as well as small clumps or clusters. Background blood and cells will appear greenish in color [27].

*EM Examination*

A portion of tissue can be placed in 3% phosphate-buffered glutaraldehyde and processed for EM by routine methods [16]. Thin sections can be stained with uranyl acetate-lead citrate. Both tissue sections and smears of cultures could be examined. In tissue, organisms are usually found extracellularly amidst collagen fibrils and in areas where discontinuity of normal tissue and some cellular debris is evident. At higher magnification a partially detached outer membrane, a well-defined inner membrane, and in some areas, a thin peptidoglycan layer characteristic of Gram-negative bacilli can be easily identified. Similar morphologic features can be seen upon examination of smears of broth cultures. In addition, numerous peripheral ribosomes and fibrinous nuclear material can be seen. On some occasions, bacteria with dense granules, similar to phosphate-rich metachromatic granules, and surrounding fibrillar capsule-like material can be observed. No mesosomal structures were seen in any of the sections studied to date [16]. Obviously EM is not a suitable method for routine application but this technique can be revealing if other methods fail.

*Culture from Blood*

While blood from either routine 'manually processed' or 'automated' blood culture detection systems can be used for subculturing, it is more likely to detect *B. henselae* using an automated system such as BacT/Alert (Organon Tenika, Durham, N.C., USA), Bactec 460 or NR 660 (e.g. BD Instruments, Sparks, Md., USA) which are dependent upon an objective detection of bacterial growth via increasing levels of $CO_2$ rather than relying purely on subjective observation. In such automated systems, 'positives' are determined by algorithms programmed into the computer. Gram staining performed on such 'positive' cultures are usually negative. However, a wet-prep or phase-microscopic examination will usually yield bacilli with characteristic 'rachety' or 'twitching' motility. Routine subculture on bacteriologic media will yield no growth after a routine incubation period of about 72 h.

Using automated systems, the time to detection will vary dependent upon the initial bioload from $\leq 1$ to $> 14$ days with the mean about 9 days depending on the system used. Although numerous methods have been used to isolate *Bartonella* species from blood cultures, Tierno et al. [27] reported that the

BacT/Alert appears to be the most successful commercial detection system to grow *B. henselae* from patients not suspected of *Bartonella* bacteremia. In their study, the time to detection varied from 0.125 to 6.4 days with a mean of 4 days, which represents a substantial improvement over earlier reports. The authors found that the aerobic bottle was exclusively positive. Tierno et al. [27] reported that the peculiarity of the distinctively swift detection time of 0.125 day in one case seemed to have been an inoculum-dependent phenomenon. Excision of the patient's spleen undertaken immediately before blood sample collection may have released a substantial organism load into the bloodstream. The enlarged spleen may have been infected or may have accumulated organisms through vascular filtration. The proposal of an unusually heavy inoculum is supported by the pronounced and immediate rise in $CO_2$ demonstrated shortly after loading the bottles as well as the steeply sloped increase sustained for at least 24 h once the positive bottle was reloaded for further observation. The authors reported that early wet mounts from the bottle soon after primary detection revealed that the blood was virtually teeming with organisms. With other patients' samples, they reported that organisms were far less conspicuous on wet mounts even after substantially longer incubation periods.

In another study [25], *B. quintana* was detected using a different automated nonradiometric resin blood culture system, Bactec, after 8 days of incubation, although some nonresin Bactec bottles took as long as 28 and 42 days of incubation.

Aliquots of blood of 2–4 ml can be taken from any positive automated blood culture bottle and directly cultured, but Isolator-tube lysed preparations of blood culture blood, as described previously, is preferred. Inoculate two fresh chocolate and two fresh TSA with 5% sheep blood agar plates. The plates should be allowed to absorb the blood and then can be incubated in high humidity of about 80% at 36 °C in an atmosphere of 5% $CO_2$ for 2 h before sealing. Plates should then be sealed with Shrink Seals (Scientific Device Laboratory, Glenview, Ill., USA) to prevent drying during incubation. All plates should be examined daily for the first week, then twice weekly for 1.5 months or, until growth is evident. Both horse and rabbit blood have been reported to be superior supplements compared to sheep blood [20, 29] but in our hands any of these bloods proved satisfactory as long as plates are made fresh. Additionally, it is wise to supplement blood agar media with both hemin (250 mg/ml) and 6–8% Fildes reagent [29].

Isolator tubes contain sodium polyanethosulfonate, an anticoagulant, and saponin, a lytic agent that causes lysis of erythrocytes and leukocytes. It has been reported that *B. henselae* are intracellular inside RBCs [27, 30] as well as epicellular, and, thus, such organisms will be liberated upon lysis. A recent report [31] compared the effect of prolonged freezing on blood from *B. henselae* bacteremias using Isolator versus conventional EDTA blood collection tubes. The authors used blood specimens from *B. henselae*-infected cats collecting both EDTA and Isolator blood lysis tubes which were subsequently plated onto rabbit blood BHI agar using three different schedules: plating immediately, plating after 24 h at 25 °C, and plating after 26 days at 65 °C. In both cases (Isolator or EDTA tubes), frozen blood yielded higher numbers of *B. henselae* colonies compared to room temperature or immediate plating. The frozen EDTA tubes however, were clearly superior to frozen Isolator tubes and the authors speculated that collecting blood in tubes containing EDTA and subsequent freezing may further improve the detection of *B. henselae* [31], because *Bartonella* appear to be more sensitive to the Isolator components than it is to EDTA after freezing.

When growth does appear, it generally does not appear on semisolid media until about the third week. Small, flat or raised, dry, off-white adherent colonies will be seen on chocolate or supplemented TSA blood agar [1]. Growth is heterogeneous with respect to size and consistency. Colonies can exhibit a 'smooth and rough', as well as 'large and small' appearance. Numerous colonies are only pinpoint in size while others are several millimeters in diameter. When colonies are removed from agar, an imprint with a peripheral identation should be clearly evident [27]. In our experience, only 66% of 'positive' blood cultures grew *B. henselae* on semisolid agar. Growth can take up to 49 days before appearing and rarely at 7 days' incubation [32]. Chances of isolating *B. henselae* from blood after antibiotic therapy has begun are greatly reduced. If blood culture bottles are tilted to one side, colonies adherent to the other surface of glass may be observed. There is no typical turbidity associated with the growth of *B. henselae* in broth culture.

*Culture from Tissue*

Isolation of *B. henselae* from BA lesions has not been successful and attempts at such culture is not productive. The optimal bacteriological culture conditions for growth of *B. henselae* are listed in table 4. The greatest success in culturing *B. henselae* has come with use of specimen types such as blood, spleen or lymph. *Bartonella* species have been reported recovered by directly plating ground-up tissue specimens onto agar media but such recovery is not very efficient. To my knowledge, there has been only one strain of *B. henselae* from a patient with BA lesions that grew by such a direct plating technique [21]. However, this report is unclear as to the time origin of the culture source (i.e. BA lesion and/or spleen).

While *B. quintana* organisms can be isolated from cutaneous lesions by cocultivation with endothelial cell monolayer as described by Koehler et al.

*Table 4.* Optimal cultural conditions for growth of *B. henselae*

| |
|---|
| Freshly prepared TSA, BHI, Brucella blood agars, or chocolate agar |
| Supplemented with 250 μg/ml hemin and 8% Fildes solution |
| $pCO_2 \cong 5\%$ |
| Humidity $\cong$ 80% |
| Temperature 36 °C |
| Incubation time up to 49 days |

[21], *B. henselae* cannot. Biopsy material was washed, minced and then homogenized. These authors then inoculated CPA bovine endothelial cell monolayers with tissue homogenates, incubated at 36 °C in the presence of 6% $CO_2$ and 85% humidity in sterile candle jars until *B. quintana* growth was evident as determined by turbidity. This technique has failed to grow *B. henselae.*

*Fatty-Acid Methyl Esters (FAME) Analysis*

Whole cell fatty acids of the organisms can be analyzed as FAME by gas chromatography as previously reported [16]. Bacteria should be harvested from either 6-week-old growth in TSB or BHI broth or agar supplemented with 6–8% Fildes enrichment and hemin (250 μg/ml). Numerical data should also be performed, resulting in a dendrogram which shows the euclidean distance among strains and related species. *B. henselae* isolates should be characterized by the presence of major amounts of C18:1, C18:0 and C16:0; only *B. bacilliformis* yields >15% of C16:1 [16, 20].

*Immunofluorescence (IF) Slide Technique*

Slides can be made by air drying one drop of concentrated lysed blood culture broth from an Isolator at room temperature [27]. Once slides are prepared, goat antisera (1:1,000 dilution) should be applied and the mixtures should be incubated for 30 min at 37 °C in a moist chamber. The slides should be twice washed with PBS followed by preabsorption with rabbit serum for 30 min at 37 °C again followed by a PBS wash. Rabbit anti-goat immunoglobulin G-fluorescein isothiocyanate conjugate (1:50) can then be added, and the mixtures should be incubated for 30 min at 37 °C in a moist chamber. The slides can be twice washed with PBS. After air drying, the slides should be prepared with buffered glycerol mounting medium (pH 7.2) and coverslipped for examination by epifluorescence microscopy. Goat antiserum raised against *B. henselae*, which was first preabsorbed with rabbit antisera before adding rabbit anti-goat conjugate (Sigma, St. Louis, Mo., USA), can yield IF with *B. henselae* strains at dilutions of 1:1,000. Thus, identification of *B. henselae* can be confirmed as shown in figure 3. At the same dilution of 1:1,000, the

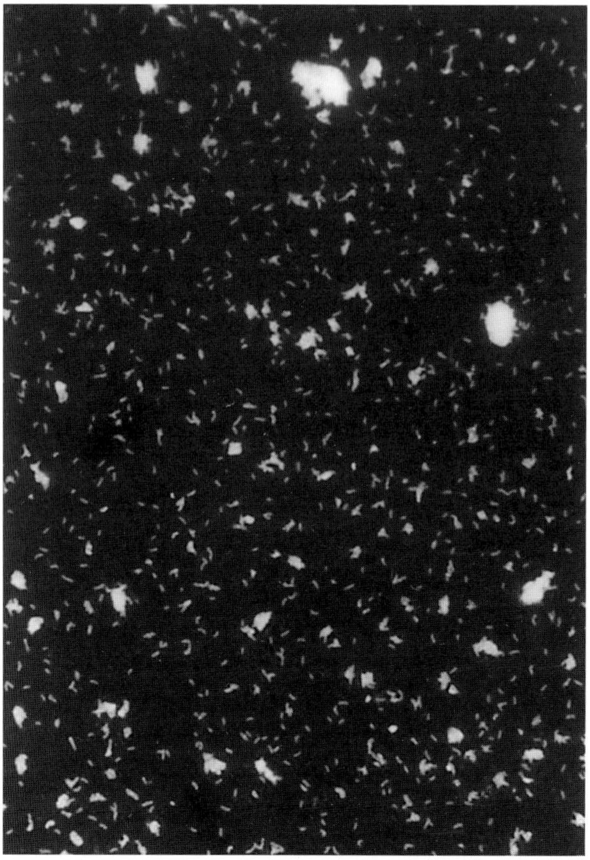

*Fig. 3.* Identification confirmation of *B. henselae* by direct immunofluorescence technique.

goat antiserum raised against *B. quintana* usually yields no fluorescence, or less fluorescence on the same isolates. For some strains, higher dilutions may be necessary in order to differentiate *B. henselae* from *B. quintana* [27]. However, at a dilution of 1:1,000, *B. quintana* is cross-reactive with *B. henselae.* As has been previously reported [13], both *B. henselae* and *B. quintana* antisera react with *Staphylococcus aureus* at the 1:1,000 dilution, likely because of nonspecific bonding of IgG to *S. aureus* protein A. However, staphylococci can easily be ruled out by morphology.

*Immunoperoxidase Slide Technique*

A variation of the IF detection technique was first reported by Dipasquale et al. [33]. Slides can be prepared as described above for the IF assay. Once slides are prepared, human antisera (Linmed Biologies, Calif., USA) diluted 1:20

should be applied and the mixture should be incubated in a sealed moist chamber at room temperature for 30 min [33], after which slides should be removed from the moist chamber and rinsed gently with PBS, then placed in a Coplin jar for at least two changes of PBS for no less than 5 min each time. Return slide to moist chamber and apply peroxidase-conjugated anti-human IgG (dilution 1:200, Sigma) to well. Incubate 30 min at room temperature, then rinse. Prepare detection solution (diaminobenzidine (DAB) and $H_2O_2$/urea; Sigma). Apply detection solution to well and incubate in dark for approximately 10 min. Stop reaction with PBS and counterstain with hematoxylin, dehydrate through ascending alcohol washes (75–100%), dip in xylene then mount with Permount and coverslip. Positive signal is dark brown granular precipitate in cytoplasm. Such a positive reaction confirms presence of *Bartonella* species.

*Polymerase Chain Reaction*

Regnery et al. [24] developed a specific PCR assay that detects DNA sequencing of both *B. henselae* and *B. quintana* in tissue. While PCR technology is useful in that, this technique can identify bacteria that cannot be grown, though PCR is not yet common to some clinical microbiology laboratories. A variety of oligonucleotide primers can be used to amplify the 16S-23S rRNA spacer regions of bacterial DNA present in clinical samples [18, 20, 24]. In general, after PCR amplification is completed, *Bartonella*-specific oligonucleotide probes can be used. The $5^1$-biotinylated oligonucleotide probe, specific for *Bartonella*, can be used to detect type-specific *Bartonella* PCR products. Relman et al. [12] designed PCR primers to amplify the 241-bp fragment from the 16S rRNA gene. These primers were designed before the sequence of the 16S rRNA gene was available for members of genus *Bartonella* other than *B. quintana*. Many complex PCR methodologies are currently available [18, 20, 24, 34] which are too numerous to delineate in this chapter.

## Serologic Detection

Certainly serologic detection of *Bartonella* specific antibodies for the diagnosis of *B. henselae* infection is advantageous because it avoids the excessive incubation time necessary for culture, or, the complexity of PCR analysis. The following are three typical serologic methods for detecting anti-*Bartonella* antibodies.

*Indirect Immunofluorescent Antibody Assay (IFA)*

Indirect immunoassay for *Bartonella*-specific antibodies is based upon the detection of an antigen-antibody complex in an appropriate test medium.

This principle is represented by the immunofluorescent antibody method introduced by Weller et al. [35], and further developed by Riggs et al. [36]. The principle of the immunofluorescent antibody procedure follows two basic reaction steps:

*Step 1*: Human serum is reacted with the antigenic substrate. Antibodies, if present, will bind to the antigen forming stable antigen-antibody complexes. If no antibodies are present, the complexes will not be formed and serum components will be washed away.

Six- or 12-well slide containing a cell culture infected with *B. henselae*. Each reaction well will contain between 10 and 50% infected cells mixed with uninfected cells. Therefore, only 10–50% of the cells will exhibit the specific fluorescent staining pattern. The uninfected cells serve as negative control cells, and as a control for nonspecific staining due to the presence of autoantibodies in the serum sample.

*Step 2*: Fluorescein-labeled antihuman IgG or IgM antibody is added to the reaction site, which will react with the antigen-antibody complexes formed in step 1. A positive staining reaction is typified by a bright apple-green fluorescence when viewed with a properly equipped fluorescence microscope. If no complexes are formed in step 1, the fluorescein-labeled antibody will be washed away exhibiting a negative staining result.

It is important to understand the generic limitations of the IFA procedure: (1) Serological test results should be used in conjunction with information available from the clinical evaluation and other diagnostic information. (2) A negative test result does not necessarily rule out current or recent infection. The specimen may have been collected too early in the disease before demonstrable antibody is present. (3) Antinuclear antibodies (ANA) present in serum may interfere with the IFA test. They can be differentiated from the specific antigen staining in that ANA will stain the nucleus of both infected and uninfected cells. However, the specific *Bartonella* antibodies will exhibit staining only in the infected cells [35–37].

*Immunoperoxidase Antibody Assay (IPA)*

IPA is in reality a modification of the IFA technique substituting immunoperoxidase staining of *B. henselae*-infected Hep-2 cells in order to detect either IgG or IgM titers in serum [33]. This procedure, first reported by Dipasquale et al. [33], utilizes the same infected slides as for IFA, the difference being the use of peroxidase-conjugated goat anti-human IgG or IgM sera and the appropriate staining reagents must be used (i.e. $H_2O_2$/urea/DAB). In addition, counterstaining with hematoxylin provides appropriate contrast. These slides are permanent unlike those from the IFA procedure. Our [33] detailed methodology follows.

Bion 12-well *B. henselae* antigen slides (Cat. No. BH-1612) are used. These slides have 12 wells covered with Hep-2 cells infected by *B. henselae*, which is detectable in approximately 20% of the cells. For IgM determination, sera were pretreated with GullSorb at 1:10 final dilution to remove any IgG interference. Twofold dilutions of dilutions of the pretreated sera (1:20, 1:40, 1:80, etc.) were then prepared. The test slides were allowed to equilibrate at room temperature before opening the sealed package. The appropriately diluted serum was then added to each well, without touching the antigen surface with the pipette tip. For IgG determination, the slides were incubated in a sealed moist chamber at room temperature for 30 min. For IgM determination, the substrate slides were incubated at 35–37 °C for 90 min. The slides were then removed from the moist chamber and rinsed gently with PBS and placed in a Coplin jar for at least two changes of PBS for no less than 5 min each time. The slides were removed one at a time from the jar and the excess PBS was shaken off. The slides were returned to the moist chamber and the appropriate peroxidase-conjugated goat anti-human IgM or IgG antibody was added to each well of the slide. For IgG detection, the incubation was 30 min in the moist chamber at room temperature, whereas for IgM detection it lasted for 60 min at 35–37 °C. At the end of the incubation, the slides were removed from the moist chamber, rinsed and washed.

The detection DAB solution was prepared just prior to use. In addition, $H_2O_2$/urea tablets were used. The detection solution was protected from direct light. A drop of the solution was added to each well and the slides were incubated in the dark for approximately 10 min. The intensity of the staining of the positive control was checked at the microscope and the reaction was stopped with PBS when appropriate. The slides were counterstained with hematoxylin, dehydrated through ascending alcohol washes (75–100%), dipped in xylene and mounted with Permount and coverslip. Positive signal is a dark brown granular precipitate in the cytoplasm of approximately 10–20% of cells, identifying intracytoplasmic *B. henselae* bacteria. The positive titer was given by the last dilution which showed positive cytoplasmic stain.

In general, the sensitivity of IPA is superior to IFA since the IPA slides can be examined more completely and thoroughly, and because they are permanent preps that do not fade out as it occurs with the IFA procedure.

*Enzyme Immunoassay (EIA)*

Extracted proteins from *B. henselae* can be applied to flat-bottom wells of microtiter plates as described by Slater et al. [38]. Patient antisera can be applied in desired dilutions. After appropriate incubation and washes, anti-human IgG or IgM-alkaline phosphatase conjugate (Sigma) can be applied. Color development is determined by addition of *p*-nitrophenol phosphate. Optical density can be read using an automated reader.

While the EIA procedure is more or less a variation of the standard EIA, both IPA and IFA are the preferred serologic methods since infected cells can be observed and thusly nonspecific cross-reactions can be minimized, if not eliminated.

## References


1 Stoler MH, Bonfiglio TA, Steigbigel RT, Pereira M: An atypical subcutaneous infection associated with acquired immune deficiency syndrome. Am J Clin Pathol 1983;80:714–718.

2 Cockerell CJ, Whitlow MA, Webster GF, Friedman-Kien AE: Epithelioid angiomatosis: A distinct vascular disorder in patients with the acquired immunodeficiency syndrome or AIDS-related complex. Lancet 1987;ii:654–656.

3 LeBoit PE, Berger TG, Egbert BM, Yet TS, Stoler MH, Bonfiglio TA, Strauchen JA, English CK, Wear DJ: Epithelioid hemangioma-like vascular proliferation in AIDS: Manifestation of cat scratch disease bacillus infection? Lancet 1988;i:960–963.

4 Koehler JE, LeBoit PE, Egbert BM, Berger TG: Cutaneous vascular lesions and disseminated cat scratch disease in patients with the acquired immunodeficiency syndrome (AIDS) and AIDS-related complex. Ann Intern Med 1988;109:449–455.

5 Angritt P, Tuur SM, Macher AM, Smith KJ, Park SC, Hobin F, Myrie-Williams C: Case for diagnosis. Milit Med 1988;153:M26–M32.

6 Angritt P, Tuur SM, Macher AM, Smith KJ, Park CS, Hobin F, Myrie-Williams C: Epithelioid angiomatosis in HIV infection: Neoplasm or cat scratch disease? (letter) Lancet 1988;i:996.

7 Hall AV, Roberts CM, Maurice PD, McClean KA, Shousha S: Cat scratch disease in patients with AIDS: Atypical manifestations (letter). Lancet 1988;ii:453–454.

8 Knobler EH, Silvers DN, Fine KC, Lefkowitch JH, Grossman ME: Unique skin lesions associated with human immunodeficiency virus. JAMA 1988;260:524–527.

9 Scholssberg D, Morad Y, Krouse TB, Wear DJ, English CK: Culture-proved disseminated cat scratch disease in acquired immunodeficiency syndrome. Arch Intern Med 1989;149:1437–1439.

10 Cockerell CJ, Bergstresser PR, Myrie-Williams C, Tierno PM: Bacillary epithelioid angiomatosis occurring in an immunocompetent individual. Arch Dermatol 1990;126:787–790.

11 Tappero JW, Koehler JE, Berger TG, Cockerell CJ, Lee TH, Busch MP, Sites DP, Mohle-Bostani J, Reingold AL, LeBoit PE: Bacillary angiomatosis and bacillary splenitis in immunocompetent adults. Ann Intern Med 1993;118:363–365.

12 Relman DA, Louitit JS, Schmidt TM, Falkow S, Tomkins LS: The agent of bacillary angiomatosis: An approach to the identification of uncultured pathogens. N Engl J Med 1990;323:1573–1580.

13 Slater LN, Welch DF, Hensel D, Coody DW: A newly recognized fastidious gram-negative pathogen as a cause of fever and bacteremia. N Engl J Med 1990;323:1587–1593.

14 Regnery RL, Anderson BE, Clarridge JE, Rodriguez-Barradas MC, Jones DC, Carr JH: Characterization of a novel *Rochalimaea* species, *R. henselae* sp nov, isolated from the blood of a febrile human immunodeficiency virus-positive patient. J Clin Microbiol 1992;30:265–274.

15 Koehler JE, Glaser CA, Tappero JW: *R. henselae* infection: A new zoonosis with the domestic cat as reservoir. JAMA 1994;271:531–535.

16 Cockerell CJ, Tierno PM, Friedman-Kien AE, Kim KS: Clinical histologic, microbiologic, and biochemical characterization of the causative agent of BEA: A rickettsial illness with features of bartonellosis. J Invest Dermatol 1991;97:812–817.

17 Garcia FU, Wojta J, Broadly KN: *Bartonella bacilliformis* stimulates endothelial cells in vitro and is angiogenic in vivo. Am J Pathol 1990;136:1125–1129.

18 Maurin M, Raoul D: *Bartonella quintana* infections. Clin Microbiol Rev 1996;9:273–292.

19 Baker JA: A rickettsial infection in Canadian voles. J Exp Med 1946;84:37–51.

20 Welch DF, Pickett DA, Slater LN: *Rochalimaea henselae* sp nov, a cause of septicemia, bacillary angiomatosis, and parenchymal peliosis. J Clin Microbial 1992;30:275–280.

21 Koehler JE, Quinn FD, Berger TG: Isolation of *Rochalimaea* species from cutaneous and osseous lesions of bacillary angiomatosis. N Engl J Med 1990;327:1625–1631.
22 Perkocha LA, Grenahan SM, Yen TSB: Clinical and pathological features of bacillary peliosis hepatitis in association with HIV infection. N Engl J Med 1990;323:1581–1586.
23 Wech DF, Hensel DM, Pickett DA: Bacteremia due to isolates in the clinical laboratory. J Clin Microbiol 1993;32:2381–2386.
24 Regnery RL, Anderson BE, Clarridge JE: Characterization of a novel *Rochalimaea* species, *R. henselae* sp nov isolated from blood of a febrile, human immunodeficiency virus-positive patient. J Clin Microbiol 1992;30:265–274.
25 Larson AM, Dougherty MY, Nowowiejski DJ: Detection of *Bartonella (Rochalimaea) quintana* by routine acridine orange staining of broth blood cultures. J Clin Microbiol 1994;32:1492–1496.
26 Spach DH, Calhs KP, Poaw DS: Endocarditis caused by *R. quintana* on a patient infected with HIV. J Clin Microbiol 1993;31:692–694.
27 Tierno PM, Inglima K, Parisi MT: Detection of *Bartonella henselae* bacteremia using BacT/Alert Blood Culture System. Am J Clin Pathol 1995;104:530–536.
28 Birtles RJ, Harrison TG, Saunders NA, Molyneux DH: Proposals to unify the genera *Grahamella* and *Bartonella*. Int J Syst Bacteriol 1995;45:1–8.
29 Swartzman WA, Nesbit CA, Baron EJ: Development and evaluation of blood free medium for determining growth curves and optimizing growth of *B. henselae*. J Clin Microbiol 1993;31:1882–1885.
30 Breitschwerdt EB, Kordick DL: Intraerythrocytic presence of *Bartonella henselae*. J Clin Microbiol 1995;33:1655–1656.
31 Brenner SA, Rooney JA, Manzewitsch P, Regnery RL: Isolation of *Bartonella henselae*: Effects of methods of blood collection and handling. J Clin Microbiol 1997;35:544–547.
32 Hensel DM, Slates LN: The genus *Bartonella*. Clin Microbiol Newslett 1995;17:9–14.
33 Dipasquale B, McMeeking AA, Cadet-Legros J, Tierno PM: IgM and IgG antibody titers to *B. henselae* in HIV-positive and healthy individuals in New York City area. Proc Am Soc Microbiol, 1997, vol 97, p 294.
34 O'Connor SP, Dorsch M, Stergerwalt AG, Brenner DJ, Stakebrandt E: 16S RNA sequences of *Bartonella bacilliformis* and CSD bacillus reveal phylogenetic relationships with alpha-Z subgroup of class Proteobacteria. J Clin Microbiol 1991;29:2144–2150.
35 Weller TH, Coons AH: Fluorescent antibody studies with agents of varicella and herpes zoster propagated in vitro. Proc Soc Exp Biol Med 1954;88:789–794.
36 Riggs JL, Siewald RJ, Burckhalter JH, Downs CM, Metcalf TG: Isothiocyanate compounds as fluorescent labeling agents for immune serum. Am J Pathol 1959;34:1081–1097.
37 Holborow EJ, Weir DM, Johnson GD: A serum factor in lupus erythematosus with affinity for tissue nuclei. Br Med J 1957;11:732–734.
38 Slater LN, Coody DW, Woobridge LK, Welch DF: Murine antibody responses distinguish *R. henselae* from *R. quintana*. J Clin Microbiol 1992;30:1722–1727.

Dr. Philip M. Tierno, Jr., New York University Medical Center, Tisch Hospital,
560 First Avenue, Microbiology Department – Room H374, New York, NY 10016 (USA)
Tel. (212) 263 5905, Fax (212) 263 7922

Schmidt A (ed): *Bartonella* and *Afipia* Species Emphasizing *Bartonella henselae*.
Contrib Microbiol. Basel, Karger, 1998, vol 1, pp 130–142

# New Approaches in Molecular Diagnostics of Human Infections Caused by *Bartonella henselae*

*Daniel Goldenberger, Martin Altwegg*

Department of Medical Microbiology, University of Zürich, Switzerland

## Introduction

It is now firmly established that *Bartonella henselae* represents one of the agents causing bacillary angiomatosis (BA; in addition to at least *B. quintana*) and that it is the primary, if not sole, causative agent of cat scratch disease (CSD) [1, 2]. However, this organism was not known until 1990 when Relman et al. [3] used the broad-spectrum polymerase chain reaction (PCR) to amplify 16S rRNA gene fragments directly from tissue samples of patients with BA. Sequencing of these fragments revealed that they belonged to a previously uncharacterized microorganism now known as *B. henselae*, which was most closely related to *Rochalimaea* (now *Bartonella*) *quintana*. Later on, the organism was successfully cultured but even today molecular techniques play a major role not only for the detection and identification but also for epidemiological studies of human infections caused by this organism [4–9].

In this chapter, we will summarize molecular approaches used for the detection and identification of *B. henselae* directly from clinical specimens whereas the methods used for identification and subtyping of isolates will be mentioned only very briefly. In addition, available gene sequences of this organism will be presented in view of their potential as new targets for molecular assays.

## Direct Detection of *B. henselae* DNA in Clinical Specimens

Isolation of *B. henselae* is typically time-consuming, requires up to 6 weeks' incubation and often fails when applied to clinical samples such as lymph node biopsies or aspirates [2]. In this context, molecular detection and identification of *B. henselae* directly from clinical specimens promises to be a specific and rapid alternative. It has been applied in only few studies all of them using the PCR followed by identification either by hybridization with a specific probe or by sequencing. Main target genes were the 16S rRNA gene [3] and the *htrA* gene of *B. henselae* [6]. In the absence of reliable cultures, molecular results are usually compared with serological findings.

### The 16S Ribosomal rRNA Gene as Target Molecule

In the pioneering work of Relman et al. [3] using broad-spectrum PCR amplification of the 16S rRNA gene with universal primers, tissue from 3 unrelated patients yielded a unique 16S gene sequence belonging to a previously uncharacterized microorganism. A sequence obtained from a fourth patient with BA differed from the other sequences at 4 of 241 base positions. Based on the sequence of a 480-bp-long fragment, specific primers p24E and p12B were designed to allow amplification of a 296-bp fragment. Sequencing the entire 16S rRNA gene from tissue mentioned above and comparing it to the sequence of *R. henselae* sp. nov., an organism cultivated from the blood of a febrile HIV-seropositive patient, provided evidence that these sequences were most probably derived from the same organism [4, 10].

The application of the same molecular methodology as described by Relman et al. [3] led to the identification of *B. henselae* DNA in the liver of a French patient with bacillary peliosis hepatis [11]. Warthin-Starry silver staining of a liver section showed clumps of bacilli. After broad-spectrum amplification of the 16S rRNA gene a 480-bp fragment was sequenced and was identical to that reported for *B. henselae*. Similarly, Hadfield et al. [12] for the first time identified *B. henselae* DNA in a patient with culture-negative infective endocarditis. On the resected aortic and tricuspid valves, small, pleomorphic Gram-negative rods were seen in Brown-Hopps tissue Gram stain and Warthin-Starry silver stains. The 176-bp sequence determined exactly matched the sequence reported by Relman et al. [3].

The broad-spectrum PCR approach was again used to demonstrate the presence of *B. henselae*-specific DNA in fine needle aspirates of axillary lymph nodes as well as in blood leukocytes in an Australian patient with CSD [13]. While the organism was successfully cultured from the blood and fleas of the incriminated cat, cultures of blood leukocytes and lymph nodes of the patient remained negative even after incubation for 6 weeks. The diagnosis was confirmed by a *B. henselae*-specific IgG titer of 1:1,024 in the patient's serum.

Evidence for the role of *B. henselae* as cause of CSD was also provided when skin test antigens prepared from purulent lymph node material aspirated from patients with CSD were analyzed by broad-spectrum PCR and sequencing [14]. Two independent sources of antigens yielded DNA sequences (>700 bp) with 99.7 and 100% similarity to 5′-half of the 16S rRNA gene sequence of *B. henselae.* The next most closely related organisms were *B. quintana* and *B. bacilliformis* with homologies between 99.5 and 98.3%, whereas *Afipia felis* was only distantly related (homologies <88%). These authors also used the *B. henselae*-specific primers previously described by Relman et al. [3]. In their hand these primers were nonspecific, reacting with all other *Rochalimaea* (now *Bartonella* species) and *B. bacilliformis.*

Only rarely the 3′-half of the 16S rRNA gene has been a target for the detection of uncultured microorganisms. Using the broad-spectrum primers previously described by Wilson et al. [15], opportunistic lung infection due to *B. henselae* was demonstrated in a renal transplantation patient with depressed cell-mediated immunity [16]. The sequence derived was identical to that of *B. henselae* and the diagnosis was confirmed histologically (clusters of bacilli in Warthin-Starry silver stains) and serologically (high antibody titers against *B. henselae, B. quintana* and *B. elizabethae*). In contrast to PCR, serological investigations did not reveal which of the *Bartonella* species was involved. Again, blood cultures (done with use of lysis-centrifugation tubes) from 8 of the patient's many cats were positive while no organisms were recovered from the patient. These negative cultures, however, may be explained by the fact that no special culture conditions for *Bartonella* had been used for the clinical specimens.

To determine the role of *Bartonella* species in CSD, Bergmans et al. [17] used the specific primers proposed by Relman et al. [3]. They successfully amplified *B. henselae, B. quintana* and *B. bacilliformis*, but only the *B. henselae* and *B. quintana* products hybridized with their *Bartonella*-specific probe RHENS. Among a total of 226 clinical samples of patients with suspected CSD, 167 were PCR-positive. Furthermore, to determine whether *B. henselae* was the predominant species present, DNA from 8 of these specimens was subjected to broad-spectrum PCR followed by sequencing. The 5′-third (nucleotides 8–575 according to the *Escherichia coli* numbering) of the 16S rRNA gene was amplified. Analysis of the partial 16S rRNA gene sequences revealed two types. One type (6 specimens) was identical to the *B. henselae* sequence described by Regnery et al. [4], accession No. M73229, and the other type (2 samples) had sequences identical to the reference sequence of a patient with BA, accession No. Z11684 [10]. In a follow-up study from the same laboratory, a PCR assay was developed to detect these two 16S rRNA gene variants of *B. henselae* without the need of sequencing [18] (fig. 1). PCR using type-

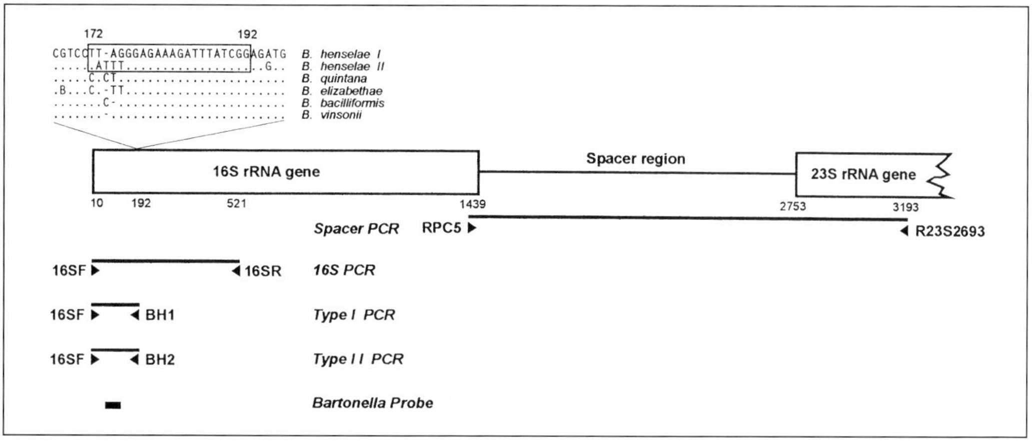


*Fig. 1.* Schematic presentation of the 16S rRNA gene, intergenic spacer region, and part of the 23S rRNA gene of *B. henselae* and positions of the primers and probe used for eubacterial and *B. henselae*-specific 16S rRNA gene PCR, eubacterial 16S-23S rRNA spacer PCR, and hybridization. The sequence of the type-specific part of the *B. henselae* 16S rRNA gene is shown and is aligned with homologous sequences of relevant *Bartonella* species. The boxed regions on the *B. henselae* type I and type II represent the target sequences for primers BH1 and BH2, respectively. Reproduced from Bergmans et al. [18], with permission.

specific primers on 41 clinical specimens known to contain *Bartonella* DNA identified 32 of type I and 7 of type II, whereas 2 specimens were negative with either primer set. In addition, restriction endonuclease analysis of the PCR-amplified 16S-23S rRNA gene spacer region was also used to investigate the prevalence of *B. henselae* variants. A 100% correlation was found between the *Alu*I spacer restriction fragment length polymorphism (RFLP) pattern and the 16S rRNA typing. The authors explain these findings with two simultaneous mutational events, one in the 16S rRNA gene and one in the 16S-23S rRNA spacer region.

Independently from the study of Bergmans et al. [17], we have used a very similar approach to analyze two lymph nodes and one subcutaneous biopsy which had been shown to contain *B. henselae* DNA using a *htrA* gene-based PCR assay (see below) [7]. The broad-spectrum primers used allowed the amplification of a fragment of about 800 bp (corresponding to nucleotides 8–806 according to the *E. coli* numbering). After semi-nested reamplification resulting in a fragment of about 525 bp, direct single-strand sequencing was performed. The alignment of the three partial 16S rRNA gene sequences revealed exactly the same variations as described by Bergmans et al. [17]. Because we were also interested in the distribution of the two variants, a

*Table 1.* Results of *B. henselae* type-specific PCR of *B. henselae*-DNA containing clinical specimens and *B. henselae* isolates from cats

| | Box et al. [19] | | Bergmans et al. [18] | |
|---|---|---|---|---|
| | type I | type II | type I | type II |
| *Clinical specimens* | | | | |
| Switzerland | 5 | 28 | | |
| Germany | 0 | 2 | | |
| USA | 4 | 0 | | |
| The Netherlands | | | 32 | 7 |
| *Cat isolates* | | | | |
| Switzerland | 0 | 2 | | |
| Germany | 0 | 15 | | |
| USA | 0 | 2 | | |

collection of human clinical samples known to contain *B. henselae* DNA and a collection of *B. henselae* strains cultured from cats was analyzed using the type-specific PCR system [18, 19].

In contrast to The Netherlands, the majority of the clinical specimens (25 of 34) and all 19 *B. henselae* strains from cats were type II (table 1). Our hypothesis, therefore, was that only type II variant is cat-associated whereas infections by *B. henselae* type I may have another yet unknown epidemiologic reservoir but this needs further confirmation [19]. Whether or not there are differences in the clinical presentations of patients infected with type I and II, respectively, is currently being evaluated. Occasionally, type-specific PCR was strongly positive for one type and very weakly positive for the other type (fig. 2, specimen 33). It is not clear whether this represents true double infections or just some nonspecific amplifications in the presence of large amounts of target DNA.

Dauga et al. [20] did not use 16S rRNA gene-based broad-spectrum but branch-specific primers for the $\alpha$ subgroup of *Proteobacteria* of which *B. henselae* is a member. Applying this PCR amplification system to clinical specimens from patients with *Bartonella*-associated infections, three different 16S rRNA gene sequences (1,210 bp) were identified: one corresponded exactly to accession number M73229 (*B. henselae*), the second was related to, but distinct from, Z11684 (referred to as *B. henselae* variant), and a third sequence was identical to M73228 (*B. quintana*). To speed up identification and to reduce costs of analysis, a nested amplification method for *B. henselae* and *B. quintana* was devised. DNA extracted from 30 unfixed lymph node biopsies,

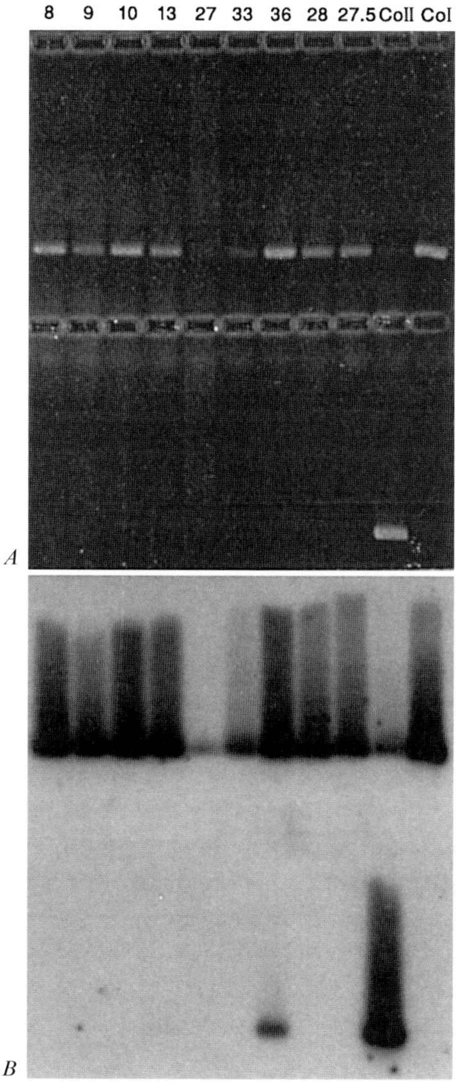


*Fig. 2.* Analysis of products of type-I and type-II specific PCRs (I and II) from clinical specimens 8, 9, 10, 13, 27, 33, 36, 28, 27, 5; specimen 27 diluted 1:5; Co II and Co I, type-specific positive controls. Agarose gel electrophoresis (*A*) and Southern blots hybridized with *Bartonella*-specific digoxigenin-labeled oligonucleotide probe (*B*). Adapted from Box et al. [19].

36 node pus samples, and 2 liver biopsies from patients with suspected CSD and 17 skin biopsies from AIDS patients with suspected BA were analyzed using this technique. *B. henselae* or *B. henselae* variant DNA were found in 42 (62%) of 68 samples from suspected CSD patients. *B. quintana* was not associated with CSD, but a *B. quintana* sequence was found in 7 (41%) of 17 samples from suspected BA patients. *B. henselae* DNA was not detected in BA specimens.

## The *htrA* Gene of *B. henselae* as Target Molecule

Another approach to identify specific gene sequences that might provide a basis for the molecular detection and identification of *B. henselae* was chosen by Anderson et al. [6]. Based on a genomic library in the vector λ ZAPII, a clone expressing a 60-kDa antigen reactive with rabbit anti-*B. henselae* serum was isolated, and the gene was sequenced. The deduced amino acid sequence was shown to have 59 and 37% homology with the HtrA stress-response protein from *Brucella abortus* and *E. coli*, respectively [6, 21]. Based on this sequence, the two primers CAT1 and CAT2 amplifying a 414-bp fragment from both *B. henselae* and *B. quintana* but not from *B. elizabethae* and *B. vinsonii* was deduced. The two species could then easily be separated by dot-blot hybridization using species-specific digoxigenin-labeled oligonucleotide probes differing in 4/20 nucleotides. This two-step assay was applied to DNA extracted from 16 fresh lymph node biopsy specimens and 9 aspirates from patients with clinical CSD, most of them with a positive serology. Twenty-one of the 25 lymph node samples (84%) were positive for *B. henselae*, while none were positive for *B. quintana*. This study showed that *B. henselae*, but not *B. quintana*, plays a central role in the etiology of CSD.

The above PCR assay has subsequently been used successfully for diagnostic applications. *B. henselae* DNA but not *B. quintana* or *A. felis* DNA was detected in the purulent material from lymph nodes in 3 children with clinical CSD [8]. All of these patients had significant antibody titers for *B. henselae* (1:64 to 1:1,024) and *B. quintana* using an indirect fluorescent antibody (IFA) test while the 2 control patients were PCR-negative in conjunction with IFA titers <1:32.

Similarly, disseminated CSD involving various organs was reported in a 9-year-old immunocompetent boy [22]. Again, elevated antibody titers to both *B. henselae* and *B. quintana* were present while PCR from the biopsied osteolytic lesion in conjunction with species-specific hybridization was positive only for *B. henselae* and not for *B. quintana*.

Using an assay essentially identical to that of Anderson et al. [6] except for replacing dot-blot by Southern blot hybridization (fig. 3), 33 clinical samples and 6 controls were investigated [9]. For proven cases of CSD as judged by a combination of clinical suspicion, histological and serological results, the sensitivity was 61%. This relatively low value may be explained by the fact that 13/18 of these samples were fixed, paraffin-embedded tissue specimens with partly degraded DNA [23]. On the other hand, *B. quintana* DNA was demonstrated in a biopsy specimen of a HIV-positive patient with subcutaneous lesions for whom the serology remained negative. Reliable differentiation between *B. henselae* and *B. quintana* was also achieved using a commercially

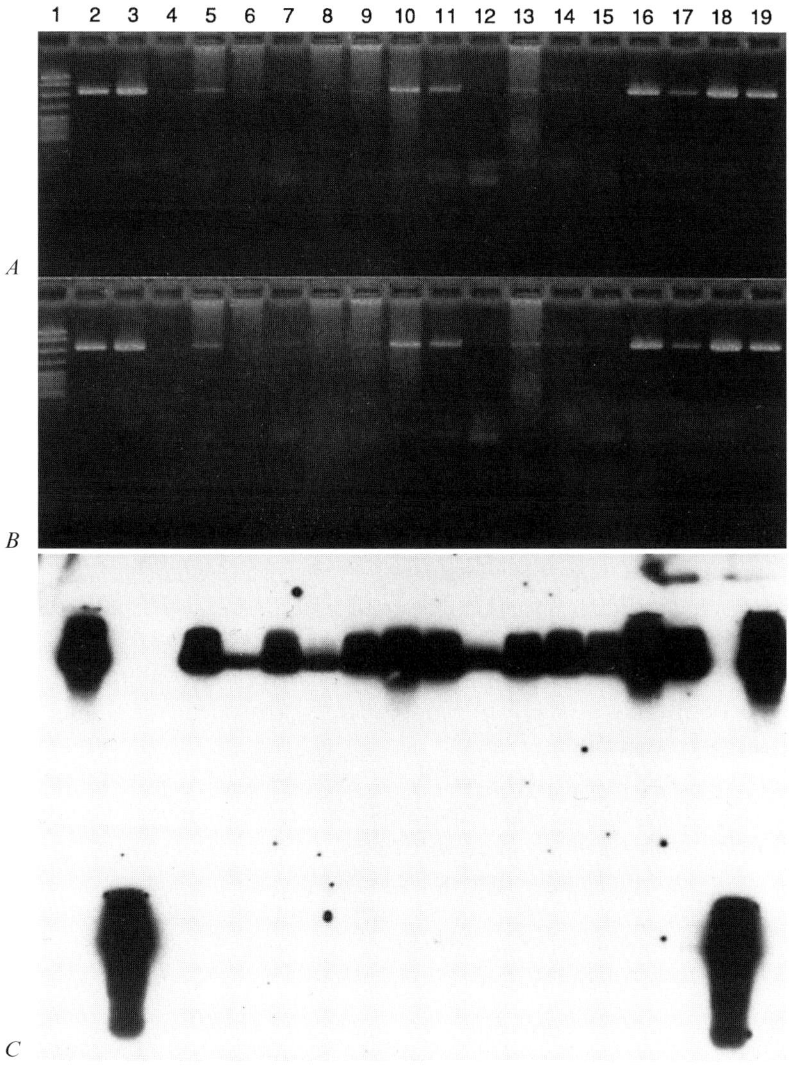


*Fig. 3.* Analysis of PCR products from clinical samples of patients with suspicion of *Bartonella*-associated infection. Agarose gel electrophoresis (*A*) and Southern blots hybridized with *B. henselae*-specific (*B*) and *B. quintana*-specific (*C*) digoxigenin-labeled oligonucleotide probe. Lane 1, molecular weight marker with DNA fragments of 622, 527, 404, 307, 242 bp and several smaller fragments; lanes 2 and 19, *B. henselae*, positive control; lanes 3 and 18, *B. quintana*, positive control; lane 4, negative control; lanes 5–17, clinical samples. Reproduced from Goldenberger et al. [9], with permission.

available, generic enzyme-linked immunoassay designed for the detection of PCR-amplified DNA [24] or by semi-nested reamplification using one common primer and the specific probes of Anderson et al. [6] as second primer [pers. unpubl. data].

#### Practical Aspects of Direct Molecular Detection of *B. henselae* DNA in Clinical Specimens

PCR is a rapid and specific but relatively expensive method to detect *B. henselae* directly in clinical specimens. In the absence of commercially available tests and considering the expertise needed for getting reliable results, the use of PCR for diagnostic purposes is mostly restricted to specialized laboratories. There are several critical issues that do apply for most molecular based tests and that shall be briefly mentioned.

Using PCR systems, and especially in conjunction with broad-spectrum primers, the risk of contamination is very high. Adequate precautions are, therefore, compulsory and have been described in detail elsewhere [25–27]. Nevertheless, only few studies have incorporated combinations of physical (e.g. separate rooms) and enzymatic procedures (e.g. the use of dUTP instead of dTTP in combination with uracil-N-glycosylase) to prevent laboratory-borne (carry-over) contaminations [7, 9]. Consequently, the specificity of diagnostic assays must be critically evaluated.

On the other edge, the sensitivity of PCR assays may be compromised by the fact that DNA from tissue of patients with suspected *Bartonella* infection resists amplification with relatively high frequency, i.e. in up to 25% of the specimens [6, 9, 20]. Diluting such samples often resulted in successful amplification. However, with such an approach the target molecule will be diluted as well and this may result in false-negative tests for specimens with a small number of bacteria present. Inhibition of amplification may be due to substances that have an adverse effect on the activity of *Taq* polymerase or may be caused by large amounts of human DNA as has been described previously for the detection of *Borrelia burgdorferi* in skin biopsy specimens [28]. In addition, the length of the amplified fragment may inversely affect the length of a given assay. This has been shown for various organisms including *Tropheryma whippelii* [29] as well as for *Bartonella* species [pers. unpubl. data]. For example, the 16S rRNA gene-based assay (amplicon size 184 bp) [19] was slightly more sensitive than the *htrA* gene-based test (amplicon size 414 bp) [9] when directly compared using 39 clinical samples of patients with suspected *Bartonella* infection but it did not allow differentiation of *B. henselae* and *B. quintana* (see above). The clinical significance of different amplicon sizes has not been

*Table 2.* List of nucleotide sequences of *B. henselae* found in GenBank and EMBL databases (April 1997)

| Gene | Accession No. | Length, bp | Reference |
|---|---|---|---|
| 16S rRNA gene | Z11684 | 1,410 | 3, 10 |
| | M59459 | 424 | 3 |
| | M73229 | 1,414 | 4 |
| 5S rRNA gene | L12403 | 119 | 42 |
| *htrA* gene of *B. henselae* | L20127 | 1,889 | 6, 21 |
| *gltA* gene (citrate synthase) | L38987 | 1,306 | 35 |
| 35 kDa protein gene, bacteriophage-like | U21304 | 1,119 | no ref. |
| 17 kDa protein gene | U23447 | 660 | 43 |
| 16S-23S intergenic spacer | L35101 | 1,351 | 32, 44 |

fully evaluated but may be more important when working with formalin-fixed than with fresh clinical specimens due to extensive degradation of the DNA upon fixation [23].

As with any other test, the positive predictive value (PPV) of molecular tests is influenced not only by its specificity but also by the prevalence of the corresponding disease [30]: in a low prevalence environment the PPV of a test with both high sensitivity and high specificity becomes relatively low. It is, therefore, important that tests are ordered on the basis of strong clinical suspicion. This does not only improve the value of a test but it also helps saving costs.

## Molecular Techniques Used for Identification and Typing of *B. henselae* Isolates

In addition to the molecular approaches described above, various methods have been used for the identification and epidemiological subtyping of *B. henselae* isolates: PCR amplification and sequencing [4, 31–33]; PCR amplification followed by RFLP [4, 34–36]; RFLP of chromosomal DNA [37], PCR fingerprinting using primers based on repetitive extragenic palindromic (REP) [38, 39] or enterobacterial repetitive intergenic consensus (ERIC) DNA sequences [38, 40]; pulse-field gel electrophoresis (PFGE) [32]; DNA-DNA hybridization [5], and SDS-PAGE [41]. Targets used were the 16S rRNA gene [4, 31–33, 37], the citrate synthase gene [4, 33, 35, 36, 39], and the 16S-23S intergenic spacer region [32], including part of the 23S rRNA gene [34]. For more details, the reader is referred to other chapters in this volume.

## Potential Targets for Molecular Diagnostics

As of April 1997, seven nucleotide sequences of *B. henselae* have been deposited in GenBank and EMBL databases (table 2). Only two of these targets have been used for the direct detection of *B. henselae* (16S rRNA gene and *htrA* gene) in clinical specimens (see above). For strain typing, the 16S rRNA gene, the *gltA* gene (citrate synthase) and the 16S-23S intergenic spacer region have been exploited. Nothing is known about the potential use of the other sequences with regard to strain typing and direct detection of the various species in clinical specimens. This needs to be addressed in future studies.

## Outlook

Molecular methods have been of paramount importance in the history of *B. henselae*. Not only did the molecular description of its 16S rRNA gene precede the first culture but even today cultures are far from being sufficiently reliable. In addition, since cross-reactivity between the various species seems to be the rule rather than the exception in serodiagnostic tests, amplification methods will remain an important factor in the diagnosis of infections related to this peculiar organism. It would not be astonishing if there existed as yet unknown *Bartonella* species of clinical significance and if the spectrum of diseases associated with these organisms were enlarged.

## References


1 Jerris RC, Regnery RL: Will the real agent of cat-scratch disease please stand up? Annu Rev Microbiol 1996;50:707–725.

2 Anderson B, Neuman MA: *Bartonella* spp as emerging human pathogens. Clin Microbiol Rev 1997; 10:203–219.

3 Relman DA, Loutit JS, Schmidt TM, Falkow S, Tomkins LS: The agent of bacillary angiomatosis. An approach to the identification of uncultured pathogens. N Engl J Med 1990;323:1573–1580.

4 Regnery RL, Anderson BE, Clarridge JE III, Rodriguez-Barradas MC, Jones DC, Carr JH: Characterization of a novel *Rochalimaea* species, *R. henselae* sp nov, isolated from blood of a febrile, human immunodeficiency virus-positive patient. J Clin Microbiol 1992;30:265–274.

5 Welch DF, Pickett DA, Slater LN, Steigerwalt AG, Brenner DJ: *Rochalimaea henselae* sp nov, a cause of septicemia, bacillary angiomatosis, and parenchymal bacillary peliosis. J Clin Microbiol 1992;30:275–280.

6 Anderson B, Sims K, Regnery R, Robinson L, Schmidt MJ, Goral S, Hager C, Edwards K: Detection of *Rochalimaea henselae* DNA in specimens from cat scratch disease patients by PCR. J Clin Microbiol 1994;32:942–948.

7 Goldenberger D, Schmidheini T, Altwegg M: Detection of *Bartonella henselae* and *Bartonella quintana* by a simple and rapid procedure using broad-range PCR amplification and direct sequencing of part of the 16S rRNA gene. Clin Microbiol Infect 1997;3:240–245.

8 Goral S, Anderson B, Hager C, Edwards KM: Detection of *Rochalimaea henselae* DNA by polymerase chain reaction of children with cat-scratch disease. Pediatr Infect Dis J 1994;13:994–997.

9 Goldenberger D, Zbinden R, Perschil I, Altwegg M: Detection of *Bartonella (Rochalimaea) henselae/B. quintana* by polymerase chain reaction (German). Schweiz Med Wochenschr 1996;126:207–213.

10 Relman DA, Lepp PW, Sadler KN, Schmidt TM: Phylogenetic relationships among the agent of bacillary angiomatosis, *Bartonella bacilliformis*, and other alpha-proteobacteria. Mol Microbiol 1992;6:1801–1807.

11 Marullo S, Jaccard A, Roulot D, Mainguene C, Clauvel JP: Identification of the *Rochalimaea henselae* 16S rRNA sequence in the liver of a French patient with bacillary angiomatosis (letter). J Infect Dis 1992;166:1462.

12 Hadfield TL, Warren R, Kass M, Brun E, Levy C: Endocarditis caused by *Rochalimaea henselae*. Hum Pathol 1993;24:1140–1141.

13 Flexman JP, Lavis NJ, Kay ID, Watson M, Metcalf C, Pearman JW: *Bartonella henselae* is a causative agent of cat scratch disease in Australia. J Infect 1995;31:241–245.

14 Anderson B, Kelly C, Threlkel R, Edwards K: Detection of *Rochalimaea henselae* in cat-scratch disease skin test antigens. J Infect Dis 1993;168:1034–1036.

15 Wilson KH, Blitchington RB, Greene RC: Amplification of bacterial 16S ribosomal DNA with polymerase chain reaction. J Clin Microbiol 1990;28:1942–1946.

16 Caniza MA, Granger DL, Wilson KH, Washington MK, Kordick DL, Frush DP, Blitchington RB: *Bartonella henselae*: Etiology of pulmonary nodules in a patient with depressed cell-mediated immunity. Clin Infect Dis 1995;10:1505–1511.

17 Bergmans AMC, Groothedde JW, Schellekens JFP, van Embden JDA, Ossewarde JM, Schouls LM: Etiology of cat scratch disease: Comparison of polymerase chain reaction detection of *Bartonella* (formerly *Rochalimaea*) and *Afipia felis* DNA with serology and skin tests. J Infect Dis 1995;171: 916–923.

18 Bergmans AMC, Schellekens JFP, van Embden JDA, Schouls LM: Predominance of two *Bartonella henselae* variants among cat-scratch disease patients in The Netherlands. J Clin Microbiol 1996;34: 254–260.

19 Box ATA, Sander A, Perschil I, Goldenberger D, Altwegg M: Cats are probably not the only reservoir for infections due to *Bartonella henselae*. J Microbiol Methods 1996;27:101–102(abstr 17).

20 Dauga C, Miras I, Grimont PAD: Identification of *Bartonella henselae* and *B. quintana* 16S rDNA sequences by branch-, genus- and species-specific amplification. J Med Microbiol 1996;45:192–199.

21 Anderson B, Jones D, Burgess A: Cloning, expression and sequence analysis of the *Bartonella henselae* gene encoding the HtrA stress-response protein. Gene 1996;178:35–38.

22 Waldvogel K, Regnery RL, Anderson BE, Caduff R, Caduff J, Nadal D: Disseminated cat-scratch disease: Detection of *Rochalimaea henselae* in affected tissue. Eur J Pediatr 1994;153:23–27.

23 Wright KD, Manos MM: Sample preparation from paraffin-embedded tissues; in Innis MA, Gelfand DH, Sninsky JJ, White TJ (eds): PCR Protocols: A Guide to Methods and Applications. Berkeley, Academic Press, 1990, pp 153–158.

24 Ritzler M, Altwegg M: Sensitivity and specificity of a commercially available enzyme-linked immunoassay for the detection of polymerase chain reaction amplified DNA. J Microbiol Methods 1996; 27:233–238.

25 Relman DA: Universal bacterial 16S rDNA amplification and sequencing; in Persing DH, Smith TF, Tenover FC, White TJ (eds): Diagnostic Molecular Microbiology. Washington, American Society for Microbiology, 1992, pp 489–795.

26 Persing DH, Cimino GD: Amplification products' inactivation methods; in Persing DH, Smith TF, Tenover FC, White TJ (eds): Diagnostic Molecular Microbiology. Washington, American Society for Microbiology, 1992, pp 105–121.

27 McCreedy BJ, Callaway TH: Laboratory design and work flow; in Persing DH, Smith TF, Tenover FC, White TJ (eds): Diagnostic Molecular Microbiology. Washington, American Society for Microbiology, 1992, pp 149–159.

28 Cogswell FB, Bantar CE, Hughes TG, Gu Y, Philipp MT: Host DNA can interfere with detection of *Borrelia burgdorferi* in skin biopsy specimens by PCR. J Clin Microbiol 1996;34:980–982.

29 Altwegg M, Fleisch-Marx A, Goldenberger D, Hailemariam S, Schaffner A, Kissling R: Spondylodiscitis caused by *Tropheryma whippelii*. Schweiz Med Wochenschr 1996;126:1495–1499.
30 Altwegg M: General problems associated with diagnostic applications of amplification methods. J Microbiol Methods 1995;23:21–30.
31 Koehler JE, Quinn FD, Berger TG, LeBoit PE, Tappero JW: Isolation of *Rochalimaea* species from cutaneous and osseous lesions of bacillary angiomatosis. N Engl J Med 1992;327:1625–1631.
32 Roux V, Raoult D: Inter- and intraspecies identification of *Bartonella (Rochalimaea)* species. J Clin Microbiol 1995;33:1573–1579.
33 Birtles RJ, Raoult D: Comparison of partial citrate synthase gene (*gltA*) sequences for phylogenetic analysis of *Bartonella* species. Int J Syst Bacteriol 1996;46:891–897.
34 Matar GM, Swaminathan B, Hunter SB, Later LN, Welch DF: Polymerase chain reaction-based restriction fragment length polymorphism analysis of a fragment of the ribosomal operon from *Rochalimaea* species for subtyping. J Clin Microbiol 1993;31:1730–1734.
35 Norman AF, Regnery R, Jameson P, Greene C, Krause DC: Differentiation of *Bartonella*-like isolates at the species level by PCR-restriction fragment length polymorphism in the citrate synthase gene. J Clin Microbiol 1995;33:1797–1803.
36 Joblet C, Roux V, Drancourt M, Gouvernet J, Raoult D: Identification of *Bartonella (Rochalimaea)* species among fastidious Gram-negative bacteria on the basis of the partial sequence of the citrate-synthase gene. J Clin Microbiol 1995;33:1879–1883.
37 Birtles RJ: Differentiation of *Bartonella* species using restriction endonuclease analysis of PCR-amplified 16S rRNA genes. FEMS Microbiol Lett 1995;129:261–266.
38 Rodriguez-Barradas MC, Hamill RJ, Houston ED, Georghiou PR, Clarridge JE, Regnery RL, Koehler JE: Genomic fingerprinting of *Bartonella* species by a repetitive element PCR for distinguishing species and isolates. J Clin Microbiol 1995;33:1089–1093.
39 Clarridge JE III, Raich TJ, Pirwani D, Simon B, Tsai L, Rodriguez-Barradas MC, Regnery R, Zollo A, Jones DC, Rambo C: Strategy to detect and identify *Bartonella* species in routine clinical laboratory yields of *Bartonella henselae* from human immunodeficiency virus-positive patient and unique *Bartonella* strain from his cat. J Clin Microbiol 1995;33:2107–2113.
40 Sander A, Bühler C, Pelz K, von Cramm E, Bredt W: Detection and identification of two *Bartonella henselae* variants in domestic cats in Germany. J Clin Microbiol 1997;35:584–587.
41 Slater LN, Welch MD, Hensel D, Coody DW: A newly recognized fastidious Gram-negative pathogen as a cause of fever and bacteriemia. N Engl J Med 1990;323:1587–1593.
42 Minnick MF, Stiegler GL: Nucleotide sequence and comparison of the 5S ribosomal RNA genes of *Rochalimaea henselae, R. quintana* and *Brucella abortus*. Nucleic Acids Res 1993;21:2518.
43 Anderson B, Lu E, Jones D, Regnery R: Characterization of a 17-kilodalton antigen of *Bartonella henselae* reactive with sera from patients with cat scratch disease. J Clin Microbiol 1995;33:2358–2365.
44 Roux V, Raoult D: The 16S-23S rRNA intergenic spacer region of *Bartonella* (*Rochalimaea*) species is longer than usually described in other bacteria. Gene 1995;156:107–111.

Dr. Daniel Goldenberger, Institut für Lebensmittelwissenschaft,
Laboratorium für Lebensmittel-Mikrobiologie, ETH-Zentrum, CH–8092 Zürich (Switzerland)
Tel. +41 (1) 632 3333, Fax +41 (1) 632 1266

Schmidt A (ed): *Bartonella* and *Afipia* Species Emphasizing *Bartonella henselae*.
Contrib Microbiol. Basel, Karger, 1998, vol 1, pp 143–153

# Characterization of Isolates of *Bartonella henselae* by Repetitive Element PCR

*Maria C. Rodriguez-Barradas*

Infectious Diseases Section and Medical Service, Veterans Affairs Medical Center, and Department of Medicine, Baylor College of Medicine, Houston, Tex., USA

## Introduction

Repetitive element sequence-based PCR (rep-PCR) refers to the general methodology involving the application of oligonucleotide primers based on families of short, extragenic repetitive sequences [1, 2], including the repetitive extragenic palindromic (REP) and the enterobacterial repetitive intergenic consensus (ERIC) sequences. The REP sequence structure consists of a 38-nucleotide consensus sequence which is a palindrome and can form a stable stem-loop structure with a 5-bp variable loop in the central region of the consensus sequence [2, 3]. The ERIC sequence is approximately 126 bp in length, includes a highly conserved central inverted repeat (potential stem-loop structure) and has no sequence similarity to the REP sequence [2, 4]. Both repetitive sequences are located in noncoding, transcribed regions of the chromosome, and their chromosomal locations differ between species. REP- and ERIC-like sequences are present in species throughout the eubacterial kingdom; the functions of these sequences are not clear [1, 2]. By using an appropriate pair of outward-facing PCR primers directed at these repeated sequences, multiple amplification products, which reflect distance polymorphisms between adjacent DNA repeats, are generated, and enable the establishment of DNA fingerprint patterns specific for individual bacterial species and strains [1, 2]. rep-PCR-generated DNA fingerprints have been useful for differentiating between species and for assessment of clonal relationships among bacterial isolates, including laboratory and clinical isolates of *Citrobacter diversus* [5], *Enterobacter aerogenes* [6], *Streptococcus pneumoniae* [7], *Acinetobacter baumannii* [8], *Burkholderia cepacia* [9], *Legionella pneumophila*

[10], and *Enterococcus* species [11, 12]. In addition, whole-cell rep-PCR methods have been developed that eliminate the need for DNA purification [13].

Definitive identification of *Bartonella* species requires the use of molecular biology techniques that include sequencing the 16S rRNA gene [14–18], restriction fragment length polymorphism (RFLP) analysis of a PCR-amplified portion of the citrate synthase gene [15, 17–20], pulsed-field gel electrophoresis (PFGE) [17, 21], or chromosomal DNA-DNA hybridization [22]. Of these methods, only sequencing of the 16S rRNA gene [23, 24] and PFGE [17, 21] have been used for subspeciation of *B. henselae* isolates. In this chapter, we describe the application of rep-PCR for the identification of *Bartonella* species and for subtyping of *B. henselae* isolates.

### Repetitive Element PCR of *Bartonella* Species

rep-PCR of *Bartonella* species can be performed from extracted DNA [25] or from whole-cell preparations [18, 26]. For the latter, colonies of *Bartonella* species isolates are scraped from the agar plate, suspended, washed once in 1 ml of 1 *M* NaCl, washed once in distilled water, and resuspended in distilled water to a final concentration of $10^7$–$10^8$ CFU/ml. The design and synthesis of the REP- and ERIC-based oligonucleotide primers have been described in detail by Versalovic et al. [1, 27]. For studying *Bartonella* species, the pair of 18-mer REP1R-Dt and REP2-Dt primers, which contain multiple nucleotides (A, C, G, or T) at ambiguous positions in the REP consensus sequence, or the set of 22-mer consensus oligonucleotides ERIC1 and ERIC2 were used in separate PCR reactions (fig. 1). Each 25-µl reaction mixture contained 50 pmol of each of the two opposing primers, 100 ng of genomic DNA or 2 µl of the whole-cell suspension as template bacterial DNA, 1.25 m*M* (each) 4-deoxynucleoside triphosphates, and 2 U of Amplitaq DNA polymerase in a buffer with 10% dimethylsulfoxide (vol/vol). PCR amplifications were performed in an automated thermal cycler (Perkin-Elmer Cetus) with an initial denaturation step (95 °C, 7 min) followed by 30 cycles of denaturation (90 °C, 30 s), annealing (REP primers, 40 °C, 1 min; ERIC primers, 51 °C, 1 min), and extension (65 °C, 8 min), followed by a single final extension (65 °C, 16 min). 7 µl of each PCR product was electrophoresed in a 1.0% agarose (Ultrapure; Gibco-BRL, Grand Island, N.Y., USA) gel at 100 V 2.5 h in 1 × Tris-borate-EDTA buffer and stained with 0.5 mg of ethidium bromide per ml. Agarose gels were visualized and photographed under UV transillumination. DNA fingerprints of isolates are compared for similarity by visual inspection of band patterns [18, 25] or by computer-assisted analysis [18, 26].

| | |
|---|---|
| REP consensus | 5'-GCC$^{G}_{T}$GATGNCG$^{G}_{A}$CG$^{C}_{T}$NNNNN$^{G}_{A}$CG$^{C}_{T}$CTTATC$^{C}_{A}$GGCCTAC -3' |
| REP1R - Dt | ← 3'-CGGNCTACNGCNGCNIII -5' |
| REP2 - Dt | 5'-NCGNCTTATCNGGCCTAC -3' → |

*a*

| | |
|---|---|
| ERIC consensus | 5'-GTGAATCCCCAGGAGCTTACATAAGTAAGTGACTGGGGTGAGCG-3' |
| ERIC1R | ← 3'-CACTTAGGGGTCCTCGAATGTA-5' |
| ERIC2 | 5'-AAGTAAGTGACTGGGGTGAGCG-3' → |

*b*

*Fig. 1.* Repetitive sequence-based oligonucleotide primers [1, 27]. *a* Alignment of REP degenerate primers with respect to the REP consensus sequence. REP oligonucleotides were designed from each half of the conserved stem of the palindrome in opposite orientations such that the 3′ ends are directed outwardly from each REP sequence. Since one side of the stem sequence is shorter, three inosines are added to the 5′ end of the REP1R-Dt primer so that REP1R-Dt primer lengths match the 18-mer length of REP2-Dt primer. Total degeneracy is represented by one of the four common bases (N = A, G, C, or T) at specific positions. *b* Alignment of ERIC oligonucleotide primer sequences with respect to the central inverted repeat of the ERIC consensus sequence. Arrows indicate the direction of polymerase extension.

Fingerprints are considered highly similar when all visible bands represented in each isolate have the same apparent migration distance. For complex fingerprints, such as those obtained by REP-PCR, the absence of 1–2 bands from one isolate when all other visible bands in the fingerprints had matching positions was allowed before isolates were considered different by visual inspection. For less complex fingerprints (< 10 bands), such as those obtained by ERIC-PCR, the presence or absence of a distinct band was considered a difference [25].

### *Identification of* Bartonella *Species by rep-PCR*

DNA fingerprints obtained from rep-PCR of extracted genomic DNA or from preparations of whole cells yielded comparable patterns [25]; consequently, subsequent studies were done using preparations of whole cells as

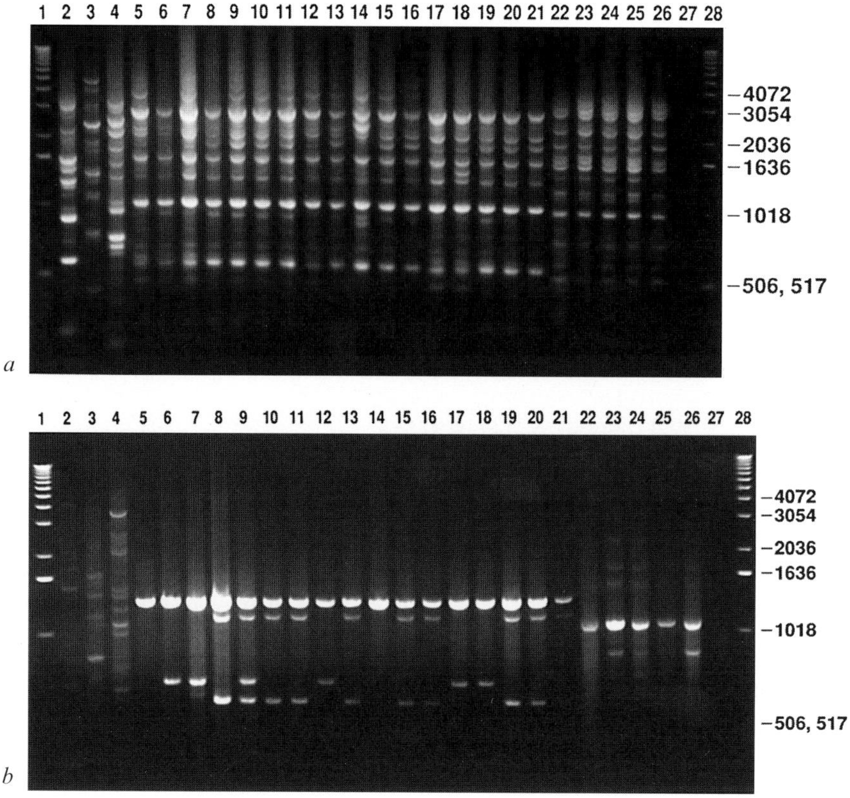


*Fig. 2.* Whole-cell based DNA fingerprints generated by Rep-PCR (*a*) and ERIC-PCR (*b*) of *Bartonella* species. Lanes 1 and 28, 1-kb ladder, marker sizes in base pairs; lane 2, *B. bacilliformis*; lane 3, *B. elizabethae*; lane 4, *B. vinsonii*. Lanes 5–21, *B. henselae* isolates: lane 5, CA-1; lane 6, SA-2; lane 7, Houston-1; lane 8, GA; lane 9, Goldie; lane 10, Tiger; lane 11, JK-13; lane 12, Krystal; lane 13, JK-9; lane 14, Bridges; lane 15, Riggs; lane 16, Placerville; lane 17, JK-33; lane 18, JK-34,; lane 19, JK-38; lane 20, JK-41; lane 21, JK-42. Lanes 22–26, *B. quintana* isolates: lane 22, D-perm; lane 23, Sh-perm; lane 24, OK-90; lane 25, WA; lane 26, JK-35. Lane 27, negative control [with permission from 25].

template [18, 26]. PCR amplification with REP or ERIC primers (REP-PCR and ERIC-PCR, respectively) revealed species-specific DNA patterns of amplification products for the various *Bartonella* isolates [25, 26] (fig. 2a, b). As described previously for other bacteria for which this technique has been used [6, 8–10], related organisms shared some bands. REP-PCR amplification with degenerate primers produces DNA patterns having approximately 10–15 bands per isolate. These bands range in size from 0.5 to 4.0 kb. *B. henselae* and

*B. quintana* share a prominent band at 1 kb but differ in other landmark bands at around 0.5, 1.6 and 3 kb. Neither *B. bacilliformis, B. elizabethae, B. vinsonii* or *B. clarridgeiae* isolates shared more than one of these landmark bands [25, 26]. For *B. henselae*, fingerprints obtained by ERIC-PCR are less complex than those obtained by REP-PCR with degenerate primers [25]. Each of the *Bartonella* species yields very distinct fingerprints with a common band present at 1.3 kb for *B. henselae* isolates and 1.1 kb for *B. quintana* isolates and not apparent in the *B. bacilliformis, B. elizabethae, B. vinsonii* or *B. clarridgeiae* strains. Isolates of *B. henselae* and *B. quintana*, in which species and genus identification had been previously determined by PCR-RFLP analysis of the citrate synthase gene and/or sequencing of a 300-bp region of the genes coding for 16 rRNA, have been correctly identified on the basis of the REP-PCR and ERIC-PCR fingerprint patterns [25].

After initial isolation of *Bartonella* organisms, identification to the species level in a routine clinical laboratory is difficult [26, 28]. The gold standard for species identification has been based on complex molecular biologic techniques such as sequencing of the 16S rRNA gene after PCR amplification [14–18], PCR-RFLP analysis of the citrate synthase gene [15, 17–20], PFGE [17, 21], and chromosomal DNA-DNA hybridization [22], studies that are usually performed in research laboratory settings. However, correct identification of *Bartonella* isolates to the species level was made in a clinical laboratory on the basis of REP-PCR generated DNA banding patterns from whole-cell preparations [26]. Clarridge et al. [26] compared REP-PCR to two other rapid systems utilized in a clinical laboratory for species identification, biochemical characterization with a RapID ANA II system panel (Innovative Diagnostic Systems, Inc.) and whole-cell fatty acid analysis (CFCA). CFCA and the RapID ANA panel were useful for genus identification, but did not consistently differentiate between *B. quintana* and *B. henselae*, while, REP-PCR was able to discriminate all known species of *Bartonella*. In addition, REP-PCR allowed the identification of a unique isolate of *Bartonella* (i.e. not one of the five previously recognized species) in the clinical laboratory within a few days of isolation. This unique isolate, later described as *B. clarridgeiae*, was corroborated as a unique species by RFLP pattern of the citrate synthase gene, sequence analysis of the citrate synthase gene, and sequence analysis of the 16S rRNA [29].

For use in the clinical laboratory, rep-PCR has the advantage of being easy to perform as compared to other PCR- or sequence-based techniques utilized for identification of *Bartonella* species. Whole-cell preparations needed for controls can be prepared and stored up to 1 year at 4 °C [26], and longer at −70 °C [unpubl. observations]. This technique, as it has been described [25, 26], has the disadvantage of requiring growth of the organism in solid

*Table 1.* Characteristics and PCR results of *B. henselae* human isolates evaluated by repetitive element PCR

| Reference | Isolate | Geographic area of origin | Clinical diagnosis | Specimen cultured | PCR pattern | | |
|---|---|---|---|---|---|---|---|
| | | | | | REP | ERIC | subtype |
| 25 | Houston-1 | Texas | HIV | Blood | 1 | B | II |
| | SA-2 | Texas | CSD | Lymph node | 1 | B | II |
| | GA-1 | Georgia | CSD | Lymph node | 1 | C | III |
| | JK-13 | Georgia | HIV | Tissue-BA | 1 | C | III |
| | CA-1 | California | HIV | Blood | 1 | A | I |
| | JK-9 | California | HIV | Tissue-BA | 1 | C | III |
| | JK-33[a] | California | HIV | Tissue-BA | 1 | B | II |
| | JK-34[a] | California | HIV | Blood | 1 | B | II |
| | JK-41[b] | Oregon | HIV | Lymph node | 1 | C | III |
| 26 | Houston-2 | Texas | HIV | Blood | 1 | ND | NA |
| | Houston-3 | Texas | HIV | Blood | 1 | ND | NA |
| 18 | Patient 1[c] | California | HIV | Blood | 1 | B | II |
| | Patient 2[d] | California | HIV | Blood | 1 | C | III |
| | Patient 3[e] | California | HIV | Tissue-BA | 1 | C | III |

HIV = Human immunodeficiency virus infection; CSD = cat scratch disease; BA = bacillary angiomatosis; ND = not done; NA = not applicable.

[a, b, c, d, e] Isolates belonging to a patient-cat(s) pair (data on corresponding cat isolates is shown in table 2).

media, which can take up to 42 days. Other PCR-based methods had been proposed that overcome this limiting factor, and allow identification of *B. henselae* directly from extracted DNA from blood culture broths [20] or from infected tissue [23, 30] in cases from which *Bartonella* species infection is suspected.

*Subtyping of* Bartonella *Species by rep-PCR*

In contrast to previous observations for other bacterial species, REP-PCR fingerprints are not sensitive in subtyping *Bartonella* species. In the evaluation of 31 isolates from different geographic locations in the United States (California, Florida, Georgia, Oregon, South Carolina, and Texas), cultured from humans (table 1) or cats (table 2), all of the isolates but one had the same DNA banding pattern (fig. 2a). ERIC-PCR, however, demonstrated four different patterns based on the presence of one to four distinct bands (fig. 2b). As expected, organisms obtained from the same patient but

*Table 2.* Characteristics and PCR results of *B. henselae* cat isolates evaluated by repetitive element PCR

| Reference | Isolate | Geographic area of origin | Owner's clinical diagnosis | Specimen cultured | PCR pattern | | |
|---|---|---|---|---|---|---|---|
| | | | | | REP | ERIC | subtype |
| 25 | Goldie-1 | Georgia | CSD | Blood | 1 | D | IV |
| | Bridges | Georgia | NA | Blood | 2 | A | V |
| | Tiger-2 | South Carolina | CSD | Blood | 1 | C | III |
| | Riggs-1 | South Carolina | NA | Blood | 1 | C | III |
| | Krystal | Florida | NA | Blood | 1 | B | II |
| | Placerville | California | NA | Blood | 1 | C | III |
| | JK-38[a] | California | BA-peliosis | Blood | 1 | C | III |
| | JK-42[b] | Oregon | BA-peliosis | Blood | 1 | C | III |
| 18 | Patient 1-cat[c] | California | BA-peliosis | Blood | 1 | B | II |
| | Patient 2-cat[d] | California | BA-peliosis | Blood | 1 | C | III |
| | Patient 3-cats (n = 7)[e] | California | BA-peliosis | Blood | 1 | C | III |

CSD = Cat scratch disease; NA = not applicable; BA-peliosis = bacillary angiomatosis-peliosis.

[a, b, c, d, e] Isolates belonging to a patient-cat(s) pair (data on corresponding human isolates is shown in table 1).

from different specimens, i.e. blood and lymph node, had identical fingerprints with either set of primers. Five different banding profile patterns or subtypes were identified when results of REP-PCR and ERIC-PCR were combined [25]. Subtype III was the most prevalent one, being recovered from 55% of the infected patients and 76% of the bacteremic cats, while subtype II was recovered from 36 and 12% of patients and cats, respectively. Subtypes I, IV and V were represented by one isolate each. It is noteworthy that subtypes I (a patient isolate) and V (a cat isolate) shared the same ERIC-PCR-derived DNA pattern, but REP-PCR yielded a unique fingerprint for the subtype V isolate. No geographic clustering could be identified for any of the *B. henselae* isolates as the most prevalent patterns (II and III) were obtained from a variety of locations. Likewise, no association between a specific subtype and clinical presentation could be made. Subtypes II and III were retrieved both from immunocompetent patients with a clinical diagnosis of cat scratch disease, as well as from immunocompromised patients with persistent bacteremia, and/or bacillary angiomatosis-peliosis.

In contrast to *B. henselae* isolates, *B. quintana* isolates yielded indistinguishable patterns both by REP-PCR and ERIC-PCR [25]. This methodology has not been used for subspeciation of other *Bartonella* species.

rep-PCR has not been compared to other molecular methods utilized for subtyping *B. henselae*. It is interesting to note, however, that by sequencing the 16S rRNA, two distinct variants of *B. henselae* have been described among patients with cat scratch disease in The Netherlands [23] and among stray cats in Paris [24]. One of these variants corresponded to one of the prevalent variants (subtype II) by our rep-PCR composite typing system (represented by the Houston-1 isolate, the ATCC-type strain). The other variant is represented by isolates with the BA-TF sequence reported by Relman et al. [14], which we have not tested. Using RFLP analysis of the 16S-23S spacer region PCR products, a larger variety of *B. henselae* subtypes have been identified [31, 32]. However, RFLP analysis of the spacer PCR products revealed only two *B. henselae* subtypes among 27 samples from Dutch patients with cat scratch disease [32]. In contrast to rep-PCR, this latter technique has been applied directly to infected tissue [32], obviating the need for culturing the organism.

rep-PCR has been demonstrated to be a useful tool in the epidemiologic evaluation of *Bartonella* species obtained from infected patients and their cats. Of 6 patients reported, 1 subject and his only cat were infected with different *Bartonella* species [26]; *B. clarridgeiae* was cultured from that cat, as well as from 1 of the 8 bacteremic cats of another patient [18]. Subspeciation of *B. henselae* isolates from the other 5 patients and their 11 cats (4 patients with 1 infected cat each, and 1 patient with 7 infected cats) was performed by PCR with REP and ERIC primers. For 4 patients, their subtype (3 patients with subtype III and 1 with subtype II) matched the subtype obtained from the cats to which the patient was exposed. However, 1 patient was infected with a subtype II (isolates JK-33 and JK-34) while the cat was infected with a subtype III (isolate JK-38). In 1 case [18], the subtype III isolate for a patient-cat pair was consistently distinguishable from the subtype III isolates of another patient-cat pair to whom it was compared by the presence of a distinct band at 910 bp using REP-PCR. Although this finding did not meet the criteria for a different genomic fingerprint [25], it allowed matching of the isolates when they were initially run as blinded samples.

## Summary and Conclusion

Repetitive element PCR yields characteristic and reproducible DNA fingerprints that allows differentiation among *Bartonella* species. Furthermore, rep-PCR with whole organisms in place of purified genomic DNA gives patterns comparable with those obtained with extracted DNA, obviating the step of DNA extraction in order to perform the procedure. For members of the family *Enterobacteriaceae*, REP-PCR seems to be a more powerful discriminatory subtyping technique compared with the corresponding ERIC-PCR-derived DNA patterns. This has not been the case among *B. henselae* isolates, for which ERIC-PCR, although yielding less complex fingerprints, has proved to be more discriminatory than REP-PCR. Five different banding profile patterns or subtypes were identified when results of REP-PCR and ERIC-PCR were combined, subtypes II and III were the most frequently recovered both among patients and cats with *B. henselae* infection. No geographic clustering or association with a clinical spectrum could be demonstrated for the most prevalent subtypes. Once an isolate is identified as a *Bartonella* species, rep-PCR is a useful technique to obtain the identification to the species level. In the clinical laboratory, rep-PCR was able to distinguish all known species of *Bartonella* and allowed the identification of a unique strain of *Bartonella* within a few days of isolation. In addition, rep-PCR is a useful method in the evaluation of the epidemiology of *Bartonella* infections since it allows the subspeciation of *B. henselae* isolates and the matching of patient's and their cats' isolates.

## References


1 Versalovic J, Koeuth T, Lupski JR: Distribution of repetitive DNA sequences in eubacteria and application to fingerprinting of bacterial genomes. Nucleic Acids Res 1991;19:6823–6831.

2 Lupski JR, Weinstock GM: Short, interspersed repetitive DNA sequences in prokaryotic genomes. J Bacteriol 1992;174:4525–4529.

3 Gilson E, Clement J-M, Brutlag D, Hofnung M: A family of dispersed repetitive extragenic palindromic DNA sequences in *E. coli*. EMBO J 1984;3:1417–1421.

4 Hulton CSJ, Higgins CF, Sharp PM: ERIC sequences: A novel family of repetitive elements in the genomes of *Escherichia coli, Salmonella typhimurium* and other enterobacteria. Mol Microbiol 1991; 5:825–834.

5 Woods CR, Versalovic J, Koeuth T, Lupski JR: Analysis of relationships among isolates of *Citrobacter diversus* by using DNA fingerprints generated by repetitive sequence-based primers in the polymerase chain reaction. J Clin Microbiol 1992;30:2921–2929.

6 Georghiou PR, Hamill RJ, Wright CE, Versalovic J, Koeuth T, Watson DA, Lupski JR: Molecular epidemiology of infections due to *Enterobacter aerogenes*: Identification of hospital outbreak-associated strains by molecular techniques. Clin Infect Dis 1995;20:84–94.

7 Versalovic J, Kapur V, Mason EO, Shah U, Koeuth T, Lupski JR, Musser JM: Penicillin-resistant *Streptococcus pneumoniae* strains recovered in Houston: Identification and molecular characterization of multiple clones. J Infect Dis 1993;167:850–856.

8 Reboli AC, Houston ED, Monteforte JS, Wood CA, Hamill RJ: Discrimination of epidemic and sporadic isolates of *Acinetobacter baumannii* by repetitive element PCR-mediated DNA fingerprinting. J Clin Microbiol 1994;32:2635–2640.

9 Hamill RJ, Houston ED, Georghiou PR, Wright CE, Koza MA, Caddle RM, and the Outbreak Investigation Team: *Burkholderia (Pseudomonas) cepacia* respiratory tract colonization and infection associated with nebulized albuterol therapy. Ann Intern Med 1995;122:762–766.

10 Georghiou PR, Doggett AM, Kielhofner MA, Stout JE, Watson DA, Lupski JR, Hamill RJ: Molecular fingerprinting of *Legionella* species by repetitive element PCR. J Clin Microbiol 1994; 32:2989–2994.
11 Hamill R, Byers P, Houston E, Koza M, Young E: Repetitive element polymerase chain reaction (rep-PCR) analysis of a nosocomial vancomycin-resistant enterococci (VRE) outbreak (abstract C20). Abstracts of the 36th Interscience Conference on Antimicrobial Agents and Chemotherapy, New Orleans, La. Washington, American Society for Microbiology, 1996.
12 Malathum K, Singh KV, Weinstock GM, Murray BE: Repetitive sequence-based versus pulsed-field gel electrophoresis for typing of *Enterococcus faecalis* at the subspecies level. J Clin Microbiol 1998;36:211–215.
13 Woods CR, Versalovic J, Koeuth T, Lupski JR: Whole-cell repetitive element sequence-based polymerase chain reaction allows rapid assessment of clonal relationship of bacterial isolates. J Clin Microbiol 1993;31:1927–1931.
14 Relman DA, Loutit JS, Schmidt TM, Falkow S, Tompkins LS: The agent of bacillary angiomatosis: An approach to the identification of uncultured pathogens. N Engl J Med 1990;323:1573–1580.
15 Regnery RL, Anderson BE, Clarridge JE III, Rodriguez-Barradas MC, Jones DC, Carr JH: Characterization of a novel *Rochalimaea* species, *R. henselae* sp. nov., isolated from blood of a febrile, human immunodeficiency virus-positive patient. J Clin Microbiol 1992;30:265–274.
16 Koehler JE, Quinn FD, Berger TG, LeBoit PE, Tappero JW: Isolation of *Rochalimaea* species from cutaneous and osseous lesions of bacillary angiomatosis. N Engl J Med 1992;327:1625–1631.
17 Maurin M, Roux V, Stein A, Ferrier F, Viraben R, Raoult D: Isolation and characterization by immunofluorescence, sodium dodecyl sulfate-polyacrylamide gel electrophoresis, Western blot, restriction fragment length polymorphism-PCR, 16s rRNA gene sequencing, and pulsed-field gel electrophoresis of *Rochalimaea quintana* from a patient with bacillary angiomatosis. J Clin Microbiol 1994;32:1166–1171.
18 Koehler JE, Sanchez MA, Garrido CS, Whitfeld MJ, Chen FM, Berger TG, Rodriguez-Barradas MC, LeBoit PE, Tappero JW: Molecular epidemiology of *Bartonella* infections in patients with bacillary angiomatosis-peliosis. N Engl J Med 1997;337:1876–1883.
19 Norman AF, Regnery R, Jameson P, Greene C, Krause DC: Differentiation of *Bartonella*-like isolates at the species level by PCR-restriction fragment length polymorphism in the citrate synthase gene. J Clin Microbiol 1995;33:1797–1803.
20 Joblet C, Roux V, Drancourt M, Gouvernet J, Raoult D: Identification of *Bartonella (Rochalimaea)* species among fastidious Gram-negative bacteria on the basis of the partial sequence of the citrate-synthase gene. J Clin Microbiol 1995;33:1879–1883.
21 Roux V, Raoult D: Inter- and intraspecies identification of *Bartonella (Rochalimaea)* species. J Clin Microbiol 1995;33:1573–1579.
22 Welch DF, Pickett DA, Slater LN, Steigerwalt AG, Brenner DJ: *Rochalimaea henselae* sp. nov., a cause of septicemia, bacillary angiomatosis, and parenchymal bacillary peliosis. J Clin Microbiol 1992;30:275–280.
23 Bergmans AM, Groothedde J-W, Schellekens JFP, van Embden JDA, Ossewaarde JM, Schouls LM: Etiology of cat scratch disease: Comparison of polymerase chain reaction detection of *Bartonella* (formerly *Rochalimaea*) and *Afipia felis* DNA with serology and skin tests. J Infect Dis 1995;171:916–923.
24 Heller R, Artois M, Xemar V, De Briel D, Gehin H, Jaulhac B, Monteil H, Piemont Y: Prevalence of *Bartonella henselae* and *Bartonella clarridgeiae* in stray cats. J Clin Microbiol 1997;35:1327–1331.
25 Rodriguez-Barradas MC, Hamill RJ, Houston ED, Georghiou PR, Clarridge JE, Regnery RL, Koehler JE: Genomic fingerprinting of *Bartonella* species by repetitive element PCR for distinguishing species and isolates. J Clin Microbiol 1995;33:1089–1093.
26 Clarridge JE, Raich TJ, Pirwani D, Simon B, Tai L, Rodriguez-Barradas MC, Regnery R, Zollo A, Jones DC, Rambo C: Strategy to detect and identify *Bartonella* species in routine clinical laboratory yields *Bartonella henselae* from human immunodeficiency virus-positive patient and unique *Bartonella* strain from his cat. J Clin Microbiol 1995;33:2107–2113.
27 Versalovic J, Schneider M, de Bruijn FJ, Lupski JR: Genomic fingerprinting of bacteria using repetitive sequence-based polymerase chain reaction. Methods Mol Cell Biol 1994;5:25–40.

28 Welch DF, Hensel DM, Pickett DA, San Joaquin VH, Robinson A, Slater LN: Bacteremia due to *Rochalimaea henselae* in a child: Practical identification of isolates in the clinical laboratory. J Clin Microbiol 1993;31:2381–2386.
29 Lawson PA, Collins MD: Description of *Bartonella clarridgeiae* sp. nov. isolated from the cat of a patient with *Bartonella henselae* septicemia. Med Microbiol Lett 1996;5:64–73.
30 Anderson B, Sims K, Regnery R, Robinson L, Schmidt MJ, Goral S, Hager C, Edwards K: Detection of *Rochalimaea henselae* DNA in specimens from cat scratch disease patients by PCR. J Clin Microbiol 1994;32:942–948.
31 Matar GM, Swaminathan B, Hunter SB, Slater LN, Welch DF: Polymerase chain reaction-based restriction fragment length polymorphism analysis of a fragment of the ribosomal operon from *Rochalimaea* species for subtyping. J Clin Microbiol 1993;31:1730–1734.
32 Bergmans AM, Schellekens JFP, van Embden JDA, Schouls LM: Predominance of two *Bartonella henselae* variants among cat-scratch disease patients in The Netherlands. J Clin Microbiol 1996; 34:254–260.

Maria C. Rodriguez-Barradas, MD, Infectious Diseases Section and Medical Service,
Veterans Affairs Medical Center, Department of Medicine, Baylor College of Medicine,
2002 Holcombe Boulevard, Houston, TX 77030 (USA)
E-Mail rodriguez-barradas.maria@houston.va.gov

Schmidt A (ed): *Bartonella* and *Afipia* Species Emphasizing *Bartonella henselae*.
Contrib Microbiol. Basel, Karger, 1998, vol 1, pp 154–163

# Characterization of Isolates of *Bartonella henselae* by Restriction Endonuclease Analysis of the PCR-Amplified 16S-23S rRNA Gene Spacer Region

*Anneke M.C. Bergmans*[a], *Leo M. Schouls*[b]

[a] St. Elisabeth Hospital Tilburg, Laboratory of Molecular Microbiology, Tilburg, and
[b] National Institute of Public Health and the Environment, Research Laboratory for Infectious Diseases, Bilthoven, The Netherlands

## Introduction

*Bartonella henselae* has been implicated in a wide spectrum of symptoms and infectons. To study the correlation between particular clinical symptoms and different *B. henselae* types, or to analyze the geographic spread of *B. henselae* variants, intraspecies subtyping tools may be of critical importance. Additionally, these tools may be useful to determine the involvement of the cat as a reservoir and of fleas and other vectors in the transmission of *B. henselae*. Because of the fastidious character of *B. henselae*, little is known about the prevalence of different *B. henselae* variants in patients and animals. Because culture of *B. henselae* from pus aspirates and lymph node biopsy specimens from patients with cat scratch disease (CSD) is extremely difficult, typing of the strains from those samples cannot easily be performed.

Regnery et al. [1] described restriction fragment length polymorphism (RFLP) analysis of PCR fragments of the citrate synthase gene of *Bartonella* as a useful method for species identification of cultured *B. henselae, B. quintana* and *B. vinsonii* organisms, but attempts to differentiate within the *B. henselae* species have not been successful by this method [2].

## The 16S-23S rRNA Intergenic Spacer Region

In many, but not all bacterial species, the genes coding for 16S ribosomal RNA (rRNA), 23S rRNA, and 5S rRNA are located in one operon. In some bacterial species, such as *Borrelia burgdorferi*, the genes coding for 5S rRNA and 23S rRNA are closely linked, whereas the 16S rRNA gene is located in a more remote region of the chromosome [3]. The 16S-23S rRNA intergenic spacer regions of *Bartonella* species are longer than usually described in other bacteria: 1,211, 1,262, 1,258, 1,529 and 906 base pairs (bp), respectively, for *B. quintana, B. henselae, B. vinsonii, B. elizabethae* and *B. bacilliformis* [4, 5]. In most bacterial species, the size of the spacer region is between 250 and 500 bp. Examples are *Mycoplasma hyopneumoniae, Enterococcus faecalis, Streptococcus pneumoniae, Mycobacterium avium* complex bacteria, *Bacillus subtilis* and *Escherichia coli* [6–11]. The organization of the 16S-23S rRNA spacer region is variable and in some bacteria several configurations can be detected. For example, in *Enterococcus faecalis* the spacer can either be short or long, depending on the presence or absence of an alanine-tRNA ($tRNA^{Ala}$) encoding gene [7]. *Bacillus subtilis* has two spacer regions which include $tRNA^{Ala}$ and isoleucine-tRNA ($tRNA^{Ile}$) genes, and eight which include no tRNA gene [10]. *E. coli* has three operons with $tRNA^{Ala}$ and $tRNA^{Ile}$ genes, and four operons with a glutamate-tRNA ($tRNA^{Glu}$) gene [11]. 16S-23S rRNA spacer regions in *M. hyopneumoniae* and *M. avium* complex do not contain tRNA genes [6, 9]. The spacer regions of *Bartonella* species are expected to exist in only one configuration, as only one PCR fragment is obtained by PCR amplification of this region [5]. All known *Bartonella* spacers contain the genes encoding $tRNA^{Ile}$ and $tRNA^{Ala}$ [4, 5]. As the major part of the spacer region of *Bartonella* species is currently considered to be nonfunctional, there is little selective pressure in this region, and thus, intraspecies sequence divergence in the spacer region is expected to be higher than the divergence in the 16S rRNA gene.

## The 16S-23S Spacer RFLP Typing Method

In 1993, Matar et al. [12] developed a PCR-based RFLP method for the characterization of cultured *Bartonella* isolates, using the intergenic spacer region between the genes encoding 16S rRNA and 23S rRNA. A schematic presentation of the principle of the 16S-23S rRNA spacer PCR-RFLP method is shown in figure 1. Broad host-range primers are used, located at the 3′ end of the 16S rRNA gene (RPC5: 5′-AAGTCGTAACAAGGT-3′), and 440 bases from the 5′ end of the 23S rRNA gene (R23S2693: 5′-TACTGGTTCAC-TATCGGTCA-3′), resulting in a PCR fragment of approximately 1,700 bp

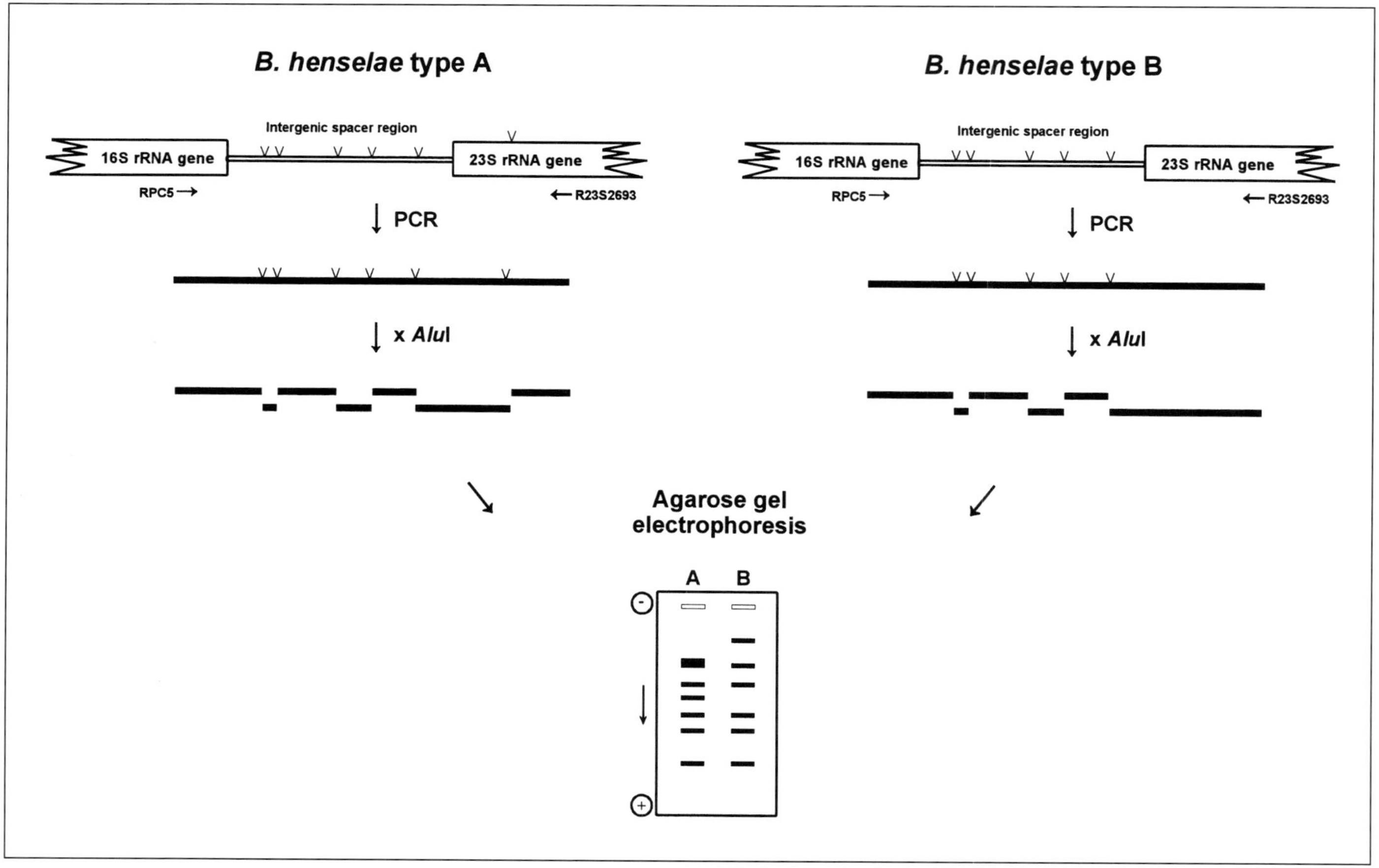


*Fig. 1.* Schematic presentation of the PCR-RFLP analysis of *Bartonella*, using the 16S-23S rRNA intergenic spacer region. V, *Alu*I endonuclease recognition site. RPC5 and R23S2693 are primers used to amplify the 16S-23S spacer region and part of the 23S rRNA gene. The 1,700-bp PCR products are digested with *Alu*I, and the resulting fragments are separated by agarose gel electrophoresis. Different spacer RFLP patterns are obtained with *B. henselae* strains A and B.

[12]. The PCR fragments are subsequently digested with a restriction endonuclease, and the restriction fragments are separated by agarose gel electrophoresis. It is expected that the number and locations of restriction endonuclease recognition sites vary between different strains within a species. As a consequence, digestion of spacer PCR products of different strains will result in different restriction fragments, and thus in different patterns on an agarose gel.

### 16S-23S Spacer RFLP Typing of *Bartonella* Strains from Bacillary Angiomatosis (BA) Patients

Matar et al. [12] combined the results of *Alu*I spacer RFLP analysis with those of *Hae*III spacer RFLP analysis, and demonstrated the existence of seven composite PCR-RFLP types in eleven *B. henselae* strains cultured from patients with BA, septicemia and parenchymal bacillary peliosis. Furthermore, they showed that *B. quintana* has a characteristic RFLP pattern which is distinct from those of *B. henselae* isolates.

### 16S-23S Spacer RFLP Typing of *Bartonella* in Clinical Material from CSD Patients

To investigate the prevalence of *B. henselae* variants in patients with CSD, we applied the 16S-23S rRNA intergenic spacer RFLP method described by Matar et al. [12] directly to clinical material from patients with CSD without cultivation of the bacteria that were present [13]. The rationale for applying the broad-host-range primers came from a previous study in our laboratory, in which it was shown by PCR and sequence analysis that pus aspirates and lymph nodes from patients with CSD did not contain any detectable DNA from bacterial species other than *Bartonella* [14]. Total DNA was extracted from pus aspirates and lymph node biopsy specimens obtained from Dutch and North American patients with clinically diagnosed CSD. All samples contained *Bartonella* DNA, as determined by a *Bartonella*-specific PCR-hybridization assay [14]. Additionally, six strains of *B. henselae* (cultured from North American patients with BA), two strains of *B. quintana*, and one strain of *B. bacilliformis* were analyzed. PCR-RFLP analysis of all specimens revealed unambiguous RFLP patterns after agarose gel electrophoresis (fig. 2) [13].

The six *B. henselae* strains from North American BA patients yielded four different *Alu*I RFLP patterns: A, B, C and D (fig. 2A). The four patterns differed from each other in only one or two bands. The difference between

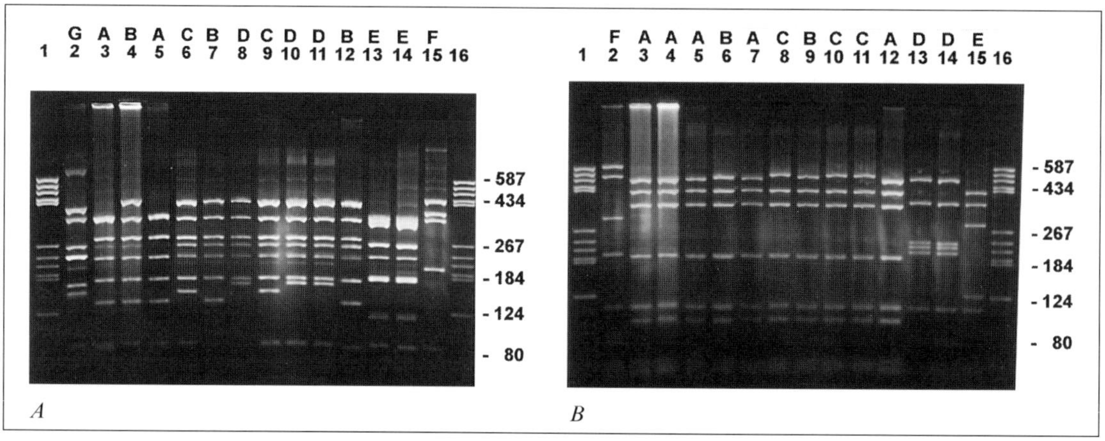


*Fig. 2.* *Alu*I (*A*) and *Sau*3A (*B*) RFLP patterns of PCR-amplified 16S-23S spacer regions from *Bartonella* species present in clinical material from patients with CSD and from *B. henselae, B. quintana* and *B. bacilliformis* strains. Lanes 1 and 16, molecular size standards (in base pairs); lane 2, blood sample from a cat; lanes 3 and 4, clinical samples from patients with CSD; lanes 5–12, *B. henselae* strains; lane 5, *B. henselae* ATCC 49882; lane 6, *B. henselae* ATCC 49793; lane 7, isolate 91-148; lane 8, isolate 92-967; lane 9, *B. henselae* ATCC 49793; lane 10, 91-100; lane 11, isolate 90-782; lane 12, isolate CAT5 (cultured from a Dutch cat); lane 13, *B. quintana* 90-268; lane 14, *B. quintana* 92-263; lane 15, *B. bacilliformis* KC583.

pattern A and pattern B is caused by the presence of one additional *Alu*I restriction site in the PCR fragment. As a result, a 430–bp fragment of pattern B is cleaved into two fragments of approximately 350 and 80 bp in pattern A. Digestion of the spacer product obtained from two *B. quintana* strains resulted in identical patterns (pattern E), and were clearly distinct from all *B. henselae* patterns, which is in accordance with the results described earlier by Matar et al. [12]. Additionally, the *Alu*I RFLP pattern (pattern F) obtained from *B. bacilliformis* KC583 DNA clearly differed from the patterns obtained from all *B. henselae* and *B. quintana* isolates (fig. 2A). The six *B. henselae* strains yielded three very similar *Sau*3A RFLP patterns (A, B and C) which could be distinguished from each other only by very small differences in the sizes of the upper band (fig. 2B). *Sau*3A RFLP did not give any additional information, because all strains with *Alu*I RFLP patterns A and B gave *Sau*3A RFLP pattern A, all strains with *Alu*I pattern C gave *Sau*3A pattern B, and all strains with *Alu*I pattern D gave *Sau*3A pattern C. As in the *Alu*I analysis, both *B. quintana* strains yielded identical *Sau*3A RFLP patterns (pattern D) which were clearly distinct from the *B. henselae* patterns. The *Sau*3A RFLP pattern (pattern E) obtained from *B. bacilliformis* KC583 was unique and differed completely from the patterns obtained from all other *Bartonella* isolates (fig. 2B).

Digestion of spacer PCR fragments from clinical samples from Dutch patients with CSD with the restriction endonuclease *Alu*I resulted in two RFLP patterns, patterns A and B (fig. 2A). Of the 27 samples from CSD patients, 20 yielded *Alu*I RFLP pattern A (74%), whereas seven samples yielded pattern B (26%). Analysis of three samples from North American patients with CSD showed that these samples contained *B. henselae* RFLP pattern B. RFLP analysis using *Sau*3A resulted in identical RFLP patterns in all 30 clinical samples (fig. 2B). Thus, *Alu*I has more potency than *Sau*3A for discriminating *B. henselae* isolates present in clinical samples from patients with CSD.

It was shown that samples from Dutch patients with CSD contain a limited number of *B. henselae* variants, suggesting that only a few of the extant *B. henselae* types can cause CSD. In immunocompromised individuals and in persons living under unhygienic conditions, not only other *B. henselae* variants but even other *Bartonella* species such as *B. quintana* are found [15].

### 16S-23S Spacer RFLP Typing of *Bartonella* in Domestic Cats

Pet animals may also carry a variety of bartonellas. Dutch cats have recently been shown to contain only three *Bartonella* variants, including *Alu*I RFLP types A, B, and a totally different type G [16]. The latter type had *Alu*I and *Sau*3A RFLP patterns that had few bands in common with those of the RFLP patterns described above; two of eight bands with *Alu*I and one of five bands with *Sau*3A, respectively, were identical in size to those of *Alu*I and *Sau*3A RFLP patterns A (fig. 2) [16]. The 16S rRNA gene sequence of *Bartonella* type G showed 99.3% identity with that of *Bartonella clarridgeiae*, a newly recognized *Bartonella* species found in North American domestic cats, and recently also shown to cause CSD [16–18]. Therefore, *Bartonella* type G may represent a *B. clarridgeiae* subspecies or another species closely related to *B. clarridgeiae*. An important finding was the existence of mixtures of different *Bartonella* species in cats: 4 of 25 bacteremic cats contained *B. henselae* of *Alu*I RFLP type B and *Bartonella* of type G, and 1 cat had *B. henselae* of type A and *Bartonella* of type G. No mixtures of types A and B were found in the cats. The prevalence of type B among Dutch bacteremic cats (56%) showed to be higher than the prevalence of A (28%) and G (36%). However, the majority of Dutch CSD patients contained type A. Maybe type A is more virulent for man than type B. It is also possible that (some) patients with *B. henselae*-related infections acquire the organism from other reservoirs than the cat, and from other vectors. Indications for the involvement of other reservoirs or vectors in *B. henselae* infection are the fact that *B. henselae AluI* RFLP types C and D (isolated from patients with BA; fig. 2) are not detected in cats so far, and the reporting of 2 patients suffering from bacteremia with *B. henselae* after sustaining tick bites [16, 19]. Therefore, the spectrum of *Bartonella* (sub)species in other animals, especially arthropods, needs to be determined.

## Consideration of the 16S-23S Spacer RFLP Method

We have applied a PCR-based RFLP method described by Matar et al. [12] to clinical samples from patients with CSD that contained *Bartonella* DNA as determined by a PCR-hybridization assay [14]. The PCR-RFLP method has been shown to be quite useful in discriminating *B. henselae* strains in clinical material. Although the primer set used in the study produces 16S-23S rRNA spacer PCR fragments with most eubacterial species, it is shown that these broad-host-range primers can also be used to type *Bartonella* species present in clinical material from CSD patients. The major advantage of the *Bartonella* PCR-RFLP typing method is the fast and easy performance without the need to culture these fastidious organisms from clinical samples. RFLP analysis of the spacer PCR products revealed only two *B. henselae* RFLP variants among Dutch patients with CSD. Matar et al. found six distinct *Alu*I RFLP types in eleven culture-grown *B. henselae* strains [12]. However, virtually all of the strains used in the latter study originated from patients with BA. This would suggest that *B. henselae* strains causing disease in immunocompromised hosts are more heterogeneous and may have other reservoirs than strains causing CSD in immunocompetent individuals. Differences in the geographic origins of the strains may also explain the differences between our results and those of Matar et al. [12]. However, we analyzed three clinical samples originating from North American patients with CSD and found that these belong to one of the two *Alu*I RFLP types (B) that we found in Dutch patients with CSD. More samples from CSD patients from various countries will have to be analyzed to determine the extent to which the variations correlate with the geographic spread of the organism.

In a previous report [14] we described that partial sequencing of the 16S rRNA genes of *B. henselae* present in eight samples from patients with CSD revealed the presence of two *B. henselae* variants, which may be designated as two subspecies. A 100% correlation between 16S rRNA type and *Alu*I spacer RFLP type has been found, which is striking, because each typing method uses polymorphism in different parts of the bacterial genome.

16S-23S spacer RFLP typing may be improved by several modifications. By using combinations of restriction enzymes in the spacer RFLP method, more variable RFLP patterns could be obtained. Additionally, end labeling of digested spacer PCR fragments will lower the detection level of the RFLP method and increase the range of fragment sizes to be used for analysis, and thus, smaller amounts of *B. henselae* DNA could also be analyzed by spacer RFLP.

## Other Typing Methods

Recently, other methods have been described for distinguishing *Bartonella* species and isolates, such as sequence analysis of the 16S-23S spacer region, pulsed-field gel electrophoresis (PFGE), repetitive element PCR (REP-PCR), and enterobacterial repetitive intergenic consensus PCR (ERIC-PCR) [20, 21].

Sequence analysis of the 16S-23S spacer region has shown a frequency of mutation of 0.5–4% within the *B. henselae* species [20]. This degree of divergence is probably too low to obtain much restriction site polymorphism. Thus, sequencing of spacer regions will be necessary to establish a greater degree of differentiation within the *B. henselae* species. Because sequence analysis is rather laborious, other methods such as single-strand conformation polymorphism (SSCP), denaturing-gradient gel electrophoresis (DGGE), or temperature-gradient gel electrophoresis (TGGE) should be optimized for use in epidemiological studies [22–24].

With PFGE, specific profiles were obtained for each of the species that were analyzed (*B. vinsonii, B. elizabethae, B. quintana* and *B. henselae*). Comparison of genomic fingerprints of three isolates of *B. henselae* and seven isolates of *B. quintana* by PFGE showed polymorphism in DNA restriction patterns, and a specific profile was obtained for each isolate [20]. The phylogenetic relationships between different *B. quintana* isolates established from PFGE profiles did not appear to correlate with geographical distribution. Similarly, there were no apparent correlations between clinical data for people infected with *B. quintana* and genotypic characterization of the organism.

Rodriguez-Barradas et al. [21] examined 17 isolates of *B. henselae* cultured from tissue and blood of HIV-infected patients, from patients with CSD, and from cats by REP-PCR and ERIC-PCR. By combining results of both PCRs, they identified five different fingerprint profiles. With REP/ERIC-PCR, no association could be made between a specific *B. henselae* strain and a clinical presentation. These PFGE and REP/ERIC-PCR data suggest that the broad spectrum of clinical manifestations caused by *Bartonella* is determined more by host factors than by the organism.

Both PFGE and REP/ERIC-PCR could be useful for *Bartonella* isolate identification, but a major disadvantage of both typing methods is the need to culture the organism. Therefore, these methods are not directly applicable to clinical material.

Another typing method which is applicable to clinical material is reverse line blotting (RLB), a rapid and sensitive method by which bacteria are detected and typed simultaneously by hybridization of PCR products with an array of specific probes [25, 26]. RLB is already successfully used for detection and identification of *Mycobacterium tuberculosis* complex strains in clinical material of patients with tuberculosis, using polymorphism in the direct repeat (DR) locus, and of *Borrelia burgdorferi* isolates in clinical material of patients with Lyme disease, using polymorphism in the spacer region between the genes coding for 5S rRNA and 23S rRNA [26, 27].

## References


1 Regnery RL, Anderson BE, Clarridge JE, Rodriguez-Barradas MC, Jones DC, Carr JH: Characterization of a novel *Rochalimaea* species, *R. henselae* sp nov, isolated from blood of a febrile, human immunodeficiency virus-positive patient. J Clin Microbiol 1992;30:265–274.

2 Norman AF, Regnery RL, Jameson P, Greene C, Krause DC: Differentiation of *Bartonella*-like isolates at the species level by PCR-restriction fragment length polymorphism in the citrate synthase gene. J Clin Microbiol 1995;33:1797–1803.

3 Schwartz JJ, Gazumyan A, Schwartz I: rRNA gene organization in the Lyme disease spirochete, *Borrelia burgdorferi*. J Bacteriol 1992;174:3757–3765.

4 Minnick MF, Strange JC, Williams KF: Characterization of the 16S-23S rRNA intergenic spacer of *Bartonella bacilliformis*. Gene 1994;143:149–150.

5 Roux V, Raoult D: The 16S-23S rRNA intergenic spacer region of *Bartonella (Rochalimaea)* species is longer than usually described in other bacteria. Gene 1995;156:107–111.

6 Taschke C, Herrmann R: Analysis of transcription and processing signals of the 16S-23S rRNA operon of *Mycoplasma hyopneumoniae*. Mol Gen Genet 1986;205:434–441.

7 Hall LMC: Are point mutations or DNA rearrangements responsible for the restriction fragment length polymorphisms that are used to type bacteria. Microbiology 1994;140:197–204.

8 Bacot CM, Reeves RH: Novel tRNA gene organization in the 16S-23S intergenic spacer of the *Streptococcus pneumoniae* rRNA gene cluster. J Bacteriol 1991;173:4234–4236.

9 Frothingham R, Wilson KH: Sequence-based differentiation of strains in the *Mycobacterium avium* complex. J Bacteriol 1993;175:2818–2825.

10 Vold BS: Structure and organization of genes for transfer ribonucleic acid in *Bacillus subtilis*. Microbiol Rev 1985;49:71–80.

11 Fournier MJ, Ozeki H: Structure and organization of the transfer ribonucleic acid genes of *Escherichia coli* K-12. Microbiol Rev 1985;49:379–397.

12 Matar GM, Swaminathan B, Hunter SB, Slater LN, Welch DF: Polymerase chain reaction-based restriction fragment length polymorphism analysis of a fragment of the ribosomal operon from *Rochalimaea* species for subtyping. J Clin Microbiol 1993;31:1730–1734.

13 Bergmans AMC, Schellekens JFP, van Embden JDA, Schouls LM: Predominance of two *Bartonella henselae* variants among cat-scratch disease patients in The Netherlands. J Clin Microbiol 1996;34: 254–260.

14 Bergmans AMC, Groothedde JW, Schellekens JFP, van Embden JDA, Ossewaarde JM, Schouls LM: Etiology of cat scratch disease: Comparison of polymerase chain reaction detection of *Bartonella* (formerly *Rochalimaea*) and *Afipia felis* DNA with serology and skin tests. J Infect Dis 1995;171:916–923.

15 Drancourt M, Mainardi JL, Brouqui P, Vandenesch F, Carta A, Lehnert F, Etienne J, Goldstein F, Acar J, Raoult D: *Bartonella (Rochalimaea) quintana* endocarditis in three homeless men. N Engl J Med 1995;332:419–423.
16 Bergmans AMC, de Jong CMA, van Amerongen G, Schot CS, Schouls LM: Prevalence of *Bartonella* species in domestic cats in The Netherlands. J Clin Microbiol 1997;35:2256–2261.
17 Lawson PA, Collins MD: Description of *Bartonella clarridgeiae* sp nov isolated from the cat of a patient with *Bartonella henselae* septicemia. Med Microbiol Lett 1996;5:64–73.
18 Kordick DL, Hilyard EJ, Hadfield TL, Wilson KH, Steigerwalt AG, Brenner DJ, Breitschwerdt EB: *Bartonella clarridgeiae*, a newly recognized zoonotic pathogen causing inoculation papules, fever, and lymphadenopathy (cat scratch disease). J Clin Microbiol 1997;35:1813–1818.
19 Lucey D, Dolan MJ, Moss CW, Garcia M, Hollis DG, Wenger S, Morgan G, Almeida R, Leong D, Greisen KS, Welch DF, Slater LN: Relapsing illness due to *Rochalimaea henselae* in immunocompetent hosts: Implication for therapy and new epidemiological associations. Clin Infect Dis 1992;14:683–688.
20 Roux V, Raoult D: Inter- and intraspecies identification of *Bartonella (Rochalimaea)* species. J Clin Microbiol 1995;33:1573–1579.
21 Rodriguez-Barradas MC, Hamill RJ, Houston ED, Georghiou PR, Clarridge JE, Regnery RL, Koehler JE: Genomic fingerprinting of *Bartonella* species by repetitive element PCR for distinguishing species and isolates. J Clin Microbiol 1995;33:1089–1093.
22 Orita M, Iwahana H, Kanazawa H, Hayashi K, Sekiya T: Detection of polymorphisms of human DNA by gel electrophoresis as single-strand conformation polymorphisms. Proc Natl Acad Sci USA 1989;86:2766–2770.
23 Fischer SG, Lerman LS: DNA fragments differing by single base-pair substitutions are separated in denaturing gradient gels: Correspondence with melting theory. Proc Natl Acad Sci USA 1983; 80:1579–1583.
24 Riesner D, Steger G, Zimmat R, Owens RA, Wagenhofer M, Hillen W, Vollbach S, Henco K: Temperature-gradient gel electrophoresis of nucleic acids: Analysis of conformational transitions, sequence variations, and protein-nucleic acid interactions. Electrophoresis 1989;10:377–389.
25 Kaufhold A, Podbielski A, Baumgarten G, Blokpoel M, Top J, Schouls LM: Rapid typing of group A streptococci by the use of DNA amplification and nonradioactive allele specific oligonucleotide probes. FEMS Microbiol Lett 1994;119:19–26.
26 Kamerbeek J, Schouls LM, Kolk A, van Agterveld M, van Soolingen D, Kuijper S, Bunschoten A, Molhuizen H, Shaw R, Goyal M, van Embden J: Simultaneous detection and strain differentiation of *Mycobacterium tuberculosis* for diagnosis and epidemiology. J Clin Microbiol 1997;35:907–914.
27 Rijpkema SG, Molkenboer MJCM, Schouls LM, Jongejan F, Schellekens JFP: Simultaneous detection and genotyping of three genomic groups of *Borrelia burgdorferi* sensu lato in Dutch *Ixodes ricinus* ticks by characterization of the amplified intergenic spacer region between 5S and 23S rRNA genes. J Clin Microbiol 1995;33:3091–3095.

Dr. A.M.C. Bergmans, St. Elisabeth Hospital Tilburg, Laboratory of Molecular Microbiology, PO Box 747, NL–5000 AS Tilburg (The Netherlands)
Tel. +31 13 539 2676, Fax +31 13 544 1264, E-Mail lab.med.microbiol@inter.nl.net

Schmidt A (ed): *Bartonella* and *Afipia* Species Emphasizing *Bartonella henselae*.
Contrib Microbiol. Basel, Karger, 1998, vol 1, pp 164–175

# Minimal Inhibitory Concentration Determination in *Bartonella henselae*

*M. Maurin, D. Raoult*

Unité des Rickettsies, CNRS UPRESA 6020, Université de la Méditerranée, Faculté de Médecine, Marseille, France

The genus *Bartonella* now comprises 11 recognized species, including the 4 human pathogens *B. bacilliformis* (the agent of Carrion's disease), *B.* (ex *Rochalimaea*) *quintana, B.* (ex *Rochalimaea*) *henselae* and *B. elizabethae*. In 1990, Relman et al. [52] used the PCR method to amplify bacterial 16S rRNA gene fragments of *B. henselae* directly from biopsy material taken from AIDS patients suffering from bacillary angiomatosis (BA). The isolation and characterization of *B. henselae* [32, 49] allowed the development of specific diagnostic methods for this bacterium and led to increased medical awareness of its potential pathogenicity. A number of pathologic manifestations are now associated with *B. henselae* infection, including cat scratch disease (CSD), bacteremia, endocarditis, BA, peliosis hepatitis and neurological manifestations. Renewal of the medical interest in the group of *Bartonella* (ex *Rochalimaea*) species led also to the recognition of new pathological conditions associated with the early described species *B. quintana*, as well as description of new *Bartonella* species, *B. quintana*, the agent of trench fever, is also responsible for BA, septicemia, endocarditis and chronic lymphadenopathies. *B. elizabethae* has been isolated only once from an endocarditis patient [17].

Members of the genus *Bartonella* are defined as Gram-negative, oxidase-negative, fastidious, aerobic, rod-shaped bacteria. Growth may be obtained in axenic medium, either on blood-enriched agar, rabbit blood or horse blood being more effective than sheep blood, or in broth [61]. *B. henselae* grows best at 37 °C in vitro and in the presence of increased carbon dioxide pressure, fetal calf serum, and hemin [22]. However, growth of all *Bartonella* species is slow. When using blood agar, primary isolates are obtained typically after 12–14 days, although prolonged incubation periods of up to 45 days have been reported to be necessary

[42]. First subcultures of an isolate are also difficult to obtain, with colony formation again taking 10–15 days. Repeated subculture, however, reduces this time to only 3–5 days, although significantly affects colonial morphology. Colonies are rough, adherent, pitting the agar on primary isolation and become smooth and less adherent after several passages.

*Bartonella* species were early reported to live in close association with host cells. The most striking pathological feature of *Bartonella* infection is the apparent ability of these bacteria to produce angioproliferative lesions, specifically among immunocompromised patients such as those infected with HIV. Capillary and endothelial cell proliferations are characteristic histologic findings of BA, peliosis hepatitis and the verruga peruana form of Carrion's disease [3, 34, 47]. Characteristically, on histological examination, Warthin-Starry-stained bacilli are observed within these angioproliferative lesions, and these lesions resolve on antibiotic treatment [11]. In vitro, *B. henselae* can infect a number of cell cultures, including bovine endothelial cells [32] and human umbilical vein endothelial cells [15], and the intraerythrocytic presence of *B. henselae* in cat erythrocytes has also been recently observed [33]. Recent experimental data indicate that *Bartonella* species are facultative intracellular pathogens [6, 62].

*Bartonella* infections are characterized by their propensity either to resist antibiotic therapy such as in the case of CSD or to relapse after antibiotic withdrawal such as in BA cases. The lack of in vivo bactericidal activity of antibiotics, the facultative intracellular lifestyle of bartonellae as well as the immune status of infected patients may explain the difficulty of eradication of *Bartonella* infection. The development of *Bartonella*-specific cultures in routine laboratory practice has allowed more frequent isolation of *Bartonella* strains. Recent investigations using most available *Bartonella* strains have allowed characterization of the in vitro antibiotic susceptibility of these species. In the following sections, methods for in vitro antibiotic susceptibility testing of *Bartonella* isolates will be discussed. Results of in vitro experiments will be tentatively correlated with in vivo data on antibiotic therapy efficacy in *B. henselae* infections, with special emphasis on BA, endocarditis, and CSD, for which clinical data are more widely available.

## In vitro Antibiotic Susceptibility Testing of *Bartonella* Species

A few experimental data on the antibiotic susceptibility of *Bartonella* isolates are available [39, 41, 44, 45]. Methods were elaborated to test the bacteriostatic or bactericidal activity of antibiotics either in axenic medium or in cell culture systems.

*Determination of Minimal Inhibitory Concentrations (MICs) in Axenic Medium*

Since *Bartonella* species are fastidious microorganisms, MIC determination assays as recommended by the National Committee for Clinical Laboratory Standards (NCCLS) are not suitable. In a recent study [39], we developed a modified version of the NCCLS method. We used an antibiotic agar dilution method in which the growth medium was Columbia agar base supplemented with 10% sheep blood. Plates were incubated at 37 °C, in a 5% $CO_2$-enriched atmosphere for 5 days. Such incubation time was previously determined as optimum to allow accurate visualization of bacterial growth. MICs corresponded to the minimal concentration of the antibiotic tested allowing complete inhibition of bacterial growth as compared to a drug-free control.

MICs of 3 *B. henselae* isolates, 9 *B. quintana* isolates, 1 *B. bacilliformis* isolate, and 1 *B. elizabethae* isolate, to a number of antimicrobial agents was determined [39] (table 1). It should be emphasized that according to the modifications of standard NCCLS procedure, in vitro MIC determination for the fastidious *Bartonella* species must be considered cautiously. The results indicated that all isolates of the different *Bartonella* species displayed comparable antibiotic susceptibilities. The isolates of the different *Bartonella* species were highly susceptible to penicillin G, aminopenicillins, third-generation cephalosporins, aminoglycosides, macrolides, tetracyclines and rifampin. They were less susceptible to penicillinase-resistant penicillins, first-generation cephalosporins and clindamycin. Susceptibility to fluoroquinolone compounds varied according to the compound considered, with sparfloxacin and ciprofloxacin being the most effective agents. Although vancomycin was poorly effective, MICs to this antibiotic compound were surprisingly low for Gram-negative bacteria.

*Determination of the Bactericidal Activity of Antibiotics in Axenic Medium*

The bactericidal activity of antibiotics against *B. henselae* was evaluated in broth medium [44]. Bacteria were grown in Schaedler broth medium supplemented with vitamin $K_3$, 5% defibrinated sheep blood, 300 µg/l of hemin, and 5% heat decomplemented fetal calf serum. One milliliter of a bacterial inoculum ($10^6$ CFU/ml) was incorporated into shell vials, and antibiotics were added at various concentrations. Shell vials were incubated at 37 °C in 5% $CO_2$-containing atmosphere, and bacterial counts were determined after 8 and 24 h of incubation respectively, in antibiotic-containing cultures using the CFU technique, and compared to the titer of the primary inoculum. Results showed that amoxicillin (8 µg/ml), cefotaxime (8 µg/ml), ceftriaxone (8 µg/ml), erythromycin (0.5 µg/ml), doxycycline (2 µg/ml), ciprofloxacin (1 µg/ml) and rifampin

*Table 1.* MICs of *B. henselae*, as determined by an antibiotic agar dilution method [39].

| Antibiotics | *B. henselae* | | |
|---|---|---|---|
| | Houston-1 | San Ant-2 | King |
| Penicillin G | 0.03 | 0.06 | 0.03 |
| Oxacillin | 1 | 2 | 2 |
| Amoxicillin | 0.06 | 0.12 | 0.06 |
| Cephalotin | 16 | 16 | 8 |
| Cefotaxime | 0.12 | 0.25 | 0.25 |
| Ceftriaxone | 0.12 | 0.12 | 0.25 |
| Imipenem | 0.12 | 0.25 | 0.25 |
| Gentamicin | 0.12 | 0.25 | 0.25 |
| Tobramycin | 0.5 | 1 | 1 |
| Amikacin | 2 | 4 | 2 |
| Erythromycin | 0.06 | 0.25 | 0.12 |
| Roxithromycin | 0.015 | 0.015 | 0.03 |
| Azithromycin | 0.006 | 0.006 | 0.03 |
| Clarithromycin | 0.006 | 0.006 | 0.03 |
| Doxycycline | 0.12 | 0.12 | 0.12 |
| Pefloxacin | 4 | 4 | 8 |
| Ciprofloxacin | 0.25 | 1 | 0.5 |
| Sparfloxacin | 0.06 | 0.06 | 0.06 |
| Cotrimoxazole[1] | 1/5 | 1/5 | 1/5 |
| Rifampin | 0.03 | 0.06 | 0.03 |
| Colistin | 4 | 16 | 8 |
| Vancomycin | 2 | 8 | 4 |

Columbia agar base supplemented with 10% sheep blood was used as a growth medium, and plates were incubated at 37 °C, in a 5% $CO_2$-enriched atmosphere, for 5 days.

[1] MICs are given for trimethoprim and sulfamethoxazole, respectively.

(4 µg/ml), which are bacteriostatic at such concentrations, did not display any bactericidal activity throughout the 24–hour incubation period. In contrast, the aminoglycosides gentamicin (4 µg/ml), amikacin (16 µg/ml) and tobramycin (4 µg/ml) were highly bactericidal.

*Determination of the Activity of Antibiotics in Cell Systems*

The activity of antibiotics against intracellular *B. henselae* was determined either using a murine macrophage-like cell line (ATCC TIB63) or a human endothelial cell line (ECV 304,9) [44]. Confluent cells, grown in shell vials, were inoculated with $10^7$ CFU of *B. henselae* in 1 ml of RPMI. After centrifugation of the shell vials at 10,000 *g* for 1 h at 37 °C to allow intracellular penetration of bacteria, the supernatant was removed and replaced by 1 ml of fresh RPMI. Antibiotics were added at a single concentration, including amoxicillin (8 μg/ml), cefotaxime (8 μg/ml), ceftriaxone (8 μg/ml) gentamicin (4 μg/ml), amikacin (16 μg/ml), tobramycin (4 μg/ml), erythromycin (0.5 μg/ml), doxycycline (2 μg/ml), ciprofloxacin (1 μg/ml) and rifampin (4 μg/ml). Shell vials were incubated at 37 °C in a 5% $CO_2$-containing atmosphere, and viable bacteria in the supernatant and within cells (after cell lysis) were enumerated using the CFU technique, respectively after 8 and 24 h of incubation. The bacteriostatic activity of antibiotics was determined by comparing bacterial titers in antibiotic-containing cultures to drug-free controls at the same incubation time. As for the bactericidal activity, the titer of bacteria within antibiotic-containing cultures was compared to the titer of the primary inoculum. As compared to antibiotic activity in axenic medium, cocultivation of *Bartonella* species with eukaryotic cells did not change their antibiotic susceptibilities. However, the β-lactam compounds, erythromycin, doxycycline, ciprofloxacin and rifampin did not display any bactericidal activity. In contrast, the aminoglycosides gentamicin, tobramycin and amikacin were highly bactericidal.

More recently, Ives et al. [30] described an alternative methodology to test the activity of antibiotics against the intracellular *Bartonella* species *B. quintana, B. henselae* or *B. elizabethae*. Strains were inoculated to Vero cell monolayers for 2 h at 35 °C in chamber slides as to allow intracellular penetration of bacteria. Various antibiotic concentrations were incorporated in culture media. Cell infection was revealed by an immunofluorescent assay using anti-*Bartonella* antibodies. Inhibition of *Bartonella* proliferation was determined in antibiotic-containing cultures as compared to drug-free infected controls. Intracellular growth of *Bartonella* was obtained with erythromycin, roxithromycin, azithromycin and clarithromycin, with MICs ranging from 0.0156 to 0.75 μg/ml. Azithromycin was the most effective compound with MICs of 0.0156, 0.0312 and 0.0249 μg/ml for *B. henselae, B. quintana* and *B. elizabethae*, respectively.

## Clinical Data on the Activity of Antibiotics to Treat *B. henselae* Diseases

*Bacillary Angiomatosis*

BA refers to a vascular proliferative disease most often involving the skin, but which may disseminate to other organs, including the bone marrow, spleen, liver, brain, lymph nodes or the bowel [24, 31, 43]. The diseases most often involve HIV-infected patients [10, 11, 50, 57] and organ transplant recipients [54]. *B. quintana* and *B. henselae* are both etiologic agents of BA [16, 32, 52].

Failures have been reported in the treatment of BA when using nafcillin, dicloxacillin and cephalexin, which is consistent with the poor in vitro activity of these antibiotic compounds. Erythromycin was the first antibiotic treatment regimen reported to be active in BA-affected patients. A regimen of erythromycin (250–500 mg, 4 times/day) has been advocated as the most effective method of treating cutaneous BA [47, 52–54, 60]. Although fever and cutaneous lesions resolve in almost every case, however, relapses often occur after antibiotic treatment withdrawal, particularly in HIV-infected patients on short courses of treatment of $<15$ days [54]. Clinical data suggest that other antibiotics may be effective, including amoxicillin [35], ceftriaxone [35, 54], aminoglycosides [35, 47], doxycycline [49], trimethoprim-sulfamethoxazole [9, 54], norfloxacin [54] and ciprofloxacin [35, 54], although several patients may also experience relapses after antibiotic therapy has been stopped. Antimycobacterial drugs, supposedly because of the rifampin component, were also reported to be effective in eradicating BA [47], since cutaneous BA lesions resolved when these compounds were administered to treat concomitant mycobacterial diseases. In fact, the duration of therapy may be more important than the choice of antibiotic, especially in the immunocompromised host. Fewer relapses have been noted in patients treated for more than a month, and such antibiotic duration should be considered minimal.

*Endocarditis*

*B. henselae* [20, 27, 29, 35], *B. quintana* [21, 36, 55, 56], and *B. elizabethae* [17] have been associated with bacterial endocarditis. Recently, Raoult et al. [48] diagnosed 22 new cases of culture-negative endocarditis caused by *Bartonella* species, including 5 cases attributed to *B. quintana*, 4 to *B. henselae*, and the remaining 13 to *Bartonella* species (diagnosis was based upon serological investigations which cannot clearly distinguish *Bartonella* species). All 22 cases were native-valve endocarditis. *B. quintana* endocarditis was most often observed in homeless, chronic alcoholic patients, without previous known valvulopathy, whereas *B. henselae* endocarditis most often occurred in patients with known valvulopathy, who had contact with cats. The incidence of *Bartonella* endocarditis was evaluated in patients which were tested in reference centers in three different countries, and corresponded to 3% of all cases of endocarditis diagnosed.

Data on the requirements for the effective treatment of *Bartonella*-induced endocarditis are scarce, again because so few cases have yet been reported. Successful treatment has been reported with a complex therapy regimen consisting of (a) intravenous amoxicillin combined with gentamicin [21]; (b) intravenous vancomycin with ofloxacin and netilmicin, followed by oral therapy with rifampin, ofloxacin and pristinamycin [21], and (c) intravenous ceftriaxone followed by long-term erythromycin [55]. Endocarditis due to *B. elizabethae* did not respond to treatment with nafcillin and gentamicin, but resolved after cardiac-valve replacement and a regimen of vancomycin and imipenem [17]. Intravenous antibiotic therapy was continued for 6 weeks and oral trimethoprim-sulfamethoxazole was administered for a further 5 weeks. It should be noted that *Bartonella*-induced endocarditis usually results in extensive valve damage requiring replacement [17, 21]. The high incidence of *Bartonella* endocarditis and the availability of *Bartonella*-adapted cultures in most clinical laboratory will probably increase the number of cases reported and will help to more precisely define the optimum antibiotic therapy to be administered. The combination of amoxicillin or ceftriaxone with gentamicin seems at present reasonable, both because only the aminoglycosides are highly bactericidal against *Bartonella* species, and because the combination of a β-lactam compound and an aminoglycoside is the first-line antibiotic combination to treat culture-negative endocarditis.

*Cat Scratch Disease*

Although CSD was first described in 1950 [18], *B. henselae* was first recognized as the main etiologic agent of this disease only in 1992, when Regnery et al. [51] demonstrated that 88% of sera of these patients contained antibodies specific to *B. henselae* antigens. *B. henselae* was later isolated from lymph nodes of CSD patients [19, 26, 59] and its DNA was amplified from pus preparations prepared from CSD patients which was used for skin test antigen in CSD diagnostics [46]. In 1988, a Gram-negative bacillus was isolated from infected lymph nodes of patients suffering from CSD [23]. This bacterium was then characterized as a new species, *Afipia felis* [5] and proposed as the etiologic agent of CSD. Although a mass of epidemiological, serological and molecular detection-based data implicated *B. henselae* as the main agent of CSD rather than *A. felis*, very few clinical isolates of *B. henselae* have been obtained. Furthermore, in a minority of cases of typical clinical CSD, no evidence of *B. henselae* infection can be found. Antigenic variations in *B. henselae* strains, as recently detected [20], may explain such discrepancies. Alternatively, the apparent lack of specific antigens in patients with typical clinical signs of CSD may indicate that other etiologic agents including *A. felis*, may occasionally be responsible for CSD [1].

The most frequent clinical presentation of CSD is lymphadenopathy in lymph nodes draining the site of the cat scratch [8]. Local lesions at the site of the scratch may also develop. The involved lymph nodes usually regress over a period of weeks or months, although the lymphadenopathy may proceed to suppuration in approximately 10% of the cases. Unusual presentations include Parinaud's oculoglandular syndrome [7], with preauricular lymphadenopathy and conjunctivitis when bacterial inoculation occurs via the conjunctiva; uveitis and papilloretinitis [63], encephalopathy, erythema nodosum, osteolytic lesions and disseminated diseases with visceral involvement [38, 58, 64] especially occur in immunocompromised patients.

In most cases, the lymphadenopathy of CSD regresses spontaneously within weeks or months. Comparative trials between antibiotic-treated patients and patients receiving placebo are still not available. On the other hand, large-scale studies are scarce and include only the study reported by Carithers et al. [8] on 1,200 CSD involved patients and that reported by Margileth et al. [37] on 268 patients. These reports have emphasized that the chronic lymphadenopathy of CSD does not respond to antibiotic therapy using penicillins, cephalosporins, tetracyclines, macrolides, or chloramphenicol [8, 37]. This is in sharp contrast to the efficacy of such antibiotics in the treatment of BA and other *Bartonella*-related opportunistic infections in AIDS patients. Antibiotics with potential activity included rifampin, ciprofloxacin, gentamicin and cotrimoxazole [37]. Other anecdotal reports indicate that cotrimoxazole [13, 14] and ciprofloxacin [28] may prevent evolution of the chronic lymphadenopathy to local suppuration. However, antibiotic therapy is considered not indicated in immunocompetent patients with typical presentation of CSD. Antibiotic therapy may be indicated in case of local complications or generalized diseases [37, 38], although clinical data indicate that most immunocompetent patients will recover spontaneously without sequelae. Pus aspiration may aid to cure local suppurative complications. Gentamicin has been reported as effective in several patients involved with local or systemic complications of CSD [2, 4, 12]. These data correlate well with the in vitro bactericidal activity of aminoglycosides. Anecdotal reports indicate that rifampin was effective in a patient suffering from hepatosplenic involvement of CSD [25]. Gentamicin (3 mg/kg/day), used intravenously, represents the current recommendation for antibiotic therapy of CSD patients suffering from local or systemic complications, especially in immunocompromised patients. Interestingly, this antibiotic regimen may also be effective in case of *A. felis* coinfection [40]. More clinical data are needed to more precisely define the role of antibiotic therapy in the management of CSD patients. Since, in most cases, CSD resolves spontaneously within weeks or months, comparative clinical trials are needed to determine the optimum antibiotic choice.

The poor efficacy of the β-lactams in the treatment of *Bartonella*-induced illness and the frequency of relapses when antibiotic therapy is withdrawn despite high in vitro susceptibility of bartonellae to antibiotics are striking.

As discussed earlier, several observations and experiments have indicated that *Bartonella* species are also found intracellularly in infected tissue [6]. On the other hand, recent in vitro experiments have shown that most antibiotics, except the aminoglycosides, do not display any bactericidal activity against bartonellae [44], and a bactericidal activity may be more important in vivo especially in immunocompromised patients or patients with chronic infections or endocarditis. Although the formulation of a standard antibiotic regimen for antibiotic treatment of *Bartonella*-related diseases remains hazardous, both the use of aminoglycosides and prolonged administration of the antibiotic therapy should be advocated.

## References


1 Alkan S, Morgan M, Sandin R, Moscinski L, Ross C: Dual role for *Afipia felis* and *Rochalimaea henselae* in cat-scratch disease. Lancet 1995;345:385.

2 Apalsch AM, Nour B, Jaffe R: Systemic cat-scratch disease in a pediatric liver transplant recipient and review of the literature. Pediatr Infect Dis J 1993;12:769–773.

3 Arias-Stella J, Lieberman PH, Erlandson RA: Histology, immunochemistry, and ultrastructure of the verruga in Carrion's disease. Am J Surg Pathol 1986;10:595–610.

4 Bogue CW, Wise JD, Gray GF, Edwards KM: Antibiotic therapy for cat-scratch disease. JAMA 1989;262:813–816.

5 Brenner DJ, Hollis DG, Moss CW, English CK, Hall GS, Vincent J, Radosevic J, Birkness KA, Bibb WF, Quinn FD, Swaminathan B, Weaver RE, Reeves MW, O'Connor SD, Hayes PS, Tenover FC, Steigerwalt AG, Perkins BA, Daneshvar MI, Hill BC, Washington JA, Woods TC, Hunter SB, Hadfield TL, Ajello GW, Kaufmann AF, Wear DJ, Wenger JD: Proposal of *Afipia* gen nov, with *Afipia felis* sp nov (formerly the cat scratch disease Bacillus), *Afipia clevelandensis* sp nov (formerly the Cleveland Clinic Foundation Strain), *Afipia broomeae* sp nov and three unamed genospecies. J Clin Microbiol 1991;29:2450–2460.

6 Brouqui P, Raoult D: *Bartonella quintana* invades and multiplies within endothelial cells in vitro and in vivo and forms intracellular blebs. Res Microbiol 1996;147:719–731.

7 Carithers HA: Oculoglandular disease of Parinaud. Am J Dis Child 1978;132:1195–1200.

8 Carithers HA: Cat-scratch disease. An overview based on a study of 1,200 patients. Am J Dis Child 1985;139:1124–1133.

9 Cockerell CJ, Berghstresser PR, Myrie-Williams C, Tierno PM: Bacillary epithelioid angiomatosis occurring in an immunocompetent individual. Arch Dermatol 1990;126:787–790.

10 Cockerell CJ, Leboit PE: Bacillary angiomatosis: A newly characterized, pseudoneoplastic, infectious cutaneous vascular disorder. J Am Acad Dermatol 1990;22:501–512.

11 Cockerell CJ, Webster GF, Whitlow MA, Friedman-Kien AE: Epithelioid angiomatosis: A distinct vascular disorder in patients with the acquired immunodeficiency syndrome and AIDS-related complex. Lancet 1987;ii:654–656.

12 Cohen-Abbo A, Cheatham S, Edwards KM: Disseminated cat-scratch disease simulating neuroblastoma. Pediatr Infect Dis J 1992;11:1058–1060.

13 Collip PJ: Cat-scratch disease therapy. Am J Dis Child 1989;143:1261.

14 Collip PJ: Cat-scratch disease: Therapy with trimethoprim-sulfamethoxazole. Am J Dis Child 1992; 146:397–399.

15 Conley T, Slater L, Hamilton K: *Rochalimaea* species stimulate human endothelial cell proliferation and migration in vitro. J Lab Clin Med 1994;124:521–528.

16 Cotell S, Noskin G: Bacillary angiomatosis. Clinical and histologic features, diagnosis, and treatment. Arch Intern Med 1994;154:524–528.

17 Daly JS, Worthington MG, Brenner DJ, Moss WC, Hollis DG, Weyant RS, Steigerwalt AG, Weaver RE, Daneshvar MI, O'Connor SP: *Rochalimaea elizabethae* sp nov isolated from a patient with endocarditis. J Clin Microbiol 1993;31:872–881.

18 Debré R, Lamy M, Jammet ML, Costil L, Mozziconacci P: La maladie des griffes du chat. Soc Med Hôp Paris 1950;66:76–79.

19 Dolan MJ, Wong MT, Russel L, Regnery RL, Jorgensen JH, Garcia M, Peters J, Drehner D: Syndrome of *Rochalimaea henselae* adenitis suggesting cat scratch disease. Ann Med Intern 1993; 118:331–336.

20 Drancourt M, Birtles R, Chaumentin G, Vandenesch F, Etienne J, Raoult D: A new serotype of *Bartonella henselae* causes endocarditis and cat-scratch disease. Lancet 1996;347:441–443.

21 Drancourt M, Mainardi J, Brouqui P, Vandenesch F, Carta A, Lehnert F, Etienne J, Goldstein F, Acar J, Raoult D: *Bartonella (Rochalimaea) quintana* endocarditis in three homeless men. N Engl J Med 1995;332:419–423.

22 Drancourt M, Raoult D: Routine identification of *Rochalimaea* species. Eur J Clin Microbiol Infect Dis 1993;12:710–713.

23 English CK, Wear DJ, Margileth AM, Lissner CR, Walsh GP: Cat scratch disease: Isolation and culture of the bacterial agent. JAMA 1988;259:1347.

24 Fagan WA, Skinner SM, Ondo A, Williams JT, Anthony K, De Villez RL, Pulitzer DR: Bacillary angiomatosis of the skin and bone marrow in a patient with HIV infection. J Am Acad Dermatol 1995;32:510–512.

25 Golden SE: Hepatosplenic cat-scratch disease associated with elevated anti-*Rochalimaea* antibody titers. Pediatr Infect Dis J 1993;12:868–871.

26 Gradon JD, Stein DS: Association between *Rochalimaea* infection and cat-scratch disease. Clin Infect Dis 1993;17:287–288.

27 Hadfield TL, Warren R, Kass M, Brun E, Levy C: Endocarditis caused by *Rochalimaea henselae*. Hum Pathol 1993;24:1140–1141.

28 Holley HP: Successful treatment of cat-scratch disease with ciprofloxacin. JAMA 1991;265:1563–1565.

29 Holmes AH, Greenough TC, Balady GJ, Regnery RL, Anderson BE, Okeane JC, Fonger JD, McCrone EL: *Bartonella henselae* endocarditis in an immunocompetent adult. Clin Infect Dis 1995; 21:1004–1007.

30 Ives TJ, Manzewitsch P, Rechery RL, Butts JD, Kebede M: In vitro susceptibilities of *Bartonella henselae, B. quintana, B. elizabethae, Rickettsia rickettsii, R. conorii, R. akari* and *R. prowazekii* to macrolide antibiotics as determined by immunofluorescent-antibody analysis of infected Vero cell monolayers. Antimicrob Agents Chemother 1997;41:578–582.

31 Koehler JE, Cederberg L: Intra-abdominal mass associated with gastrointestinal hemorrhage: A new manifestation of bacillary angiomatosis. Gastroenterology 1995;109:2011–2014.

32 Koehler JE, Quinn FD, Berger TG, Leboit PE, Tappero JW: Isolation of *Rochalimaea* species from cutaneous and osseous lesions of bacillary angiomatosis. N Engl J Med 1992;327:1625–1631.

33 Kordick DL, Breitschwerdt EB: Intraerythrocytic presence of *Bartonella henselae*. J Clin Microbiol 1995;33:1655–1656.

34 Leboit PE, Berger TG, Egbert BM, Beckstead JH, Yen BTS, Stoler MH: Bacillary angiomatosis. The histopathology and differential diagnosis of a pseudoneoplastic infection in patients with human immunodeficiency virus disease. Am J Surg Pathol 1989;13:909–920.

35 Lucey D, Dolan MJ, Moss CW, Garcia M, Hollis DG, Weigner S: Relapsing illness due to *Rochalimaea henselae* in immunocompetent hosts: Implication for therapy and new epidemiological associations. Clin Infect Dis 1992;14:683–688.

36 Mainardi JL, Drancourt M, Roland JM, Gestin JL, Raoult D, Acar JF, Goldstein FW: *Bartonella (Rochalimaea) quintana* endocarditis in an Algerian farmer. Clin Microbiol Infect 1996;1:275–276.

37 Margileth AM: Antibiotic therapy for cat-scratch disease: Clinical study of therapeutic outcome in 268 patients and review of the literature. Pediatr Infect Dis J 1992;11:474–478.

38 Margileth AM, Wear DJ, English CK: Systemic cat scratch disease: Report of 23 patients with prolonged or recurrent severe bacterial infection. J Infect Dis 1987;155:390–404.

39 Maurin M, Gasquet S, Ducco C, Raoult D: MICs of 28 antibiotic compounds for 14 *Bartonella* (formerly *Rochalimaea*) isolates. Antimicrob Agents Chemother 1995;39:2387–2391.

40 Maurin M, Lepocher H, Mallet D, Raoult D: Antibiotics susceptibility of *Afipia felis* in axenic medium and in cells. Antimicrob Agents Chemother 1993;37:1410–1413.
41 Maurin M, Raoult D: Antimicrobial susceptibility of *Rochalimaea quintana, Rochalimaea vinsonii* and the newly recognized *Rochalimaea henselae.* J Antimicrob Chemother 1993;32:587–594.
42 Maurin M, Roux V, Stein A, Ferrier F, Viraben R, Raoult D: Isolation and characterization by immunofluorescence, SDS-PAGE, Western blot, RFLP-PCR, 16S rRNA gene sequencing and pulsed-field gel electrophoresis of *Rochalimaea quintana* from a French patient with bacillary angiomatosis. J Clin Microbiol 1994;33:1166–1171.
43 Milam MW, Balerdi JF, Toney JF, Foulis PR, Milam CP: Epithelioid angiomatosis secondary to disseminated cat scratch disease involving the bone marrow and skin in a patient with acquired immune deficiency syndrome: A case report. Am J Med 1990;88:180–183.
44 Musso D, Drancourt M, Raoult D: Lack of bactericidal effect of antibiotics except aminoglycosides on *Bartonella (Rochalimaea) henselae.* J Antimicrob Chemother 1995;36:101–108.
45 Myers WF, Grossman DM, Wisseman CL Jr: Antibiotic susceptibility patterns in *Rochalimaea quintana*, the agent of trench fever. Antimicrob Agents Chemother 1984;25:690–693.
46 Perkins BA, Swaminathan B, Jackson LA, Brenner DJ, Wenger JD, Regnery RL, Wear DJ: Case 22-1992. Pathogenesis of cat scratch disease. N Engl J Med 1992;327:1599–1601.
47 Perkocha LA, Geaghan SM, Yen TSB, Nishimura SL, Chan SP, Garcia-Kennedy R, Honda G, Stoloff AC, Klein HZ, Goldman RL, van Meter S, Ferrel LD, Leboit PE: Clinical and pathological features of bacillary peliosis hepatitis in association with human immunodeficiency virus infection. N Engl J Med 1990;323:1581–1586.
48 Raoult D, Fournier PE, Drancourt M, Marrie TJ, Etienne J, Cosserat J, Cacoub P, Poinsignon Y, Leclercq P, Sefton AM: Diagnosis of 22 new cases of *Bartonella* endocarditis. Ann Intern Med 1996;125:646–652.
49 Regnery RL, Anderson BE, Clarridge JE, Rodriguez-Barradas MC, Jones DC, Carr JH: Characterization of a novel *Rochalimaea* species, *R. henselae* sp nov, isolated from blood of a febrile, human immunodeficiency virus-positive patient. J Clin Microbiol 1992;30:265–274.
50 Regnery RL, Childs JE, Koehler JE: Infections associated with *Bartonella* species in persons infected with human immunodeficiency virus. Clin Infect Dis 1995;21:S94–S98.
51 Regnery RL, Olson TG, Perkins BA, Bibb W: Serological response to *Rochalimaea henselae* antigen in suspected cat-scratch disease. Lancet 1992;339:1443–1445.
52 Relman DA, Loutit JS, Schmith TM, Falkow S, Tompkins LS: The agent of bacillary angiomatosis. An approach to the identification of uncultured pathogens. N Engl J Med 1990;323: 1573–1580.
53 Rudikoff D, Phelps RG, Gordon RE, Bottone EJ: Acquired immunodeficiency syndrome-related bacillary vascular proliferation (epithelioid angiomatosis): Rapid response to erythromycin therapy. Arch Dermatol 1989;125:706–707.
54 Slater L, Welch DF, Hensel D, Coody DW: A newly recognized fastidious gram-negative pathogen as a cause of fever and bacteremia. N Engl J Med 1990;323:1587–1593.
55 Spach DH, Callis KP, Paauw DS, Houze YB, Schoenknecht FD, Welch DF, Rosen H, Brenner DJ: Endocarditis caused by *Rochalimaea quintana* in a patient infected with human immunodeficiency virus. J Clin Microbiol 1993;31:692–694.
56 Spach DH, Kanter AS, Daniels NA, Nowowiejski DJ, Larson AM, Schmidt RA, Swaminathan B, Brenner DJ: *Bartonella (Rochalimaea)* species as a cause of apparent 'culture-negative' endocarditis. Clin Infect Dis 1995;20:1044–1047.
57 Stoler MH, Bonfiglio TA, Staigbigel MT, Pereira M: An atypical subcutaneous infection associated with acquired immune deficiency syndrome. Am J Clin Pathol 1983;80:714–718.
58 Tan TQ, Wagner ML, Kaplan SL: *Bartonella (Rochalimaea) henselae* hepatosplenic infection occurring simultaneously in two siblings. Clin Infect Dis 1996;22:721–722.
59 Waldvogel K, Regnery RL, Anderson BE, Caduff R, Caduff J, Nadal D: Disseminated cat-scratch disease: Detection of *Rochalimaea henselae* in affected tissue. Eur J Pediatr 1994;153:23–27.
60 Welch DF, Pickett DA, Slater LN, Steigerwalt AG, Brenner DJ: *Rochalimaea henselae* sp nov, a cause of septicemia, bacillary angiomatosis, and parenchymal bacillary peliosis. J Clin Microbiol 1992;30:275–280.

61 Wong MT, Thornton DC, Kennedy RC, Dolan MJ: A chemically defined liquid medium that supports primary isolation of *Rochalimaea (Bartonella) henselae* from blood and tissue specimens. J Clin Microbiol 1995;33:742–744.
62 Zbinden R, Höchli M, Nadal D: Intracellular location of *Bartonella henselae* cocultivated with Vero cells and used for an indirect fluorescent-antibody test. Clin Diagn Lab Immunol 1995;2: 693–695.
63 Zhao X, Ge B: Treatment of papillo-retinitis and uveitis associated with cat-scratch disease by combination of TCM and modern drugs. J Tradit Chin Med 1991;11:184–186.
64 Zinzindohoue F, Guiard-Schmid JB, La Scola B, Frottier J, Parc R: Portal triad involvement in cat-scratch disease. Lancet 1996;348:1178–1179.

M. Maurin, Unité des Rickettsies, CNRS UPRESA 6020, Université de la Mediterranée,
Faculté de Médecine, 27, Blvd Jean-Moulin, F–13385 Marseille Cedex 05 (France)

Schmidt A (ed): *Bartonella* and *Afipia* Species Emphasizing *Bartonella henselae*.
Contrib Microbiol. Basel, Karger, 1998, vol 1, pp 176–182

# Therapy of *Bartonella henselae*-Associated Human Disease

*Christina Krasemann*

Department of Medical Microbiology and Immunology, Rheinische Friedrich Wilhelms University Bonn, Germany

## Introduction

Recommendations for antibiotic therapy in defined infections are usually based on two different types of observations: adequate in vitro investigations and well-documented clinical studies. The combination of both findings normally results in guidelines for sensitivity testing and in the definition of critical MIC values for 'sensitive' and 'resistant' strains, even though these definitions are not unanimously accepted. For *Bartonella henselae*, unfortunately, none of these prerequisites is fulfilled. This unsatisfactory situation can be explained by the fact that the relation between this pathogen and cat-scratch disease (CSD) or bacillary angiomatosis (BA) was only recently established. In 1950, Debré et al. [5] described CSD and in 1983, Stoler et al. [18] found by a special staining method bacilli in the lesions of an HIV-positive patient presenting with BA. But the isolation of the pathogen was only described in 1992 in BA [11] and 1993 in CSD [6]. Furthermore, the pathogen is very fastidious and it is not surprising that hitherto only a limited number of strains has been isolated and identified or sensitivity tests have been performed. Under the conditions of a routine laboratory, the pathogen presumably is overlooked in many cases, e.g. positive blood cultures might only be identified applying unusual methods after at least one week of incubation or longer.

## In vitro Sensitivity of *B. henselae* and Related Organisms to Antibiotics

As *B. henselae* is a fastidious organism, standard methods for MIC determination and interpretation according to NCCLS (National Committee for

*Table 1.* MIC ranges (μg/ml) with three strains of *Bartonella henselae* [14]

| | MIC range | | MIC range | | MIC range |
|---|---|---|---|---|---|
| *β-Lactams* | | *Macrolides* | | *Aminoglycosides* | |
| Penicillin | 0.03–0.06 | Erythromycin | 0.06–0.25 | Gentamicin | 0.12–0.25 |
| Amoxicillin | 0.06–0.12 | Roxithromycin | 0.015–0.03 | Tobramycin | 0.5–1 |
| Amoxicillin +clavulanic acid | 0.06–0.12 | Clarithromycin | 0.006–0.03 | Amikacin | 2–4 |
| | | Azithromycin | 0.006–0.015 | | |
| Ticarcillin | 0.25 | | | *Others* | |
| Oxacillin | 1–2 | | | Doxycylcine | 0.12 |
| Cefalotin | 8–16 | *Quinolones* | | Rifampin | 0.03–0.06 |
| Cefotetan | 0.25–0.5 | Pefloxacin | 4–8 | TMP/SMX | 1/5 |
| Cefotaxime | 0.12–0.25 | Ciprofloxacin | 0.25–1 | Clindamycin | 2–4 |
| Ceftriaxone | 0.12–0.25 | Sparfloxacin | 0.06 | Vancomycin | 2–8 |
| Ceftazidime | 0.25–0.5 | | | Fosfomycin | 16–32 |
| Imipenem | 0.5 | | | Colistin | 4–16 |

Clinical Laboratory Standards) or comparable organizations are not applicable and recommendations for this recently recognized pathogen are not available. Therefore, it is not astonishing that different approaches have been described in the literature and they yield contradictory results. Maurin et al. [14] tested a total of 14 strains, belonging to the species *B. quintana, B. vinsonii, B. henselae* and *B. elizabethae*, performing the agar dilution method. As this approach still is the basic and predominant technique for sensitivity testing, the results for *B. henselae* are shown in detail in table 1. With regard to the β-lactams, benzylpenicillin, amoxicilin, ticarcillin, cefotaxime, ceftriaxone, ceftazidime and imipenem were highly effective, according to conventional definitions. The same is true for all macrolides as well as doxycycline and rifampin. The lowest MICs for quinolones were observed with sparfloxacin, followed by ciprofloxacin and pefloxacin. The least active compounds were fosfomycin, vancomycin and colistin. The other *Bartonella* species showed almost identical sensitivity pattern.

In 1993, Dolan et al. [6] reported the susceptibility of 3 isolates of *B. henselae* with the broth microdilution method. The MICs are comparable to the results shown in table 1. Wolfson et al. [20] tested 10 isolates of *B. henselae* against erythromycin, azithromycin, doxycycline, ciprofloxacin, rifampicin and vancomycin with the E-test. They basically found the same results as reported with the agar dilution test. The isolates were resistant to vancomycin and sensitive to all other compounds. Good agreement between E-test and agar dilution was also found by Picket and Welch [16].

Even though *B. henselae* can be grown with completely cell-free agar or broth media, this species has the capability to adhere and penetrate into cells [3]. Therefore, sensitivity testing with cell culture systems seems a reasonable approach. Musso et al. [15] compared the activity of several β-lactams and aminoglycosides, doxycycline, rifampicin, erythromycin and ciprofloxacin, using two different cell lines and an axenic medium. Bactericidal activity against the *B. henselae* strain ATCC 49882 after at least 24 h exposure to the antibiotics was observed only with the aminoglycosides. There was no difference between the cell culture systems and the axenic medium. The authors conclude that aminoglycosides may be an effective therapy against *B. henselae* infections.

Ives et al. [7] found good activity of all macrolides investigated. The known efficacy of tetracycline was used as control. They claim that the good intracellular penetration of the antibiotic might be an important factor for the efficacy against *Bartonella* strains because they are facultative intracellular pathogens.

## In vitro Testing as Guide to Therapy

It seems reasonable to conclude that compounds with high MICs will not be effective in vivo and therefore they should be precluded from therapy. With regard to *B. henselae* this is true for oxacillin, cefalotin and other cephalosporins of the first generation, clindamycin, vancomycin, fosfomycin and colistin. Possibly the E-test is the most practical approach to sort out ineffective antibiotics or to see whether a clinical isolate with this chronic type of infection shows an unusual resistance pattern, e.g. in recurrent septic episodes. More sophisticated methods like cell cultures presumably are too time-consuming and too expensive to be performed for individual infections, but they yield useful information when performed periodically by specialized reference laboratories with larger collections of the most recent isolates. Trends of changing sensitivity patterns could be recognized and communicated.

## Clinical Observations

Low MICs do not ensure clinical success. The outcome of well-designed clinical studies or at least well-documented observations in single cases are the only reliable guide for selecting the appropriate antibiotic. But here again the current situation is still unsatisfactory.

Infections due to *B. henselae* can be divided into two groups:

(1) *Localized self-limiting lymphadenitis* is observed in immunocompetent persons (CSD sensu strictu). The symptoms might persist for 2–6 months until spontaneous resolution is completed. Fortunately, the vast majority of cases belongs to this category, where observation and conservative symptomatic treatment is sufficient. In this situation it is extremely difficult to judge the effect of an antibiotic therapy. The course of the lymphadenopathy is not clearly shortened; it is possible that the predominant cell-mediated immunologic response to the antigen continues, even after viable bacteria are no longer present [1, 8, 9]. Reports about antibiotic therapy are biased by this circumstance. In 1992, two retrospective comprehensive compilations of antibiotic treatment in CSD were published. Magileth [13] reports a retrospective uncontrolled study over 24 months with 268 patients. 202 of them were treated with one or two substances separately for at least 3–5 days. Effectiveness of therapy was controlled by follow-up examinations and telephone calls. Main criterion was clinical improvement, and in 90 patients the sedimentation rate was measured. As many as 18 different antibiotics were given to these patients. Only 4 substances were judged as beneficial: the efficacy rates were 87% for rifampin, 84% for ciprofloxacin, 58% for trimethoprim-sulfmethoxazole and 73% for intramuscular gentamicin. Collipp [4] summarizes 101 cases, observed from 1984 to 1990. 71 patients received trimethoprim-sulfmethoxazole, 25 oral first-generation cephalosporins, 3 other antibiotics and 2 no antibacterials. According to his experience, only in the trimethoprim-sulfmethoxazole group the infection healed promptly without suppuration or drainage from the nodules, whereas in 7 other patients the process progressed steadily. From September 1991 through November 1993, Wong et al. [21] prospectively identified 26 patients with *B. henselae* infections either by serology (IFA) or culture. They showed different clinical symptoms, 11 of them lymphadenitis alone. The authors observed that therapy with either penicillins or cephalosporins did not prevent the progression of the symptoms. But therapy with erythromycin or doxycycline, eventually in combination with rifampin, for 4 weeks showed good clinical results.

(2) *Severe disseminating infections* with or without bacteremia mainly occur in immunocompromised patients and especially endanger HIV-positive persons. They can affect all organs. Here, in contrast to the self-limiting lymphadenopathy, the benefit of antimicrobial therapy is undebated. The clinical response is rapid and untreated infections might be fatal. But again systematic studies are lacking and therapy can only be based on clinical experience. According to the review articles of Adal et al. [2] and Koehler and Tappero [10], cutaneous and bacillary angiomatosis and bacillary peliosis hepatis should

be treated either with erythromycin or, in case of intolerance, with doxycycline. It has been recommended to start antibiotic therapy in severely ill patients intravenously with a combination of erythromycin or doxacyclin with rifampin or gentamicin. A Jarisch-Herxheimer reaction after initiation of therapy is possible [11].

Severe infections both in immunocompetent and in immunocompromised patients might need an extremely long duration of antibiotic therapy. Wong et al. [21] describe 3 cases of neuroretinitis and 1 case of chronic fatigue syndrome in immunocompetent adult patients. Therapy with oral doxycycline and rifampin was given for 4 weeks. In 3 cases either symptoms persisted or bacteremia recurred, necessitating antibiotic therapy for 4 more weeks until resolution. The regimen was modified to ofloxacin plus rifampin or azithromycin plus rifampin. Liston and Koehler [12] report a case of granulomatous hepatitis and necrotizing splenitis in a patient with cancer. Therapy with doxycycline in combination with rifampin was given for as long as 4 months. On the other hand, monotherapy with rifampin at a dose of 15 mg/kg/day for only 2 weeks might be sufficient even in hepatosplenic manifestations. Tan et al. [19] observed 2 cases in immunocompetent brothers aged 5.5 and 4 years respectively.

The difficulty to eradicate the bacteria in severe infections is confirmed by recently published data with experimental infections in cats [17]. The authors investigated amoxicillin, the veterinary quinolone enrofloxacin, tetracycline and erythromycin. The β-lactam and quinolone antibiotic showed no effect. Only tetracycline and erythromycin depressed the bacteremia. However, even with these antibiotics the duration of bacteremia remained similar to that in untreated cats.

## Conclusions

In immunocompetent patients only severe infections with *B. henselae* require antibiotic treatment. With regard to the choice of the suitable drug, the situation in CSD seems far less clear as compared to severe infections in immunocompromised patients. Recent case reports based on actual diagnostic methods and comparing different substances are lacking. In immunocompromised patients either erythromycin or doxycycline in combination with rifampin or gentamicin are established therapies. The efficacy of both tetracycline and erythromycin is further substantiated by experimental infection in cats. However, actually it seems impossible to define the duration of therapy precisely. It can only be based on the observation of the clinical symptoms and might need several months. Severe infections in immunocompetent patients should be treated with the same regimen.

Keeping in mind the in vitro activity against *B. henselae* and pharmocokinetic properties of newer macrolides such as azithromycin, clarithromycin or roxithromycin, these substances merit further systematic evaluation for the treatment of infections due to this microorganism. Perhaps newer quinolones are of interest as well.

Until further data are available, it seems reasonable to apply the same antibiotics (macrolides, tetracyclines and/or rifampin) in CSD as it is recommended for BA in immunocompromised patients.

## References


1 Adal KA: *Bartonella*: New species and new diseases. Rev Med Microbiol 1995;6:155–164.

2 Adal KA, Cockerell CJ, Petri WA: Cat scratch disease, bacillary angiomatosis, and other infections due to *Rochalimea*. N Engl J Med 1994;330:1509–1515.

3 Batterman HJ, Peek JA, Loutit JS, Falkow S, Tompkins LS: *Bartonella henselae* and *Bartonella quintana* adherence to and entry into cultured human epithelial cells. Infect Immun 1995;63:4553–4556.

4 Collipp PJ: Cat-scratch disease: Therapy with trimethoprim-sulfmethoxazole. Am J Dis Child 1992; 146:397–399.

5 Debré R, Lamy M, Lammet ML, Costil L, Mozziconacci P: La maladie des griffes de chat. Bull Mem Soc Méd Hed Hôp Paris 1950:66;76–79.

6 Dolan MJ, Wong MT, Regnery RL, Jorgensen JH, Garcia M, Peters J, Drehner D: Syndrome of *Rochalimaea henselae* adenitis suggesting cat scratch disease. Ann Intern Med 1993;118:331–336.

7 Ives TJ, Manzewitsch P, Regnery RL, Butts JD, Kibede M: In vitro susceptibilities of *Bartonella henselae, B. quintana, B. elizabethae, Rickettsia rickettsii, R. conorii, R. akari,* and *R. prowazekii* to macrolide antibiotics as determined by immunofluorescent-antibody analysis of infected Vero cell monolayers. Antimicrob Agents Chemother 1997;41:578–582.

8 Jerris RC, Regnery RL: Will the real agent of cat scratch disease please stand up? Annu Rev Microbiol 1996;50:707–725.

9 Koehler JE: *Bartonella* infections. Adv Pediatr Infect Dis 1996;11:1–27.

10 Koehler JE, Tappero JW: Bacillary angiomatosis and bacillary peliosis in patients infected with human immunodeficiency virus. Clin Infect Dis 1993;17:612–624.

11 Koehler JE, Quinn FD, Berger TG: Isolation of *Rochalimea* species from cutaneous and osseous lesions of bacillary angiomatosis. N Engl J Med 1992;327:1625–1631.

12 Liston TE, Koehler JE: Granulomatous hepatitis and necrotizing splenitis due to *Bartonella henselae* in a patient with cancer: Case report and review of hepatosplenic manifestations of *Bartonella* infection. Clin Infect Dis 1996;22:951–957.

13 Magileth AM: Antibiotic treatment for cat scratch disease: Clinical study of therapeutic outcome in 268 patients and review of the literature. Pediatr Infect Dis J 1992;11:474–478.

14 Maurin M, Gasquet S, Ducco C, Raoult D: MICs of 28 antibiotic compounds for 14 *Bartonella* (formerly *Rochalimaea*) isolates. Antimicrob Agents Chemother 1995;39:2387–2391.

15 Musso D, Drancourt M, Raoult D: Lack of bactericidal effect of antibiotics except aminoglycosides on *Bartonella henseale*. J Antimicrob Chemother 1995;36:101–108.

16 Picket DA, Welch DF: Susceptibility testing of *Bartonella* spp. Abstr Gen Meet Am Soc Microbiol, 1995, p 18, abstr C-102.

17 Regnery RL, Rooney JA, Johnson AM, Nesby SL, Manzewitsch P, Bever K, Olson JG: Experimentally induced *Bartonella henselae* infections followed by challenge exposure and antimicrobial therapy in cats. Am J Vet Res 1996;57:1714–1719.

18 Stoler MH, Bonfiglio TA, Steigbigel RT, Pereira M: An atypical subcutaneous infection associated with acquired immune deficiency syndrome. Am J Clin Pathol 1983;80:714–718.

19 Tan TQ, Wagner ML, Kaplan SL: *Bartonella (Rochalimea) henselae* hepatosplenic infection occurring simultaneously in two siblings. Clin Infect Dis 1996;22:721–722.
20 Wolfson C, Branley J, Gottlieb T: The E-test for antimicrobial susceptibility testing of *Bartonella henselae*. J Antimicrob Chemother 1996;38:963–968.
21 Wong MT, Dolan MJ, Lattuada CP, Regnery RL, Garcia ML, Mokulis EC, LaBarre RC, Ascher DP, Delmar JA, Kelly JW, Leigh DR, McRae AC, Reed JB, Smith RE, Melcher GP: Neuroretinitis, aseptic meningitis, and lymphadenitis associated with *Bartonella henselae* infection in immunocompetent patients and patients infected with human immunodeficiency virus type 1. Clin Infect Dis 1995; 21:352–360.

Christina Krasemann, apl. Prof. for Medical Microbiology and Immunology,
Rheinische Friedrich Wilhelms University Bonn, Friedenstrasse 12, D–40724 Hilden (Germany)

Schmidt A (ed): *Bartonella* and *Afipia* Species Emphasizing *Bartonella henselae*.
Contrib Microbiol. Basel, Karger, 1998, vol 1, pp 183–200

# Infections and Carriership of *Bartonella* and *Afipia* Species in Veterinary Medicine

*Dorsey L. Kordick, Edward B. Breitschwerdt*

Department of Companion Animal and Special Species Medicine,
College of Veterinary Medicine, North Carolina State University,
Raleigh, N.C., USA

The genera *Afipia* and *Bartonella* have important relationships to veterinary medicine. In the late 1980s, English et al. [1] observed argyrophilic bacilli in the lymph nodes of several cat scratch disease (CSD) patients. Subsequent isolation and culture of the organism from affected lymph nodes resulted in the description of the genus *Afipia*, including *Afipia felis*, belived to be the elusive causative agent of CSD [2]. In 1992, two groups reported the isolation of *Bartonella* (previously called *Rochalimaea*) from patients with and without underlying disease [3, 4]. Shortly thereafter, Regnery et al. [5] developed an indirect fluorescent antibody (IFA) test to detect *Bartonella*-specific serum immunoglobulins. Utilizing the IFA technique to analyze samples from people with assorted disorders, investigators observed that most sera from CSD patients were strongly reactive against *Bartonella* but not *Afipia* antigens. This observation initiated further research into the etiology of CSD. Since that time, several studies have begun to define the incidence of *Bartonella* infections in domestic cats and have initiated a search for *Bartonella* species in other animals.

Only one species of *Afipia, A. felis*, has been associated with animal contact. These Gram-negative, argyrophilic organisms belong to the $\alpha 2$ subgroup of proteobacteria and are catalase-negative, oxidase-positive, urease-positive, and motile using monotrichous flagella. These pleomorphic bacteria are approximately $0.2–0.5 \times 0.2–2.5$ µm in size and can be isolated from environmental surface water. Laboratory cultivation of *A. felis* is best achieved on buffered charcoal yeast extract medium under aerobic conditions at incubation temperatures of 25–30 °C. Genotypic analysis of the genus *Afipia* has revealed a close relationship to nitrogen fixing bacteria that live in the soil; however, tolerance of higher salt concentrations by *A. felis* permits its survival at physiological conditions.

Systemic infection and subsequent recovery of *A. felis* from animals has been accomplished in experimentally-inoculated hamsters, mice, guinea pigs, rats, and nine-banded armadillos [1]. Mice and rats maintained subclinical infections for 22 days at which time *A. felis* was recovered from spleen and liver of mice and lymph nodes of rats. Lymph node cultures from guinea pigs were positive 30 days postinoculation while brain tissue from hamsters was culture-positive at 31 and 60 days postinoculation. Only the armadillo developed clinical evidence of infection in the form of dermal lesions reminiscent of those observed in people. Histologic examination of biopsied skin revealed degenerative bundles of collagen containing *Afipia* organisms and viable *A. felis* were recovered from cultured lesional tissue. Experimental, intracutaneous inoculation of rabbits with *A. felis* for polyclonal antibody production did not result in readily apparent signs of infection [6]. Since the investigators assumed infection was not established, the rabbits were bled weekly to evaluate seroreactivity but bacteremia was not assessed. Following the initial inoculation, the rabbits produced undetectable to low levels of *Afipia*-specific antibodies. Six weeks after rechallenge, the antibody titer against *A. felis* was higher, but cross-reactivity with *Bartonella* antigens was also reported.

The medical literature contains numerous cases of CSD attributed to infection with *A. felis*. Diagnoses have been based upon serology, culture, and PCR amplification of *A. felis* DNA from tissue specimens. However, to the best of our knowledge, the isolation of *A. felis* from blood or other tissues of naturally-infected animals has not been reported. Recent microbiologic studies involving dogs and cats associated with CSD patients have been optimized to enhance the recovery of *Bartonella* species, but have not utilized media or conditions appropriate for cultivation of *Afipia*. *Afipia* species grow best aerobically at 25–30 °C, while *Bartonella* prefer 28–37 °C with 5% $CO_2$. Cultures for both *Afipia* and *Bartonella* may require prolonged incubation. *Afipia* colonies are usually visible within 2–9 days, while *Bartonella* colonies are often not evident until after 2 weeks of incubation. Although a chemically-defined liquid medium that supports growth of *B. henselae, B. quintana*, and *A. felis* has been described, only one blood culture attempt which resulted in the isolation of *B. henselae* from a cat has been reported [7]. Analysis of sera from pet cats and dogs owned by CSD patients in Hawaii revealed seroreactivity against *A. felis* in 1/30 cats and 1/27 dogs [8]. As blood cultures were not obtained, the significance of this observation is unknown. Other canine and feline serosurveys have been performed with antigen derived from *Bartonella* species, but in responders and nonresponders, reactivity against *A. felis* was not tested. Although recent investigations have not adequately addressed the potential for cats or dogs to act as biological vectors of *A. felis*, there is some evidence to warrant consideration of their role as a mechanical vector for human exposure. Given the ability of *A. felis* to survive in the environment, its presence in the mouth or claws of cats and dogs could conceivably lead to human infection following close or traumatic contact.

In contrast to observations indicating that *A. felis* is an infrequent cause of CSD, *Bartonella* species have emerged as important human pathogens. Several isolates of *Bartonella* have been characterized in recent years, increasing the number of recognized species and subspecies to twelve. Many apparently unique strains await taxonomic classification. *Bartonella* are Gram-negative, argyrophilic capnophiles that also belong to the $\alpha$ subgroup of proteobacteria. Biochemically, they are minimally reactive, although some species (those previously called *Grahamella*) are Voges-Proskauer-positive. Most *Bartonella* are nonmotile, however, *B. bacilliformis* and *B. clarridgeiae* possess lophotrichous flagella and have been observed to have a twitching movement. In the presence of exogenous $CO_2$, growth can be achieved on blood agar at 28–37 °C, depending upon the species. Phylogenetic analyses using the DNA sequence of the 16S ribosomal RNA, citrate synthase (gltA), or heat-shock protein (groEL) genes have identified *Bartonella* as close relatives of *Brucella* and *Agrobacterium*, intracellular pathogens of animals and plants, respectively. The natural host range of *Bartonella* species is wide and vectorial transmission by fleas, lice, ticks, mites and flies is common to members of the genus.

*B. vinsonii* subspecies *vinsonii* was originally isolated from voles in Grosse Isle, Canada in the mid-1900s during a scrub typhus study [9]. When captured, voles had enlarged spleens, but splenomegaly was not necessarily associated with positive organ cultures or bacteremia. No other gross abnormalities or signs of illness were evident. Baker [9] experimentally inoculated hamsters, mice, guinea pigs, monkeys and rabbits with a suspension of yolk sacs infected with the 'vole agent'. The hamsters and mice developed subclinical bacteremia that persisted until sacrifice 75 days postinoculation. Some bacteremic guinea pigs became slightly febrile, lost weight, and developed low complement-fixing antibody titers (1:8–1:16). In contrast, monkeys and rabbits that received inoculum did not develop clinical signs of infection or bacteremia. In order to investigate the possibility of intrauterine transmission or transmission through casual cage contact, ectoparasites were removed from pregnant naturally-infected voles and subsequent litters were evaluated for bacteremia. Transfer of infection was not detected.

Since Baker's study [9], no additional isolations of *B. v. vinsonii* have been reported. However, field-caught rodents and other small mammals in Europe,

Africa and the USA comprise a large reservoir for numerous *Bartonella* species, many of which are currently being speciated. Birtles et al. obtained several *Bartonella* isolates from fat sand rats in Tunisia [unpubl. data] and small woodland mammals in England and France [10]. Methanol-fixed blood smears were stained by the Giemsa method and up to 2% of erythrocytes were infected, with each cell containing from 1 to 20 organisms. Careful analysis of these isolates and a review of closely related *Grahamella* species, led to the reclassification of *Grahamella* species into the genus *Bartonella* [11]. Cultures of *B. peromysci* and *B. talpae* are no longer available for study. *B. taylorii, B. doshiae* and *B. grahamii* are recognized as commensals in a variety of Old and New World rodents and small mammals. As a group, these rodent isolates can be diffentiated from other *Bartonella* species by a positive Voges-Proskauer test. Recently, Kosoy et al. [12] described *Bartonella* strains cultured from various rodents in the USA. These strains have not yet been recovered from people or other animals, but they appear to be closely related to *B. grahamii* and *B. elizabethae* (a species associated with a single case of human endocarditis). Although not host-specific with regard to a particular type of rodent, polyclonal bacteremia appears to be uncommon. Infected rodents usually harbor only one species of *Bartonella* at a time, perhaps indicating vector specificity. *Bartonella* isolates were more often obtained in late summer and early autumn, probably due to the prevalence of arthropod vectors. Carriership of heavy bacterial loads in rodents appears to be asymptomatic, and postmortem examination of infected animals did not reveal macroscopic abnormalities. A unique *Bartonella* species was recently isolated from asymptomatic warren rabbits in France [Heller et al., unpubl. data].

Experimental intraperitoneal inoculation of CD-1 mice with $10^5$–$10^7$ CFU of *B. henselae* or *B. quintana* (a species not yet found in mice) results in the production of immune sera without apparent morbidity [13]. However, despite the absence of overt clinical signs, experimental infection of SCID and Balb/C mice with $10^8$–$10^9$ CFU of *B. henselae* or *B. clarridgeiae* will induce bacteremia and neutrophilic inflammation in the spleen and liver of both immunocompetent and immunocompromised mice, and microabscess formation in the lungs of immunocompromised mice [Brown et al., unpubl. data]. Similarly, rabbits infected for polyclonal antibody production have not developed gross lesions, or morbidity or mortality following *Bartonella* inoculation [6].

Besides rodents, *Bartonella* species can also infect other feral animal species. Heller et al. [unpubl. data] recently isolated a previously uncharacterized *Bartonella* from roe deer in France. Similarly, healthy, black-tail deer in the western US were also bacteremic with a *Bartonella* [Chomel et al., unpubl. data]. Paradoxically, although the black-tailed deer were bacteremic, very few were seroreactive when tested against antigens derived from *B. henselae* or from isolates obtained from the deer. During the same survey, investigators also isolated bartonellae from coyotes. In addition, limited studies have identified bacteremic and/or seroreactive free-ranging mountain lions and bobcats, and captive felids. Isolates appear to be closely related to *B. henselae*. Chomel et al. [unpubl. data] observed that heavy tick infestation was associated with bacteremia in free-roaming felids, while flea infestation and often ear mites were associated with seroreactivity of zoo animals. A convenience survey of various felids kept at a nonprofit trust in the southeastern US detected *Bartonella*-specific seroreactivity in caracals, tigers and snow leopards [Kordick and Breitschwerdt, unpubl. data]. Although organisms were not recovered by blood culture, *Bartonella*-specific DNA was amplified from caracal blood samples. The captive cats were housed outdoors and therefore exposed to potential arthropod vectors such as fleas, ticks, or mites that could serve as vectors for bartonellae from the rodent or domestic cat populations.

Dogs can be naturally infected with *B. vinsonii* subspecies *berkhoffii*. The type strain was isolated from the blood of a dog with vegetative, valvular endocarditis [14, 15], and preliminary data suggests its association with additional cases of culture-negative endocarditis in dogs [Breitschwerdt, unpubl. data]. The dog from which the type strain was recovered had been diagnosed with and treated for ehrlichiosis and systemic lupus erythematosus during the preceding 5 months. Although not unique to *Bartonella* infection, clinical abnormalities included mild anemia, thrombocytopenia, hyperproteinemia, recurrent epistaxis, shifting leg lameness, weight loss, and suppurative vasculitis. In addition to the amplification of *B. v. berkhoffii* DNA from the aortic valve, organisms were visualized in the valve tissue by transmission electron microscopy. *B. v. berkhoffii* has also been implicated as a cause of granulomatous lymphadenitis and peliosis hepatis in dogs [Breitschwerdt, unpubl. data]. *B. v. berkhoffii* has also been cultured from subclinically bacteremic dogs [14, 16]. Although chronic, asymptomatic *Bartonella* infection does not appear to be as common in dogs as in cats, *B. v. berkhoffii* was cultured repeatedly from a healthy dog during a 14-month observation period [16]. This dog was housed indoors with 7 cats, of which 1 was infected with *B. henselae* and 1 with *B. clarridgeiae*. Despite continued close contact, and the occasional presence of fleas, the dog did not become bacteremic with *B. henselae* or *B. clarridgeiae*, nor did the cats become bacteremic with or seroconvert to *B. v. berkhoffii* antigen. Dogs appear to be preferentially susceptible to *B. v. berkhoffii* and attempts by Chomel [17] to infect dogs with *B. henselae* were unsuccessful. Although seroconversion to *B. henselae* occurred, infection was not believed to be established, since subsequent isolation of the organism by blood culture was not accomplished.

An ecologic source of *B. v. berkhoffii* has not been found, but ticks should be considered as likely vectors. A seroepidemiologic study performed in the southeastern US detected seroreactivity to *B. v. berkhoffii* in 3.6% (69/1,920) of the sick dogs tested [18]. Seroreactivity was strongly associated with tick rather than flea exposure. Simultaneous transmission of *B. vinsonii* along with other vector-borne organisms such as *Ehrlichia canis* or *Babesia canis* probably occurs in endemic regions. Epidemiologic analysis suggested a role for *Rhipicephalus sanguineus* in the transmission between dogs, while other ticks such as *Dermacentor variabilis, Amblyoma americanum* and *Ixodes scapularis* should be considered as potential vectors from a wildlife reservoir.

During the past few years, a substantive amount of data has been generated with regard to the prevalence and persistence of *Bartonella* infections in cats. It has become quite apparent that bartonellosis occurs more frequently in cats than in dogs. Many healthy cats carry *Bartonella*, and feline infections are unequivocally endemic in domestic cat populations throughout the world. Two species have been cultured from cats (*B. henselae* and *B. clarridgeiae*) and potentially unique strains have been reported [19, 20]. *Bartonella* organisms have been isolated from cats living in the USA, the UK, Switzerland, Germany, France, The Netherlands, Australia, New Zealand, Japan and Israel [20–29; Baneth et al., unpubl. data]. Seroreactivity has also been reported in cats from Egypt, Portugal and southern Africa [30, 31]. The degree of *Bartonella* endemicity appears to correspond with regional climates. Jameson et al. [32] performed a serosurvey encompassing numerous regions of the USA utilizing samples obtained from commercial diagnostic labs. The authors concluded that seroreactivity was positively correlated with estimated cat flea populations, which are associated with warmer temperatures and increased precipitation. Ueno et al. [33] made similar observations during a study performed in Japan.

Bergmans et al. [34] observed differences in the DNA sequence of the 16S rRNA gene of *B. henselae* isolates from human patients and from a cat in The Netherlands. This observation led to the distinction of subtypes I and II. When cultivated on solid media, morphologic differences between types I and II are not obvious. Furthermore, no correlation was found between the types and disease presentation in people; however, investigations are underway to determine if strain variations are associated with pathogenicity in animals. In Germany, researchers have also detected genotypic variations among cat isolates of *B. henselae* that may eventually lead to recognition of biological relevance associated with further subtyping of *Bartonella* species [23].

Concomitant infection with different types of *B. henselae* or *B. henselae* and *B. clarridgeiae* can occur. The authors inoculated specific-pathogen-free (SPF) cats with blood from a donor naturally coinfected with *B. henselae* and *B. clarridgeiae* [unpubl. data]. At times, recipient cats became bacteremic with *B. henselae*, and at other times, recipients became bacteremic with *B. clarridgeiae*. In France, Gurfield et al. [25] reported coinfection with *B. henselae* and *B. clarridgeiae* in 5/436 blood cultured cats, while 2/436 were concurrently bacteremic with *B. henselae* types I and II. Based upon currently used techniques, it is probable that coinfection with *Bartonella* species has been underrecognized in studies to date. Dual infection implies a lack of cross-protection between some *Bartonella* species and subtypes, but whether certain types or species are predominant over others during coinfection is unknown.

Although sex of the cat does not appear to be a risk factor for *Bartonella* infection, there appears to be a correlation between bacteremia and age of the cat [21, 23, 24]. Sander et al. [23] reported an 18% (11/60) rate of culture positivity in cats less than 2 years of age and a 5% (2/40) rate of culture positivity in cats older than 2 years of age. Similarly, Heller et al. [24] found that 69% (18/26) of cats sampled at 1 year of age or less were bacteremic, while 47% (32/68) of cats greater than 1 year of age were bacteremic. Two studies that compared the incidence of *Bartonella* infection in feral and pet cats found feral cats were more likely to be seroreactive or bacteremic [21, 27]. In The Netherlands, a region with less flea exposure, there was no difference in the prevalence of *Bartonella* infection between shelter and pet cats [26]. These observations are important since feral cats constitute a substantial portion (estimates of 50%) of the cat population. Although Bergmans et al. [26] did not find evidence of *Bartonella* infection in 25 SPF cats from The Netherlands, anecdotal reports of *Bartonella*-seroreactive or bacteremic SPF cats in the USA are not surprising since screening for these organisms in commercial catteries was not performed until recently.

Despite the heightened susceptibility of retroviral-infected cats to various other infectious agents, the authors did not find an increased incidence of *Bartonella* infection within this subpopulation [unpubl. data]. These observations have been substantiated by several other investigators [21, 24, 30]. In one study, however, prevalence of *Bartonella*-specific seroreactivity was associated with the presence of antibodies to *Toxoplasma gondii* [35].

Experimental transmission of *B. henselae* and *B. clarridgeiae* is easily accomplished following intravenous or intramuscular injection of infected blood, raising the concern for iatrogenic transmission of *Bartonella* during blood transfusion therapy [36]. Cats infected in this manner developed a prolonged infection with recrudescent episodes of bacteremia. Transmission of *B. henselae* has also been accomplished following intravenous, intramuscular, intradermal and oral administration of lab-cultivated bacteria or exposure to fleas previously fed on bacteremic cats [37–41]. In general, parenteral inoculation with laboratory-cultivated bacteria resulted in a transient bacteremia that persisted for 4–6 months without relapse. Fever, of 1–2 days' duration was reported, and some cats developed abscesses at intradermal inoculation sites. Oral administration of $10^9$ CFU of *B. henselae* to kittens (5–14 days old) resulted in subclinical bacteremia that persisted until they were sacrificed at 16 weeks of age [Guptill et al., unpubl. data]. Interestingly, unlike kittens that received inoculum intradermally, those kittens that received oral *Bartonella* inoculum did not seroconvert despite becoming bacteremic. In another study, experimental transmission was not accomplished after intramuscular inoculation of urine sediment from infected cats [36]. Although urine cultures of bacteremic cats have been negative [36, 41], *Bartonella* species can remain viable for at least 48 h following experimental inoculation in cat urine [Kordick and Breitschwerdt, unpubl. data].

Higgins et al. [42] recently verified the ability of cat fleas (*Ctenocephalides felis*) to become infected with and support replication of *B. henselae.* Organisms were visible in dissected flea guts and viable bartonellae were cultured from flea feces up to 9 days after being fed infected blood. In addition, a recent seroepidemiologic study showed that many *Bartonella*-infected cats were concurrently seroreactive to *Rickettsia felis*, an organism that is also carried by the cat flea [Breitschwerdt et al., unpubl. data]. These and other epidemiologic data suggested a flea-borne mode of transmission for *B. henselae* which has been substantiated in experiments performed by Chomel et al. [40]. Since utilization of an invertebrate vector is a common feature of the genus *Bartonella*, it is likely that *B. clarridgeiae* is similarly transmitted by cat fleas, however, the precise method(s) by which transfer of *B. henselae* or *B. clarridgeiae* to a susceptible host occurs, remains unclear. Self-inoculation of infected flea feces while scratching or ingestion of infected fleas during grooming are potential routes by which cats become infected. Epidemiological studies indicate that direct flea transmission to people is an uncommon occurrence. Combining experimental results that verify oral transfer of infection to cats and multiplication of *B. henselae* in cat fleas, oral transmission following ingestion of infected fleas or flea feces seems plausible. Furthermore, the apparent lack of seroreactivity observed in many bacteremic cats may possibly be explained by a state of tolerance that results from infection by a mucosal route. Although fleas are important vectors of *B. henselae* and presumably *B. clarridgeiae*, anecdotal reports of human CSD following tick exposure suggest that at least occasionally, ticks may be involved in the transmission of bartonellae among cats. Ticks, however, are infrequently found on cats as compared to dogs.

Placentation in cats is endotheliochorial, therefore, it would be reasonable to expect transplacental transmission of *Bartonella* species. The blood parasites, *Eperythrozoon felis* and *Haemobartonella felis* are transferred from queens to kittens by this route. An attempt to experimentally transmit *B. henselae* from highly bacteremic, experimentally-infected queens to kittens was not successful [Guptill et al., unpubl. data]. Although maternal IgG antibodies were present in the kittens, levels of *Bartonella*-specific immunoglobulin were diminished by 10 week's postpartum. Therefore, antibodies detected before 10 weeks of age most probably reflect the presence of passively transferred maternal antibody. Although ingestion of cultured bacteria can effectively establish infection in cats, lactogenic transfer has not been documented. Colostrum and milk from infected queens were negative for *Bartonella* DNA when analyzed by PCR, indicating that bacteria were probably not shed via the milk or perhaps milk contains PCR inhibitors [Guptill et al., unpubl. data]. Transmission did not occur when a breeding pair, consisting of a bacteremic queen and an SPF male were housed together and periodically tested for bacteremia during a 6-month evaluation period [37]. Seminal fluid from bacteremic males has not been tested for the presence of *Bartonella* nor has the opportunity for veneral transfer via semen been investigated.

Using *B. henselae*-specific PCR, two groups of investigators have attempted to amplify *Bartonella* DNA from the buccal cavity of bacteremic cats [8, 23]. Only 1 kitten out of 94 had evidence of *Bartonella* in saliva. Given the fact that *Bartonella* species are hemotropic bacteria, stomatitis or traumatic rupture of mucous membranes after chewing sharp objects could potentially result in saliva becoming contaminated with these organisms. The presence or absence of oral lesions was not mentioned in either study. Although cat bites and licking are occasional historical events in some cases of human infection, these mechanisms do not appear to be primary methods of exchange among cats as occurs with the feline immunodeficiency virus. This premise is supported by the observation that retroviral-infected cats are no more likely than nonretroviral-infected cats to be bacteremic with *Bartonella*.

Normal daily contact via food dishes, litter boxes, play behavior and sharing beds does not apparenty facilitate transmission [16, 37]. Abbott et al. [37] housed 5 naive kittens with 2 bacteremic kittens for 20 weeks, but transfer of infection to the naive kittens did not occur. In fact, multicat households can contain only one bacteremic or seroreactive cat [20, 43]. Investigators in Germany, however, observed that cats from the same household were uniformly culture-positive or -negative [23].

Little is known about the cellular predilection or habitat of *B. henselae* or *B. clarridgeiae* in cats. Using transmission electron microscopy, the authors observed bartonellae within erythrocytes of naturally-infected cats [44]. In vitro infection of feline erythrocytes with *B. henselae* was recently accomplished following 8–24 h of incubation [Mehock et al., unpubl. data]. Temperature-dependent invasion was inhibited by KCN pretreatment of bacteria, but trypsin, neuraminidase, or immune cat serum failed to prevent bacterial adherence or invasion. Confocal microscopy of acridine orange-stained blood smears revealed intracellular bartonellae in $<10\%$ of the cocultivated erythrocytes.

Diagnosis of *Bartonella* infection can be elusive. With the exception of *B. bacilliformis* and previous *Grahamella* species, organisms are usually not demonstrable in blood films. Since cats are poor delayed-type hypersensitivity responders, intradermal inoculation of skin test antigen does not appear to be a feasible method to identify carrier cats [Kordick and Breitschwerdt, unpubl. data]. Serologic testing has been extensively employed to determine the extent of *Bartonella* exposure in cats, but the correlation of serology with infection is questionable. In addition, the IFA technique as well as many ELISA-based serodiagnostics lack specificity. Unpredictable cross-reactivity can exist among antigens derived from different *Bartonella* species or types [45]. *Bartonella* reactive human sera can contain cross-reacing antibodies to *Coxiella burnetii* or *Chlamydia* species [46]. The extent to which cross-reactivity influences canine or feline serologic results is unknown. Absorption techniques used by Baneth et al. [45] revealed that *B. henselae*-reactive cat sera from Israel reacted preferentially and nonspecifically by IFA to antigens derived from *B. quintana*. For these reasons, serologic determination of the infecting *Bartonella* species is not yet possible. In some instances, utilization of antigens derived from regional isolates may be necessary to detect seroreactivity. Drancourt et al. [22] detected antibodies to a locally derived *B. henselae* isolate in 18/113 human patients previously determined to be seronegative to the Houston-1 strain of *B. henselae*. Similarly, the authors observed several naturally- and experimentally-infected bacteremic cats without detectable antibody levels to homologous and heterologous *Bartonella* isolates. However, serology may be a useful indicator for the absence of bacteremia. Based upon correlation with culture results, Bergmans et al. [26] reported a positive predictive value of 39% and negative predictive value of 96%, and Chomel et al. [21] reported a positive predictive value of 46% and negative predictive value of 90%, respectively. Therefore, with current methods, the interpretation of positive or negative serologic results can be misleading. At any one point in time, a cat can be bacteremic and seropositive, bacteremic and seronegative, abacteremic and seropositive, or abacteremic and seronegative, yet still be a *Bartonella* carrier [36].

Blood cultures, when positive, are diagnostic, and facilitate molecular characterization of the infecting species. In addition, a variety of methods including species-specific PCR, gene sequencing, PCR-RFLP, ERIC-PCR, REP-PCR and DNA-DNA hybridization have been developed to identify *Bartonella* to the species level. However, the natural history of persistent *Bartonella* infection includes unpredictable relapses of bacteremia which renders definitive interpretation of negative bacteriologic tests impossible [36, 37]. *B. henselae* and *B. clarridgeiae* can remain a part of the microbial flora of healthy cats for months to years. Prolonged infection with *Bartonella* has been documented for up to 24 months in naturally-infected cats, but given our inability to detect or quantitate unculturable levels of bacteremia, the maximum period of persistence is unknown [20, 37]. The authors have successfully transmitted *B. henselae* from a culture-negative cat by blood transfusion [unpubl. data]. The analytical sensitivity of molecular diagnostic techniques, such as PCR, has enhanced our ability to identify some infected cats that are negative by serologic testing and blood culture [Kordick et al., unpubl. data]. The 'abacteremic' carrier state is an incompletely characterized phenomenon in which the immune system may be sufficient to prevent bacteremia, but does not eliminate all infectious organisms from the body. Although the medical implications associated with occult *Bartonella* infection are still unknown, it is possible that the cat as well as other species, pays a biological price for chronic insidious infection. Glaus et al. [43] observed an increased frequency of stomatitis or renal disease in *Bartonella*-seroreactive sick cats from Switzerland and southern Germany. If substantiated by future studies, *Bartonella* infection may prove to be contributory to chronic progressive renal disease in cats.

Little is known about the clinical manifestations, pathophysiology, or the utility of treatment of *Bartonella* infections in cats. Cats appear to be evolutionarily adapted hosts for *B. henselae* and *B. clarridgeiae* in nature and generally maintain quiescent infections. The extent to which bartonellae function as a contributor or cofactor in clinical disease is unknown. For example, whether incidental infection with *Bartonella* in retroviral-infected cats results in more severe morbidity, as has been observed in humans, is unknown. Future controlled coinfection studies should address these issues.

Despite the isolation of *B. henselae* or *B. clarridgeiae* from seemingly healthy cats, evidence is slowly accumulating to support a pathogenic role for *Bartonella* in cats (table 1). Brief febrile periods have been documented during the acute stage of experimental infections [36, 41; O'Reilly et al., unpubl. data]. In addition, transient anemia and persistent eosinophilia were observed in one group of cats following inoculation with blood from *Bartonella*-infected donors [36, 41]. Recurrent episodes of bacteremia in these cats, however, were not accompanied by recurrent fever or anemia. Although well documented with other infectious agents, the effect of splenectomy on *Bartonella*-infected cats has not been exammined. Similarly, the role of surgical stress or effect of exogenous steroid administration on recrudescence of latent *Bartonella* infection or exacerbation of active infection is uncertain. The authors have observed naturally-infected cats that became transiently febrile after sterilization surgery [unpubl. data]. Evidence is also accumulating to implicate *B. henselae* as a

*Table 1.* Abnormalities observed in cats infected with *B. henselae* or *B. clarridgeiae*

| Experimental infection | Reference | Natural infection | Reference |
|---|---|---|---|
| Fever | 36, 41, O'Reilly, unpubl. data | Fever | 20 |
| Anemia | 36 | Lymphadenomegaly | 20 |
| Eosinophilia | 41, Kordick et al., unpubl. data | Uveitis | Lappin et al., unpubl. data |
| Lymphadenomegaly | 36, 41 | Lymphadenomegaly | 20 |
| Cataracts | Kordick et al., unpubl. data | Renal disease | 43 |
| Cholangitis | Kordick et al., unpubl. data | Neurologic dysfunction | 20, 36 |
| Reproductive failure | 37, Guptill et al., unpubl. data | | |
| Renal lesions | 41 | | |
| Neurologic dysfunction | 36, O'Reilly, unpubl. data | | |
| Cardiac lesions | Kordick et al., unpubl. data | | |

cause of reproductive failure in cats. Abbott et al. [37] and Guptill et al. [unpubl. data] observed that bacteremic queens experienced decreased conception rates and abortions until levels of circulating bartonellae decreased.

Since *Bartonella* colony counts often reach high levels despite the presence of substantial immunoglobulin titers, natural antibodies are not protective. CD4 and CD8 T-cell populations remained unaltered in cats experimentally infected with laboratory-cultivated *B. henselae* [37, 41], and lymphocyte stimulation assays performed on one group would indicate that *B. henselae* is not immunosuppressive to cats [41]. However, when interpreting these data derived from experimentally-infected cats, one must carefully consider the source and strain of inoculum and mode of inoculation. Furthermore, the effect of *B. clarridgeiae*, concurrent *B. henselae* and *B. clarridgeiae* infection, or other *Bartonella* coinfections on immunologic status has not been reported.

Lymphadenopathy is not consistently observed in cats following experimental inoculation. In some cats, regional lymphadenomegaly occurred postinoculation, even with administration of uninfected inocula, and probably reflects a nonspecific immunologic response to a foreign substance [36]. In contrast, Guptil et al. [41] reported generalized lymphadenopathy in all cats that received *B. henselae* inoculum intravenously. Kirkpatrick et al. [47] described silver-staining bacteria morphologically similar to *Bartonella* in enlarged lymph nodes from cats, but definitive identification of the argyrophilic organism has not been made. A recent attempt to characterize the organisms as *Bartonella* by immunohistochemistry, using paraffin-embedded tissues archived at the Armed Forces Institute of Pathology, was not successful [Hadfield, unpubl. data].

Cats that received infected blood inoculum have transiently displayed mild neurologic dysfunction which included disorientation, lack of response to environmental stimuli, and lethargy [36]. O'Reilly et al. [unpubl. data] observed depression, anorexia, lethargy and hyperesthesia in SPF or pound cats that received $10^6$–$10^7$ CFU of *B. henselae* (derived from a naturally-infected pound cat) intramuscularly or intravenously. These clinical signs, briefly accompanied by fever at the onset, began 7–10 days postinoculation and continued for approximately 10–20 days.

Systemic *Bartonella* infection in people can result in a variety of ocular manifestations including uveitis. During a continuing investigation of cats with uveitis, *Bartonella*-specific antibodies were detected in the serum and aqueous humor. In addition, *Bartonella* DNA was amplified from aqueous humor of some affected cats [Lappin et al., unpubl. data]. Although uveitis was not observed, several cats experimentally-inoculated with *Bartonella*-infected blood developed cataracts after 1 year. *Bartonella*-specific antibodies and/or DNA were present in the aqueous humor of some experimentally-inoculated cats (with or without evidence of cataracts) [Kordick et al., unpubl. data]. Histologically, hematoxylin and eosin-stained sections of eyes from experimentally-infected cats were unremarkable.

Following subcutaneous inoculation of cultured organisms, hematogenous spread of bartonellae may result in persistent tissue colonization. Although no macroscopic abnormalities have been observed at necropsy, postmortem histologic findings included microabscess formation in the liver and spleen, multifocal myocarditis, and focal pyogranulomatous nephritis in experimentally-infected cats sacrificed 2–32 weeks postinfection [41]. Lymphoplasmacytic periportal infiltration was observed in chronically-infected cats inoculated by blood transfusion and necropsied between 241 and 454 days postinfection [Kordick et al., unpubl., data]. Although potentially unrelated to *Bartonella* infection, these inflammatory infiltrates were predominantly confined to the bile duct region and contained Warthin-Starry silver-staining bacteria (fig. 1). *Bartonella* DNA has also been amplified from heart and brain tissue of chronically-infected cats with nonspecific inflammatory lesions [Kordick, unpubl. data].

Antimicrobial elimination of *B. henselae* and *B. clarridgeiae* infections in cats has been attempted by several investigators, however, the optimal antimicrobial regimen to eliminate feline *Bartonella* infections has yet to be determined [38, 39, 48]. As in the human medical literature, anecdotal reports suggest responsiveness to various antimicrobials. In controlled studies, enrofloxacin, doxycycline and amoxicillin have all appeared to decrease colony count or eliminate bacteremia at some times, but not others [38, 39, 48]. In cats, treatment duration, source of inocula, bacterial load, and chronicity of

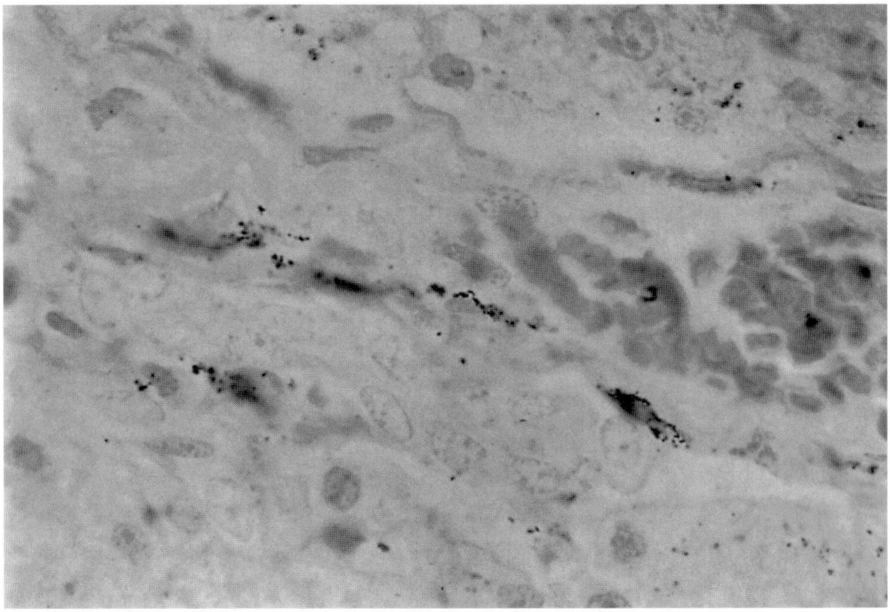

*Fig. 1.* Liver section from a cat chronically bacteremic with *B. henselae*. Note the clumps of silver-staining bacteria. Photomicrographs provided by Dr. Talmage Brown, College of Veterinary Medicine, North Carolina State University.

infection may ultimately affect the response to treatment. As an alternative to treatment, several investigators are pursuing the development of a vaccine that will prevent *Bartonella* infections in cats. Not surprisingly, substantial concern exists surrounding the potential that cats can become reinfected following successful antimicrobial elimination. The authors documented *B. clarridgeiae* transmission to a cat previously bacteremic with *B. henselae* [unpubl. data]. The cat was naturally-infected with *B. henselae*, but while maintained in a flea-free environment, appeared to spontaneously eliminate the infection. After 19 months of negative blood clutures, the cat was challenge-exposed by blood transfusion with *B. clarridgeiae* and became bacteremic. Figure 2 depicts PCR-RFLP patterns of *Bartonella* isolates recovered from the cat at various sampling times. Incomplete immunity against different strains of *Bartonella* has also been observed by others. Yamamoto et al. [unpubl. data] demonstrated the lack of cross-protective immunity among four *Bartonella* strains: *B. henselae* type I, *B. henselae* type II, a *Bartonella* strain obtained from a mountain lion, and *B. clarridgeiae*. Challenge inoculation with cultured organisms was performed after animals were culture-negative for at least 3 months, and an

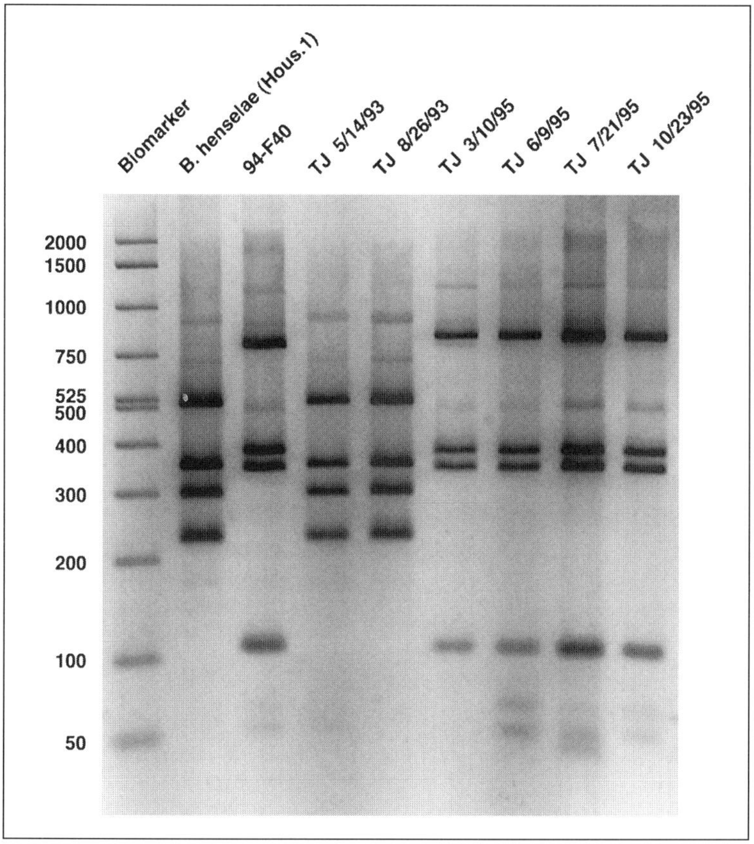


*Fig. 2.* Digestion profiles obtained following PCR-RFLP of the 16S rRNA gene from *Bartonella* isolates cultured from a cat naturally-infected with *B. henselae* and subsequently challenged with *B. clarridgeiae.*

additional challenge using a third strain was performed following another 3-month culture-negative interval. Regnery et al. [38] were also able to infect cats with *B. henselae* after previous exposure to *B. quintana*. In all studies to date, cats challenged with homologous strains did not become bacteremic, but generally experienced an increase in IgG titer.

Despite major deficiencies in our understanding of the pathogenesis of *Bartonella* infections, it appears that various animal species can tolerate chronic *Bartonella* infection without obvious clinical indications of disease. However, given recent observations derived from experimental and natural infection studies, *Bartonella* species may ultimately be identified as the cause of some idiopathic disease conditions of cats and dogs.

## References


1 English CK, Wear DJ, Margileth AM, Lissner CR, Walsh GP: Cat-scratch disease: Isolation and culture of the bacterial agent. JAMA 1988;259:1347–1352.

2 Brenner DJ, Hollis DG, Moss CW, English CK, Hall GS, Vincent J, Radosevic J, Birkness KA, Bibb WF, Quinn FD, Swaminathan B, Weaver RE, Reeves MW, O'Connor AP, Hayes PS, Tenover FC, Steigerwalt AG, Perkins BA, Daneshvar MI, Hill BC, Washington JA, Woods TC, Hunter SB, Hadfield TL, Ajello GW, Kaufmann AF, Wear DJ, Wenger JD: Proposal of *Afipia* gen nov, with *Afipia felis* sp nov (formerly the cat scratch disease bacillus), *Afipia clevelandensis* sp nov (formerly the Cleveland Clinic Foundation strain), *Afipia broomeae* sp nov, and three unnamed genospecies. J Clin Microbiol 1991;29:2450–2460.

3 Regnery RL, Anderson BE, Clarridge JE III, Rodriguez-Barradas MC, Jones DC, Carr JH: Characterization of a novel *Rochalimaea* species, *R. henselae* sp nov, isolated from blood of a febrile, human immunodeficiency virus-positive patient. J Clin Microbiol 1992;30:265–274.

4 Welch DF, Pickett DA, Slater LN, Steigerwalt AG, Brenner DJ: *Rochalimaea henselae* sp nov, a cause of septicemia, bacillary angiomatosis, and parenchymal bacillary peliosis. J Clin Microbiol 1992;30:275–280.

5 Regnery RL, Olson JG, Perkins BA, Bibb W: Serological response to *Rochalimaea henselae* antigen in suspected cat-scratch disease. Lancet 1992;339:1443–1445.

6 Engbaek K, Koch C: Antibody response in rabbits infected with *Rochalimaea henselae, Rochalimaea quintana* and *Afipia felis.* APMIS 1994;102:943–949.

7 Wong MT, Thornton DC, Kennedy RC, Dolan MJ: Defined liquid medium that supports primary isolation of *Rochalimaea* (*Bartonella*) *henselae* for blood and tissue specimens. J Clin Microbiol 1995;33:742–744.

8 Demers DM, Bass JW, Vincent JM, Person DA, Noyes DK, Staege CM, Samlaska CP, Lockwood NH, Regnery RL, Anderson BE: Cat-scratch disease in Hawaii: Etiology and seroepidemiology. J Pediatr 1995;127:23–26.

9 Baker JA: A rickettsial infection in Canadian voles. J Exp Med 1946;84:37–51.

10 Birtles RJ, Harrison TG, Molyneux DH: *Grahamella* in small woodland mammals in the UK: Isolation, prevalence, and host specificity. Ann Trop Med Parasitol 1994;88:317–327.

11 Birtles RJ, Harrison TG, Saunders NA, Molyneux DH: Proposals to unify the genera *Grahamella* and *Bartonella*, with descriptions of *Bartonella talpae* comb nov, *Bartonella peromysci* comb nov, and three new species, *Bartonella grahamii* sp nov, *Bartonella taylorii* sp nov, and *Bartonella doshiae* sp nov. Int J Sys Bacteriol 1995;45:1–8.

12 Kosoy MY, Regnery RL, Tzianabos T, Marston EL, Jones DC, Green D, Maupin GO, Olson JG, Childs JE: Distribution, diversity, and host specificity of *Bartonella* in rodents from the southeastern United States. Am J Trop Med Hyg 1997;57:578–588.

13 Slater LN, Coody DW, Woolridge LK, Welch DF: Murine antibody responses distinguish *Rochalimaea henselae* from *Rochalimaea quintana.* J Clin Microbiol 1992;30:1722–1727.

14 Breitschwerdt EB, Kordick DL, Malarkey DE, Keene B, Hadfield TL, Wilson K: Endocarditis in a dog due to infection with a novel *Bartonella* subspecies. J Clin Microbiol 1995;33:154–160.

15 Kordick DL, Swaminathan B, Greene CE, Wilson KH, Whitney AM, O'Connor S, Hollis DG, Matar GM, Steigerwalt AG, Malcolm BG, Hayes PS, Hadfield TL, Breitschwerdt EB, Brenner DJ: *Bartonella vinsonii* subsp *berkhoffii* subsp nov, isolated from dogs; *Bartonella vinsonii* subsp *vinsonii*; and emended description of *Bartonella vinsonii*. Int J Syst Bacteriol 1996;46:704–709.

16 Kordick DL, Breitschwerdt EB: Persistent infection of pets within a household with three *Bartonella* species: *Bartonella clarridgeiae, Bartonella henselae*, or *Bartonella vinsonii* subsp *berkhoffii*. Emerg Infect Dis 1998;4:in press.

17 Chomel BB: Cat-scratch disease and bacillary angiomatosis. Rev Sci Tech Off Int Epiz 1996;15:1061–1073.

18 Pappalardo BL, Correa MT, York CC, Peat CY, Breitschwerdt EB: Epidemiologic evaluation of the risk factors associated with exposure and seroreactivity to *Bartonella vinsonii* in dogs. Am J Vet Res 1997;58:467–471.

19 Lawson PA, Collins MD: Description of *Bartonella clarridgeiae* sp nov isolated from the cat of a patient with *Bartonella henselae* septicemia. Med Microbiol Lett 1996;5:64–73.
20 Kordick DL, Wilson KH, Sexton DJ, Hadfield TL, Berkhoff HA, Breitschwerdt EB: Prolonged *Bartonella* bacteremia in cats associated with cat-scratch disease patients. J Clin Microbiol 1995; 33:3245–3251.
21 Chomel BB, Abbott RC, Kasten RW, Floyd-Hawkins KA, Kass PH, Glaser CA, Pedersen NC, Koehler JE: *Bartonella henselae* prevalence in domestic cats in California: Risk factors and association between bacteremia and antibody titers. J Clin Microbiol 1995;33:2445–2450.
22 Drancourt M, Birtles R, Chaumentin G, Vandenesch F, Etienne J, Raoult D: New serotype of *Bartonella henselae* in endocarditis and cat-scratch disease. Lancet 1996;347:441–443.
23 Sander A, Buhler C, Pelz K, von Cramm E, Bredt W: Detection and identification of two *Bartonella henselae* variants in domestic cats in Germany. J Clin Microbiol 1997;35:584–587.
24 Heller R, Artois M, Xemar V, de Briel D, Gehin H, Jaulhac B, Monteil H, Piemont Y: Prevalence of *Bartonella henselae* and *Bartonella clarridgeiae* in stray cats. J Clin Microbiol 1997;35: 1327–1331.
25 Gurfield AN, Boulouis H-J, Chomel BB, Heller R, Kasten RW, Yamanoto K, Piemont Y: Coinfection with *Bartonella clarridgeiae* and *Bartonella henselae* and with different *Bartonella henselae* strains in domestic cats. J Clin Microbiol 1997;35:2120–2123.
26 Bergmans AMC, de Jong CMA, van Amerongen G, Schot CS, Schouls LM: Prevalence of *Bartonella* species in domestic cats in The Netherlands. J Clin Microbiol 1997;35:2256–2261.
27 Branley J, Wolfson C, Waters P, Gottlieb T, Bradbury R: Prevalence of *B. henselae* bacteremia, the causative agent of cat-scratch disease, in an Australian cat population. Pathology 1996;28:262–265.
28 Joseph AK, Wood CW, Robson JM, Paul SL, Morris AJ: *Bartonella henselae* bacteraemia in domestic cats from Auckland. NZ Vet J 1997;45:185–187.
29 Maruyama S, Nogami S, Inoue I, Namba S, Asanome K, Katsube Y: Isolation of *Bartonella henselae* from domestic cats in Japan. J Vet Med Sci 1996;58:81–83.
30 Childs JE, Olson JG, Wolf A, Cohen N, Fakile Y, Rooney JA, Bacellar F, Regnery RL: Prevalence of antibodies to *Rochalimaea* species (cat-scratch disease agent) in cats. Vet Rec 1995;136:519–520.
31 Kelly PJ, Matthewman LA, Hayter D, Downey S, Wray K, Bryson NR, Raoult D: *Bartonella (Rochalimaea) henselae* in southern Africa – Evidence for infections in domestic cats and implications for veterinarians. J South Afr Vet Assoc 1996;67:182–187.
32 Jameson P, Greene C, Regnery R, Dryden M, Marks A, Brown J, Cooper J, Glaus B, Greene R: Prevalence of *B. henselae* antibodies in pet cats throughout regions of North America. J Infect Dis 1995;172:1145–1149.
33 Ueno H, Muramatsu Y, Chomel BB, Hohdatsu T, Koyama H, Morita C: Seroepidemiological survey of *Bartonella (Rochalimaea) henselae* in domestic cats in Japan. Microbiol Immunol 1995; 39:339–341.
34 Bergmans AMC, Schellekens JFP, van Embden JDA, Schouls LM: Predominance of two *Bartonella henselae* variants among cat-scratch disease patients in The Netherlands. J Clin Microbiol 1996;34: 254–260.
35 Childs JE, Rooney JA, Cooper JL, Olson JG, Regnery RL: Epidemiologic observations on infection with *Rochalimaea* species among cats living in Baltimore, Md. J Am Vet Med Assoc 1994;204: 1775–1778.
36 Kordick DL, Breitschwerdt EB: Relapsing bacteremia after blood transmission of *Bartonella henselae* to cats. Am J Vet Res 1997;58:492–497.
37 Abbott RC, Chomel BB, Kasten RW, Floyd-Hawkins KA, Kikuchi Y, Koehler JE, Pedersen NC: Experimental and natural infection with *Bartonella henselae* in domestic cats. Comp Immunol Microbiol Infect Dis 1997;20:41–51.
38 Regnery RL, Rooney JA, Johnson AM, Nesby SL, Manzewitsch P, Beaver K, Olson JG: Experimentally induced *Bartonella henselae* infections followed by challenge exposure and antimicrobial therapy in cats. Am J Vet Res 1996;57:1714–1719.
39 Greene CE, McDermott M, Jameson PH, Atkins CL, Marks AM: *Bartonella henselae* infection in cats: Evaluation during primary infection, treatment, and rechallenge infection. J Clin Microbiol 1996;34:1682–1685.

40 Chomel BB, Kasten RW, Floyd-Hawkins KA, Chi B, Yamamoto K, Roberts-Wilson J, Gurfield AN, Abbott RC, Pedersen NC, Koehler JE: Experimental transmission of *B. henselae* by the cat flea. J Clin Microbiol 1996;34:1952–1956.
41 Guptill L, Slater L, Wu C-C, Lin T-L, Glickman LT, Welch DF, Hogenesch H: Experimental infection of young specific-pathogen-free cats with *Bartonella henselae*. J Infect Dis 1997;176:206–216.
42 Higgins JA, Radulovic S, Jaworski CD, Azad AF: Acquisition of the cat-scratch disease agent *Bartonella henselae* by cat fleas (*Siphonaptera: Pulicidae*). J Med Entomol 1996;33:490–495.
43 Glaus T, Hofmann-Lehmann R, Greene C, Glaus B, Wolfensberger C, Lutz H: Seroprevalence of *Bartonella henselae* infection and correlation with disease status in cats in Switzerland. J Clin Microbiol 1997;35:2883–2885.
44 Kordick DL, Breitschwerdt EB: Intraerythrocytic presence of *Bartonella henselae*. J Clin Microbiol 1995;33:1655–1656.
45 Baneth G, Kordick DL, Hegarty BC, Breitschwerdt EB: Comparative seroreactivity to *Bartonella henselae* and *Bartonella quintana* among cats from Israel and North Carolina. Vet Microbiol 1995; 50:95–103.
46 Maurin M, Eb F, Etienne J, Raoult D: Serological cross-reactivity between *Bartonella* and *Chlamydia* species: Implications for diagnosis. J Clin Microbiol 1997;35:2283–2287.
47 Kirkpatrick CE, Moore FM, Patnaik AK, Whitely HE: Argyrophilic, intracellular bacteria in some cats withidopathic peripheral lymphadenopathy. J Comp Pathol 1989;101:341–349.
48 Kordick DL, Papich MG, Breitschwerdt EB: Efficacy of enrofloxacin or doxycycline for treatment of *B. henselae* or *B. clarridgeiae* infection in cats. Antimicrob Agents Chemother 1997;41:2448–2455.

Dorsey L. Kordick, North Carolina State University College of Veterinary Medicine,
Department of Companion Animal and Special Species Medicine,
4700 Hillsborough Street at William Moore Drive, Raleigh, NC 27606 (USA)
Tel. (919) 829 4357, Fax (919) 829 4336

Schmidt A (ed): *Bartonella* and *Afipia* Species Emphasizing *Bartonella henselae*.
Contrib Microbiol. Basel, Karger, 1998, vol 1, pp 201–210

# Epidemiology and Pathology of *Bartonella henselae* in Cats

*Soichi Maruyama, Yasuji Katsube*

Laboratory of Veterinary Public Health, College of Bioresource Sciences,
Nihon University, Fujisawa, Kanagawa, Japan

The causative agent of cat scratch disease (CSD) has remained obscure for a long time. Up until the present, many kinds of microbes such as bacteria, chlamydia, or viruses have been suggested to be the putative agent of CSD. A pleomorphic fastidious Gram-negative rod bacteria has been isolated from the lymph nodes of a CSD patient and has been named *Afipia felis* [1]. Although *A. felis* has provisionally been considered to be a causative agent, the organism has only rarely been isolated from patients with CSD, and a serological investigation of these patients has shown little participation of *A. felis* in the disease.

Recent investigations suggest that *Bartonella henselae*, formerly named *Rochalimaea henselae*, is a causative agent for both bacillary angiomatosis (BA) and bacillary peliosis hepatis (BP) in HIV-positive patients [2]. It has also been reported that the symptomatology of CSD in HIV-positive patients resembles that of BA, and Warthin-Starry-stained organisms similar to those of CSD have been found in the skin and lymph node lesions of patients with BA. Furthermore, *B. henselae* has been isolated from CSD patients under immunocompetent status [3] and from healthy cats [4], and serological investigations of these patients have strongly suggested that this organism is the causative agent of CSD [5].

Although cats have been implicated in the source of CSD for a long time, the role of cats in the epidemiology of *B. henselae* infection and the pathology of the organism in cats has not yet been fully demonstrated. In this article, recent findings regarding the epidemiology and pathology of *B. henselae* infection in cats are reviewed.

*Table 1.* Prevalence of *B. henselae* bacteremia in cats

| Bacteremic animals | Note | Country (area) | Ref. |
|---|---|---|---|
| 11–46% (av. 41%) | Pet, impounded and feral cats | USA (San Francisco) | 6 |
| 4–70% (av. 40%) | Pet, impounded and feral cats<br>High rate in feral cats | USA (California) | 8 |
| 62% | 85% of positive cats were kittens | USA (Hawaii) | 16 |
| 89%<br>28% | Cats associated with CSD patients<br>Control cats | USA (North Carolina)<br>– | 7 |
| 11% | Cats around Paris | France (Paris) | 9 |
| 3% | Pet cats in the Kanto District | Japan | 11 |

## Epidemiology

*Prevalence of* B. henselae *Bacteremia in Cats.* After the lysis centrifugation method was developed for the isolation of *B. henselae* [6], several investigations into the prevalence of *B. henselae* infection (bacteremia) in cats have been conducted in the world (table 1). Most studies have been conducted in the USA, possibly because much attention has been paid to CSD and/or BA and BP in association with AIDS by physicians in that country.

The prevalence of bacteremia has varied depending upon the investigators and the source of the cats. Kordic et al. [7] have reported that 89% (17/19) of the cats owned by 14 patients diagnosed with CSD and 28% (7/25) of the cats owned by veterinary students were bacteremic with the *Bartonella* species. In addition, Koehler et al. [6] have found evidence of bacteremia with *B. henselae* in all 7 of the cats owned by 4 patients with cutaneous BA, in 41% (15/37) of the pet cats, in 41% (9/22) of the pound cats, and in 1 of 2 stray cats from the Greater San Francisco Bay Region. In northern California, 40% (81/205) of a convenience sample of cats were bacteremic, and the rate of bacteremia in pet cats (4–48%) was lower than that of the impounded (53%) or former stray (70%) cats [8]. In Hawaii, of the 31 kittens and 3 adult cats examined, 21 (62%) were blood-culture-positive for *B. henselae*, and the all blood-culture-positive cats were defined as cats less than 1 year of age [16].

In other parts of the world, the information regarding the prevalence of the bacteremia in cats is still limited. In France, 11% (7/64) of cat samples from the veterinary teaching hospital in Paris were bacteremic with *B. henselae* [9]. In Australian cat populations, 35% (27/77) harbored *B. henselae* in their blood, with 40% (24/59) of the cats being feral and 16% (3/18) being domestic cats. Most positive cats were younger than 1 year old [10]. In Japan, Maruyama et al. [11] have isolated the organism from 9% (3/33) of pet cats in the Kanto District situated in the central area of Japan. These data suggest that the organism is already distributed in domestic cats throughout the world.

In another investigation we performed, bacteremia was detected in 3% (15/462) of young and adult domestic cats, but none of the 88 newborn kittens examined were found to be bacteremic. The data suggest that vertical transmission of *B. henselae* appears to occur only rarely in cats.

Recently, a new *Bartonella* species, *B. clarridgeiae*, has been isolated from the blood of a cat owned by an HIV-positive patient [12, 13]. In the molecular epidemiological investigation of *Bartonella* isolates from the USA, France and Japan by pulsed-field gel electrophoresis, *B. clarridgeiae* was detected in the American and French isolates obtained from cats, but not among the Japanese isolates. Furthermore, it was found that some cats were reinfected and/or coinfected with different strains and/or species of *Bartonella* [14]. However, details regarding the pathogenicity of *B. clarridgeiae* in both cats or human beings remain obscure. Further investigation is necessary to clarify the detailed characteristics of the species.

*Serological Prevalence of* B. henselae *Infection in Cats.* In cats, the antibody prevalence to *B. henselae* has been examined by the indirect immunofluorescence antibody (IFA) test. *B. henselae* cocultivated with Vero cells [7,15–19] or FCWF (*Felis catus* whole fetus) [8, 9] cells, or whole organisms [20] were used as the antigen. Although the specificity has not been compared among these antigens, there seems to be little difference in the IFA results. In the IFA test, titers of $>$1:64 are considered to be positive in the literature.

Data from various serological investigations in cats are given in table 2. In 1994, Childs et al. [15] showed that an overall 15% (87/592) of the cat sera collected between 1980 and 1985 in Baltimore, Md. were seropositive to *Bartonella*. The seroprevalence in cats was similar among groups of cats with some history of human contact (12.5–14%) but was higher among feral cats (44%). In this study, the prevalence of seropositivity increased significantly with cat age, weight and seropositivity to *Toxoplasma gondii*, but did not vary according to genders. From our experience, no association between the seropositivity to *B. henselae* and *T. gondii* can be observed in cats. Furthermore, the presence of feline immunodeficiency virus (FIV) antibodies and feline leukemia virus (FeLV) antigenemia do not appear to be associated with bacteremia or seropositivity for *B. henselae* in cats [8, 21]. Of 29 kittens in Hawaii, 21 were blood-culture-positive for *B. henselae* and elevated antibody titers, 2 had a negative blood culture and positive serologic results,

*Table 2.* Seroprevalence of *B. henselae* in cats

| Seropositivity | Note | Country (area) | Ref. |
|---|---|---|---|
| 12–44% (av. 15%) | High prevalence in feral cats | USA (Baltimore) | 15 |
| 4–55% (av. 28%) | Low prevalence in cold areas<br>High prevalence in warm areas | USA | 18 |
| 62–100% (av. 81%) | Pet, impounded and feral cats | USA (California) | 8 |
| 81% | 85% of positive cats were kittens | USA (Hawaii) | 16 |
| 89%<br>48% | Cats associated with CSD patients<br>Control cats | USA (North Carolina)<br>– | 7 |
| 40%<br>40% | Cats in North Carolina<br>Cats in Israel | USA (North Carolina)<br>– | 17 |
| 36% | Pet cats around Paris | France (Paris) | 9 |
| 6–22% (av. 15%) | Low prevalence in northern part and high prevalence in central area | Japan | 20 |
| 33% | Healthy cats | Austria | 19 |
| 35% | Feral (40%) and domestic cats (16%) | Australia (Sydney) | 10 |

6 were negative in both the blood culture and the IFA findings [16]. Chomel et al. [8] have shown that 81% (166/205) of the cats in northern California are positive for *B. henselae* antibodies, and that their titers are higher than for nonbacteremic cats.

Baneth et al. [17] have shown that similar numbers of cats from Israel (40%: 45/114) and from North Carolina (40%: 46/114) are seropositive to both *B. henselae* and *B. quintana*. Breitschwerdt and Kordick [22] have evidence that 21% (109/518) of the sick cats from a veterinary teaching hospital are seropositive to *B. henselae*.

The seroprevalence of cats seems to correlate with climate. Jameson et al. [18] have examined the prevalence of serum antibody titers to *B. henselae* in 33 geographic locations throughout the USA and several areas in Canada. Overall, 28% (175/628) of the cats examined were seropositive, but a high level of seropositivity was found in the southeastern United States, Hawaii, coastal California, the Pacific Northwest, and the Central Plains (55, 47, 40, 34 and 37%, respectively). On the other hand, Alaska, the Rocky Mountain-Great Plains region, and the Midwest showed a low average prevalence of the seropositivity (5, 4 and 7%, respectively).

In Europe, Allerberger et al. [19] reported that 33% (32/96) of Austrian cats tested have antibodies to *B. henselae*. In France, seropositivity was found in 36% (23/64) of the cat samples from a veterinary teaching hospital in Paris [9].

In Japan, the overall seroprevalence in domestic cats was reported to be 15% (30/199), with 22% (13/59) in the central area and 6% (3/48) in the northeastern area [20]. In our investigation, 9% (43/471) of the cat samples collected from private veterinary hospitals in the Kanto District were seropositive to *B. henselae*. Furthermore, our preliminary study in Thailand has shown that 32% (11/34) of pet cats are seropositive to the organism.

*Cat Age.* Patients with CSD were more likely to own a kitten 12 months or younger [5]. Several investigations have also shown that cats less than 12 months old are strongly associated with bacteremia and a seropositivity to *B. henselae* [6, 8, 10, 15, 16]. Among bacteremic cats, young cats less than 1 year old are 1.7 times more likely than adult cats to be bacteremic. The seropositivity rate in young cats is also higher than that in adult cats [8].

On the other hand, no association between cat age and seropositivity was found in Japan [20]. Because the seroprevalence of cats in Japan is somewhat lower than that in other countries where bacteremia in cats is more prevalent, the cats may have fewer opportunities to acquire the infection in Japan. Therefore, in countries where the infection is more prevalent in cats, cats may acquire the infections and may develop *B. henselae* bacteremia at a young age of $<12$ months.

*Reservoir and Vectors.* As shown in the major diagnostic criteria for CSD, most cases of the disease are associated with cat scratches and/or bites. Seropositivity in cats owned by CSD patients with or without BA or BP has been shown to be higher than that of control cases. Regnery et al. [4] described *B. henselae* infection in a *Bartonella*-seropositive healthy cat for the first time and have suggested that cats may serve as a potential reservoir for *Bartonella* infections in man. Persistent *B. henselae* bacteremia has been observed in cats associated with CSD cases [7].

Most patients with CSD have been found to be persons who own a cat less than 12 months old. Kirkpatrick and Glickman [23] suggested two explanations for this fact: (1) young cats are more playful and, hence, more likely to inflict a scratch or a bite than an older cat would be; or (2) older cats develop either a specific or nonspecific immunity to the CSD agent.

The level of high seropositivity (7%: 25/351) which has been found in veterinary professionals is probably due to a greater amount of contacts with cats [24]. Overall, these data show that the cat, and especially the young kitten, is the major significant reservoir of CSD.

It has been reported that a number of CSD patients have owned kittens infested with cat fleas (*Ctenocephalides felis*), and that *B. henselae* and the DNA from fleas have been found on carrier cats [6]. Furthermore, *B. henselae* has been isolated from the blood and from the fleas of a cat of a patient with CSD in Australia, although this patient had no history of a bite or scratch from the cat and no primary lesion on the skin [25]. Furthermore, Higgins et al. [26] showed that *B. henselae* can survive in the gut of a flea up to 9 days after infection.

In our study of 10 bacteremic pet cats, 8 were reported by the owners to be infested with fleas, though unfortunately, the fleas could not be submitted to a culture for the bacteria. In the USA, flea infestation is commonly found in 90% of bacteremic cats and 69% of all cats examined [8].

Chomel et al. [27] investigated whether *B. henselae* can be experimentally transmitted to cats via fleas. A vector-mediated transmission of *B. henselae* was evaluated by removing fleas from the naturally bacteremic, flea-infested cattery cats and transferring these fleas to specific pathogen-free (SPF) kittens housed in an arthropod-free animal facility. The cat fleas removed from the bacteremic cattery cats transmitted *B. henselae* to 5 SPF kittens, although the control SPF kittens housed with highly bacteremic kittens in the absence of fleas did not become infected.

It has been shown that the rate of the seropositivity and bacteremia in impounded and feral cats is higher than that in pet cats [7, 8, 10]. This means that feral and impounded cats are more likely to come into contact with infected cats and to be infested with fleas.

Warm and humid environments are associated with higher cat seroprevalence than are cold and dry environments. These warm and humid areas which host cats with high seropositivity may correlate with a high number of potential arthropod vectors such as fleas [18]. These data strongly suggest that the transmission of *B. henselae* in both cats and humans occurs via arthropod vectors, especially cat fleas.

Lucey et al. [28] have reported 2 cases of persistent *B. henselae* bacteremia in 2 previously healthy immunocompetent men who had both experienced a tick bite. This may indicate that other arthropods such as ticks can also transmit *B. henselae*.

## Pathogenicity of *B. henselae* in Cats

Generally, no clinical manifestations have been observed in *B. henselae* bacteremic cats. Kirkpatrick and Whiteley [29] reported that a suspicious argyrophilic bacteria was detected in the lymph nodes of a cat with persistent lymphadenopathy, although no organism was isolated. It has also been reported that bacteremia persisted for a 12-month period in cats associated with CSD patients but no clinical manifestations were observed in the cats [7].

In experimentally inoculated cats, although bacteremia has been easily established and has persisted for a long period of time of 7–21 weeks, no apparent clinical manifestations have been observed [27, 30, 31]. On the other hand, Breitschwert and Kordick [22] reported a self-limiting febrile illness of 48–72 hours' duration and a transient neurologic dysfunction in 2 cats infected experimentally with *B. henselae* by blood transfusion. Ueno et al. [21] have investigated the correlation between a serological status for *B. henselae*, FIV infection, and several clinical characteristics in 170 domestic cats in Japan and have suggested that coinfection of *B. henselae* and FIV may be associated with gingivitis and lymphadenopathy in cats.

Low-passage-number, pilliated *B. henselae* adhere to and invade Hep-2 cells to a greater extent than do multiple-passaged *B. henselae* with reduced pilas expression [32]. This suggests the possibility that pili of *B. henselae* may be one pathogenic determinant for *B. henselae*. Furthermore, *B. henselae* cocultivated with Vero cells on chamber slides has been found intracellularly mainly around the nuclei of the cells [33]. Evaluation of the mechanism by which *B. henselae* enters the cells may help to clarify the pathogenicity of the organism.

## Antimicrobial Efficacy in Infected Cats

In cats, *B. henselae* bacteremia was suppressed by the oral administration of antibiotics such as doxycycline 25–50 mg twice a day, or lincomycin 100 mg twice a day [6]. Antimicrobial treatment with tetracycline, erythromycin, doxycycline, amoxicillin, or enrofloxacin has reduced the level of bacteremia, but does not completely eliminate *B. henselae* from the blood of experimentally inoculated cats. Furthermore, the duration of the bacteremia in cats treated with some antibiotics remains similar to that in untreated cats [30, 31]. The intraerythrocytic presence of the organism was demonstrated in 3 and 6% of the erythrocytes from 2 asymptomatic bacteremic cats [32], and no epicellular or extracellular organisms were observed in Vero cells by electron microscopy [34]. The intraerythrocytic presence of bacteria may provide a potential explanation for poor antimicrobial efficacy.

## Control

According to the present knowledge of the epidemiology of CSD, the principal methods for protection against CSD consist of: (1) avoiding cat scratches or bites; (2) disinfection of the area in which the cat scratch or bite has occurred; (3) general sanitation measures such as washing hands with soap and water after the contact with cats; (4) declawing the cats, and (5) control of cat fleas.

Chomel et al. [8] pointed out that seronegative cats are likely to not be bacteremic, but young kittens, especially impounded and flea-infested kittens, are more likely to be bacteremic. Therefore, people who want to own a pet cat, and especially immunocompromised individuals, should find an adult pet cat which has been raised in a flea-controlled environment. Furthermore, a serological examination for pet cats before adopting may be effective in preventing CSD. An effective vaccine for cats has not yet been developed.

## References


1 English CK, Wear DJ, Margileth AM, Lissner CR, Walsh GP: Cat scratch disease. Isolation and culture of the bacterial agent. JAMA 1988;259:1347–1352.

2 Welch DF, Pickett DA, Slater LN, Steigerwalt AG, Brenner DJ: *Rochalimaea henselae* spp. nov., a cause of septicemia, bacillary angiomatosis, and parenchymal bacillary peliosis. J Clin Microbiol 1992;30:275–280.

3 Dolan MJ, Wong MT, Regnery RL, Jorgensen JH, Garcia M, Peters J, Drehner D: Syndrome of *Rochalimaea henselae* adenitis suggesting cat scratch disease. Ann Inter Med 1993;118:331–336.

4 Regnery R, Martin M, Olson J: Naturally occurring '*Rochalimaea henselae*' infection in domestic cat. Lancet 1992;340:557–558.

5 Zangwill KM, Hamilton DH, Perkins BA, Regnery RL, Plikaytis BD, Hadler JL, Cartter ML, Wenger JD: Cat scratch disease in Connecticut. Epidemiology, risk factors, and evaluation of a new diagnostic test. N Engl J Med 1993;329:8–13.

6 Koehler JE, Glaser CA, Tappero JW: *Rochalemiaea henselae* infection. A new zoonosis with the domestic cat as reservoir. JAMA 1994;271:531–535.

7 Kordick DL, Wilson KH, Sexton DJ, Hadfield TL, Berkhoff HA, Breitschwerdt EB: Prolonged *Bartonella* bacteremia in cats associated with cat-scratch disease patients. J Clin Microbiol 1995; 33:3245–3251.

8 Chomel BB, Abbott RC, Kasten RW, Floyd-Hawkins KA, Kass PH, Glaser CA, Pedersen NC, Koehler JE: *Bartonella henselae* prevalence in domestic cats in California: Risk factors and association between bacteremia and antibody titers. J Clin Microbiol 1995;33:2445–2450.

9 Chomel BB, Gurfield AN, Boulouis HJ, Kasten RW, Piemont Y: Réservoir félin de l'agent de la maladie des griffes du chat, *Bartonella henselae*, en région parisienne: résultats préliminaires. Rec Méd Vét 1995;171:841–845.

10 Branley J, Wolfson C, Waters P, Gottlieb T, Bradbury R: Prevalence of *Bartonella henselae* bacteremia, the causative agent of cat scratch disease, in an Australian cat population. Pathology 1996; 28:262–265.

11 Maruyama S, Nogami S, Inoue I, Namba S, Asanome K, Katsube Y: Isolation of *Bartonella henselae* from domestic cats in Japan. J Vet Med Sci 1996;58:81–83.

12 Clarridge JE III, Raich TJ, Pirwani D, Simon B, Tsai L, Rodriguez-Barradas MC, Regnery R, Zollo A, Jones DC, Rambo C: Strategy to detect and identify *Bartonella* species in routine clinical laboratory yields *Bartonella henselae* from human immunodeficiency virus-positive patient and unique *Bartonella* strain from his cat. J Clin Microbiol 1995; 33:2107–2113.
13 Lawson PA, Collins MD: Description of *Bartonella clarridgeiae* sp nov isolated from the cat of a patient with *Bartonella henselae* septicemia. Med Microbiol Lett 1996;5:64–73.
14 Maruyama S, Kasten RW, Gurfield AN, Boulouis HJ, Chomel BB: Molecular epidemiological analysis of *Bartonella* isolates from the USA, France, and Japan by pulsed-field gel electrophoresis. Proc ISVEE, Paris 1997.
15 Childs JE, Rooney JA, Cooper JL, Olson JG, Regnery RL: Epidemiologic observations on infection with *Rochalimaea* species among cats living in Baltimore, Md. J Am Vet Med Assoc 1994;204: 1775–1778.
16 Dermers DM, Bass JW, Vincent JM, Person DA, Noyes DK, Staege CM, Samlaska CP, Lockwood NH, Regnery RL, Anderson BE: Cat-scratch disease in Hawaii: Etiology and seroepidemiology. J Pediatr 1995;127:23–26.
17 Baneth G, Kordick DL, Hegarty BC, Breitschwerdt EB: Comparative seroreactivity to *Bartonella henselae* and *Bartonella quintana* among cats from Israel and North Carolina. Vet Microbiol 1996; 50:95–103.
18 Jameson P, Greene C, Regnery R, Dryden M, Marks A, Brown J, Cooper J, Glaus B, Greene R: Prevalence of *Bartonella henselae* antibodies in pet cats throughout regions of North America. J Infect Dis 1995;172:1145–1149.
19 Allerberger F, Schönbauer M, Dierich MP: Prevalence of antibody to *Rochalimaea henselae* among Austrian cats. Eur J Pediatr 1995;154:165.
20 Ueno H, Muramatsu Y, Chomel BB, Hohdatsu T, Koyama H, Morita C: Seroepidemiological survey of *Bartonella* (*Rochalimaea*) *henselae* in domestic cats in Japan. Microbiol Immunol 1995; 39:339–341.
21 Ueno H, Hohdatsu T, Muramatsu Y, Koyama H, Morita C: Does coinfection of *Bartonella henselae* and FIV induce clinical disorders in cats? Microbiol Immunol 1996;40:617–620.
22 Breitschwerdt EB, Kordick DL: Bartonellosis in zoonosis update. J Am Vet Med Assoc 1995;206: 1928–1931.
23 Kirkpatrick CE, Glickman LT: Cat-scratch disease and the role of the domestic cat: Vector, reservoir, and victim? Med Hypotheses 1989;28:145–149.
24 Noah DL, Kramer CM, Verbsky MP, Rooney JA, Smith KA, Childs JE: Survey of veterinary professionals and other veterinary conference attendees for antibodies to *Bartonella henselae* and *B quintana*. J Am Vet Med Assoc 1997;210:342–344.
25 Flexman JP, Lavis NJ, Kay ID, Watson M, Metcalf C, Pearman JW: *Bartonella henselae* is a causative agent of cat scratch disease in Australia. J Infect 1995;31:241–245.
26 Higgins JA, Radulovic S, Jaworski DC, Azad AF: Acquisition of the cat scratch disease agent *Bartonella henselae* by cat fleas. J Med Entomol 1996;33:490–495.
27 Chomel BB, Kasten RW, Floyd-Hawkins K, Chi B, Yamamoto K, Roberts-Wilson J, Gurfield AN, Abbott RC, Pedersen NC, Koehler JE: Experimental transmission of *Bartonella henselae* by the cat flea. J Clin Microbiol 1996;34:1952–1956.
28 Lucey D, Dolan MJ, Moss CW, Garcia M, Hollis DG, Wegner S, Morgan G, Almeida R, Leong D, Greisen KS, Welch DF, Slater LN: Relapsing illness due to *Rochalimaea henselae* in immunocompetent hosts: Implication for therapy and new epidemiological associations. Clin Infect Dis 1992;14:683–688.
29 Kirkpatrick CE, Whiteley HE: Argyrophilic, intracellular bacteria in the lymph node of a cat: Cat-scratch disease bacilli? J Infect Dis 1987;156:690–691.
30 Greene CE, McDermott M, Jameson PH, Atkins CL, Marks AM: *Bartonella henselae* infection in cats: Evaluation during primary infection, treatment, and rechallenge infection. J Clin Microbiol 1996;34:1682–1685.
31 Regnery RL, Rooney JA, Johnson AM, Nesby SL, Manzewitsch P, Beaver K, Olson JG: Experimentally induced *Bartonella henselae* infections followed by challenge exposure and antimicrobial therapy in cats. Am J Vet Res 1996;57:1714–1719.

32 Kordick DL, Breitschwerdt EB: Intraerythrocytic presence of *Bartonella henselae.* J Clin Microbiol 1995;33:1655–1656.

33 Batterman HJ, Peek JA, Loutit JS, Falkow S, Tompkins LS: *Bartonella henselae* and *Bartonella quintana* adherence to and entry into cultured human epithelial cells. Infect Immun 1995;63:4553–4556.

34 Zbinden R, Höchli M, Nadal D: Intracellular location of *Bartonella henselae* cocultivated with Vero cells and used for an indirect fluorescent-antibody test. Clin Diagn Lab Immunol 1995;2: 693–695.

Soichi Maruyama, Laboratory of Veterinary Public Health, College of Bioresource Sciences, Nihon University, 1866 Kameino, Fujisawa, Kanagawa 252-8510 (Japan)

# Author Index

# Subject Index